More Praise for

THE PALEO MANIFESTO

"Now the definitive guide to going paleo."

—JOSHUA NEWMAN, CrossFit NYC

"Amid the mass confusion of our diet-obsessed culture, *The Paleo Manifesto* stands out as fun, refreshing, and sensible. Durant has a knack for storytelling, weaving his exploits as a modern hunter-gatherer into lessons for healthy living—all based on solid evidence from evolution and biochemistry. *The Paleo Manifesto* is the new common sense."

—MARK SISSON, author of *The Primal Blueprint* and publisher of MarksDailyApple.com

"Whether you are a skeptic or a believer, you'll admire Durant's passionate and highly personal advocacy for living a paleo lifestyle."

—DANIEL LIEBERMAN, professor of Human Evolutionary Biology at Harvard University

"Durant's provocative manifesto is bound to inspire necessary discussion about the nature of our food and the role of evolution in determining a healthy diet."

—GARY TAUBES, *New York Times* bestselling author of *Good Calories, Bad Calories* and *Why We Get Fat*

"John Durant is a bright and original thinker, and here he makes a compelling case for the health benefits of a life rooted in evolutionary principles. Insightful and inspirational, *The Paleo Manifesto* is a masterpiece."

—ERWAN Le CORRE, founder of MovNat

THE
PALEO
MANIFESTO

Ancient Wisdom for Lifelong Health

JOHN DURANT

with contributions by

Michael Malice

HARMONY

BOOKS · NEW YORK

Library of Congress Cataloging-in-Publication Data
Durant, John.
The paleo manifesto: ancient wisdom for lifelong health /
John Durant ; with contributions by Michael Malice. —
First edition.
Includes bibliographical references.
1. Health behavior—History.   2. Prehistoric peoples—Health and hygiene.
3. High protein diet.   4. Nature and civilization.   I. Malice, Michael.   II. Title.
RA776.9.D87   2013
613.2—dc23
2013017890

ISBN 978-0-307-88918-8
eBook ISBN 978-0-307-88919-5

Printed in the United States of America

Book design by Barbara Sturman
Cover design by Michael Nagin
Cover photograph: © The Trustees of the British Museum

page 35: © President and Fellows of Harvard College, Peabody Museum of
Archaeology and Ethnology, number 46-49-60/N7365.0 (digital file # 60743070)
page 193: These materials are reproduced from www.nsarchive.org with the
permission of the National Security Archive.

10 9 8 7 6 5 4 3 2 1

First Paperback Edition

To my ancestors,

for my descendants

Contents

1

BECOMING THE CAVEMAN

What would it look like if a caveman were interviewed on TV? America was about to find out. On February 3, 2010, I was backstage at *The Colbert Report*, waiting to be interviewed by the razor-sharp comedian. Colbert's interviews are among the most difficult on television—and it was going to be my first ever TV appearance.

Colbert had invited me on because of my so-called caveman diet. Admittedly, my health regimen sounds unusual at first. I attempt to mimic aspects of life during the Stone Age—or, as many people jokingly refer to it, "living like a caveman." Heck, I even look the part, with a shaggy mane and scruffy beard.

In popular culture the "caveman in civilization" is a reliable source of punch lines. In 2004 GEICO ran an award-winning series of commercials showing a pair of well-dressed cavemen offended at the insurance company's tagline, "So easy a caveman can do it." On *Saturday Night Live* in the mid-nineties, Phil Hartman played Unfrozen Caveman Lawyer, a thawed Neanderthal who enrolled in law school and won over juries by pretending to be a simpleton ("Ladies and gentlemen of the jury, I'm just a caveman!") before delivering the clinching argument.

The jokes begin as soon as people find out about my lifestyle. Whenever I use a piece of modern technology (a cell phone, a Styrofoam cup, a spoon), someone reminds me, "Cavemen didn't use those!" People tease me about the caveman approach to dating: clubbing a girl over the head and dragging her by the hair back to my apartment. And if I ever eat anything other than raw meat straight off the bone, my co-workers kindly inform me that I am doing it all wrong. Apparently, watching reruns of *The Flintstones* turns anyone into an expert paleoanthropologist.

Given the widely held cartoonish perspective of Stone Age life, I had a pretty good idea of what kind of jokes to expect from Colbert. My job was to point out that our impression of how humans lived in the Stone Age is exactly that: a cartoon. In the same way that Mickey and Minnie Mouse tell us little about the lives of real mice, *The Flintstones* tells us little about the lives of real Stone Age humans. In fact, the terms "caveman" and "Stone Age" are inaccurate and outdated. Though some early humans lived in caves, particularly in cold or mountainous climates such as Europe, our Paleolithic ancestors lived for millions of years underneath the big open sky of the African savannah.

These early humans were hunter-gatherers who foraged for a variety of wild foods, and whose lifestyle was quite different from the lives people lead today. This ancient, ancestral lifestyle is more important than we realize—especially when it comes to being healthy in the modern world.

Here's the simple truth: genetically speaking, we're all hunter-gatherers.

Of course, we're not *just* hunter-gatherers. We also carry the genes of primates; herders and farmers; factory workers and explorers; office workers and computer programmers. But at our biological core we are still largely hunters and gatherers.

My path to discovering my inner hunter-gatherer began during my junior year at college. Two important but seemingly unrelated events took place at the same time. First, I went through a long breakup with a girlfriend and watched my physical and mental health suffer. Second, I began studying under cognitive psychologist Dr. Steven Pinker, learning about the evolution of the human mind over millions of years and how that evolutionary history shapes the way our minds work today.

In the middle of the breakup I had an epiphany: If I got fewer than eight hours of sleep, it felt like my world was coming to an end. But on the days when I got more than eight hours of sleep (and exercised), I was able to put it all behind me. It blew my mind that my entire outlook on a relationship could be so noticeably influenced by my bedtime. Rather than having a mind or spirit that rose above my base body, it seemed like I was nothing more than a bunch of cells and chemicals sloshing around in a big, leaky sack.

As the geneticist Theodosius Dobzhansky said, "Nothing in biology makes sense except in the light of evolution." Pinker's course on evolutionary biology examined the capacities of the human mind through the lens of the survival and reproductive pressures faced by our ancestors. It addressed questions like "Why do many people have a visceral fear of snakes, which kill only a few people each year, but not of automobiles, which kill tens of thousands of people each year?"

Evolutionary theory points out that snakes were a real and deadly threat to our ancestors—but automobiles were not. Our ancestors with an innate fear of snakes would have been less likely to risk a deadly encounter with one, and thus would have been more likely to produce more offspring. This hypothesis wasn't just an after the fact rationalization of a fear. The fear of snakes is widespread among other primates, which share similar predators. The same line of thinking can be used to explain a variety of common fears that were past evolutionary threats, such as darkness, deep water, and heights. The power of the human mind is such that instinctual fears can be overcome (and novel fears can be imprinted), but the predisposition still looms in our minds.

Evolutionary psychology can also explain some of our moral intuitions. For example, why is there an almost universal aversion to incest? Inbreeding is far more likely to result in birth defects; just ask the owner of a purebred dog. In our evolutionary past, people with an aversion to having sex with their close kin would have been more likely to produce fertile and healthy offspring. Cultural norms almost always reinforced this instinctual aversion to incest, even though people may not have understood why the norms existed. They just worked, and the people who held such norms ended up flourishing.

This newfound perspective redirected my entire course of study halfway through college. I shifted away from my major, history, and toward evolutionary psychology, culminating in an interdisciplinary thesis advised by Pinker. I wanted to explore mankind's murky origins—and their lingering effects on us today.

Then I graduated. I moved to the urban jungle and joined the daily grind. Abstract ideas about cavemen gave way to the concrete reality of paying the rent on a cave-like apartment in New York City.

I worked long hours, including weekends, at a consulting firm. My company would buy takeout when I worked late, which meant I ate takeout almost every night. I sat most of the day and rarely found time to exercise. I didn't sleep enough, and when I had the opportunity I usually went out drinking with friends. "Work hard, play hard" meant being hard on my health all the time.

Like most others starting their first desk job, I found that my metabolism seemed to slow down in a big way. I gained about twenty pounds of solid fat. This actually didn't bother me that much. I had been lean before, and now I was "normal" (meaning, kind of hefty). To me the more important issue was my energy level: It was up and down. I often couldn't even stay awake, let alone function productively, without large amounts of caffeine.

Just like during that breakup, as my energy went, so went my mood. Low energy meant pessimism, impatience, irritability. High energy meant optimism, confidence, and an upbeat perspective. My outlook, my judgment, my decisions—things that were central to who I was as a person—seemed to be influenced by something as simple as what I had eaten for lunch (often a footlong Subway meatball sub) and whether I had made a Starbucks run.

I don't know why it took me so long to make the connection—it certainly wasn't a lack of coffee—but one day I considered the situation in a new light. Could I take control of my health and diet in order to improve my mood and outlook? Could I be "up" all the time?

I began where most people who want to get healthier begin: my diet. Maybe, as so many nutritionists advise, I needed to nibble on lots of small snacks throughout the day to keep my blood sugar up. Or maybe my metabolism was just naturally slowing down due to age. Or maybe I was eating too much fat or too many calories. Or maybe I was supposed to eat organic. Regardless, I knew I had to eat healthier—which is what most people would call "going on a diet." But I had never been on a diet in my life.

As any rugged man age eighteen to thirty-five can tell you, diets are for women and organic food is for hippies. The only time I had ever counted calories in a meal was to brag about how many I had just eaten. If I was weighing myself, it was probably because I wanted to *gain* weight (i.e., muscle). It's not as if the diet industry had a great track record of success. From an outsider's perspective, it seemed like a constant churn of celebrity-endorsed double-talk that gets renamed, repackaged, and resold to desperate women straight out of a *Cathy* cartoon. *Ack!*

I needed a scientific framework that worked and made sense. I needed something that had the power to explain *why*.

That "something" popped into my inbox at 4:01 P.M. on February 14, 2006. It came attached to an email from my older brother Clark, who sent me a twenty-six-page essay by Dr. Art De Vany, a retired economist from the University of California. De Vany titled his essay "Evolutionary Fitness." The title was an academic pun: it referred to "fitness" in the common definition of exercise, as well as "fitness" in the evolutionary biology sense of reproductive fitness, meaning an organism's overall ability to leave offspring.

The essay was based on a simple premise: *There is a mismatch between our genes and the lives that we lead today.*

Humans aren't adapted to sitting at desks all day long, eating Twinkies and drinking Pepsi. Humanity spent most of its evolutionary existence living as hunter-gatherers on the African savannah; therefore humanity was better adapted to that type of lifestyle. Many modern health problems, such as obesity, diabetes, heart disease, and cancer, are rare to nonexistent among contemporary hunter-gatherers. Our hunter-gatherer ancestors were healthier and lived longer than most people realize. If we wanted to be healthy, then we might be able to learn a thing or two from them.

Old knowledge didn't need to be wrong knowledge.

The general mismatch hypothesis wasn't original to De Vany. A wide variety of academics and authors had written about a disconnect between our ancestral lifestyles and our current ones, but in the age-old scientific tradition of self-experimentation, De Vany was one of the first to take it out of the classroom, apply it to his own diet and exercise, and then share his experience with others online.

Because I had studied evolutionary psychology, the general evolutionary approach to health immediately struck a chord with me. Instead of reading a diet book to learn about what to eat, I could find out what humans naturally ate. Lions are well adapted to a carnivorous diet. Gorillas are well adapted to an herbivorous diet. Humans are well adapted to an omnivorous diet, based on the foods eaten by hunter-gatherers.

Online I discovered a small but growing group of people who were "eating paleo," and, more broadly, following a paleo lifestyle. But what did that actually mean?

Not only did eating paleo imply avoiding processed foods, as most conventional health authorities recommend, but it also meant casting a skeptical eye on allegedly "healthy" agricultural foods like whole grains and legumes (wheat, corn, soy) and dairy (milk, yogurt, cheese), which didn't enter the human diet in any meaningful amount until the Agricultural Revolution roughly 10,000 years ago. Also suspect were two common approaches to healthy eating—low fat and vegetarianism—since humans have been eating animals for millions of years.

As for exercise, other animals don't "exercise" so much as they either play or just do what is required to survive. Birds fly. Fish swim. Humans are well adapted to moving in our own natural ways: ranging across the savannah, hunting, gathering, fighting, and procreating.

Modern humans are more sedentary than ever, and the evolutionary perspective agreed with the modern conventional wisdom. Want to be healthier? Move more. Yet many people exercise in highly routinized and monotonous ways, like running on a treadmill in a gym. They focus on abstract goals, like burning calories, and lose sight of functional, goal-oriented movements such as sprinting away from a threat or carrying an animal carcass back to camp. At a minimum, the evolutionary approach implied injecting variety into the types of movements and intensity level; hunter-gatherers did not do the elliptical for thirty minutes a day, four days a week. But there were limits to this line of thinking. The hunter-gatherer's source of motivation was running from a lion; the closest modern analogue is chasing down a cab—and no matter what we tell ourselves, there's hardly the same sense of urgency.

There were specifics to fill in, but the general evolutionary approach was sound. It was the appropriate starting point for any intelligent discussion on how to be healthy—even if it wasn't the last word.

Theories are nice, but would it work? Things were going to get real Darwinian real fast.

I started eating paleo in September of 2006.*

I stopped eating industrial foods: no ketchup, mac and cheese, mozzarella sticks, or sweets. I stopped eating grain products like wheat, corn, and rice; legumes like soy, peanuts, and beans; and dairy. I also eliminated starchy foods like potatoes (though I would come to learn that roots and tubers are a staple in many hunter-gatherer diets, both Paleolithic and contemporary).

Surprisingly (to me), there was still a wide range of foods available

---

*My current diet has "evolved" from my initial experiment at eating paleo. A longer discourse on food can be found in Chapters 7 and 8, and a summary is located in the Resources and Recommendations section (pages 291–292).

to eat. My status as an "omnivore" was not in question. I ate meat, seafood, fresh vegetables, and a modest amount of fruit, nuts, seeds, and eggs—basically any category of food that seemed like it would have been available in the wild that also happened to be available in my local grocery store.

I moved away from "three square meals a day" and interjected a little variation into my eating routines. I even fasted once a week for the first three months, skipping dinner and going roughly eighteen hours from lunch to the following breakfast.

I never counted calories or measured macronutrients (fat, protein, and carbs). Relative to what is considered "normal," I ended up with a high-fat, moderate protein, low-carbohydrate diet.

I found it hard to give up alcohol entirely, but I completely cut out sweet mixers and cut back on beer, which is grain-based. I reduced my coffee intake to about a cup a day, only in the morning.

I did my best to get at least seven hours of sleep at night, and I got more sunshine during the day.

After about ten days of eating paleo, I knew I had something. My "diet" was working.

I had much more consistent energy throughout the day. There was no more "head on the desk" after lunch. My mood improved, too. I felt more confident and optimistic. When something negative occurred in my life, I found that I was able to weather it with greater ease. The energy and mood gains in and of themselves were enough to tell me that I was on the right track.

I lost twenty-two pounds, getting back to my college weight. I lost virtually all of it within the first two and a half months. My waist dropped two to three inches, from a 34- or 35-inch waist to an easy-fitting 32-inch waist. I had to buy new pants.

Due to the low sugar content in my diet, I stopped getting a thin, filmy residue on my teeth. Industrial food started tasting way too sweet, and I came to enjoy natural flavors more. I lost the cravings for refined carbs—cookies, cupcakes, pasta, muffins, and bagels—and I found bready foods to be both salty and bland.

My immune system improved dramatically. I went through the entire winter without getting a single cold or the flu. In prior years I would often get the feeling that I was coming down with something. I'd take some vitamin C or Airborne to try to fight it off. But I never actually remember winning any of those fights. Now my body actually won. I registered something coming on, sneezed a bit, felt tired for a day, slept a lot—but then my immune system actually beat out the standard winter illnesses.

The most unexpected but well-received change was the improvement in my complexion. My skin was the best it had been since going through puberty. It was noticeably more resilient during those high-stress periods when I used to nearly always get a gigantic zit right on the same area of my nose.

Overall, it felt like waking up from a perpetual state of hangover. And once I knew what "good" felt like, it made "bad" feel a whole lot worse.

Family, friends, and co-workers started flooding me with questions:

- Wait a second, isn't this just Atkins? Have you checked your cholesterol?
- Didn't cavemen die when they were thirty?
- Haven't humans adapted to agricultural foods like dairy?
- Don't you realize that there is no such thing as one single hunter-gatherer diet?
- Have you studied nutrition? You're telling me that the federal dietary guidelines are wrong?
- If we are intended to eat so much meat, then why are our teeth small and not that sharp?
- Aren't you romanticizing life in the wild a little bit? Didn't life used to be "solitary, poor, nasty, brutish, and short"?
- Hey caveman, did you give up antibiotics?

Initially, I didn't have answers to all these questions. Besides, I wasn't even sure how much of my improvement was simply due to the fairly mainstream health advice to eat less processed food and exercise more. How much did avoiding grains, legumes, and dairy actually have to do with it? I didn't have all the answers yet, but I couldn't argue with the results. Besides, I was having fun.

Eating paleo remained a quirky hobby for the next year or two—but one that slowly started to creep into other aspects of my life. Among my social circle I was becoming known as "The Caveman." Even so, when I met new people, no one knew about it unless I told them. I could still go on dates without the topic coming up. I may have been "The Caveman" to people who knew me, but to the rest of the world I was just a hairy guy.

That was about to change.

I decided there couldn't possibly be any harm in formalizing my status as a "modern caveman" by starting an official organization of like-minded "cavepeople." I founded Paleo NYC, a Web-based Meetup group that brought together people who ate paleo for meals and various events.

Unbeknownst to me, one of the guests at our first potluck dinner was a freelance journalist. He thought it was fascinating, and apparently so did someone at the *New York Times,* who asked him to write a feature on our group. Over the next month or two the reporter tagged along to various Paleo NYC events. We made homemade jerky in my oven. A group of us ran barefoot across the Brooklyn Bridge in the middle of winter. We held Paleo Happy Hours where we would devise elaborate justifications for drinking alcohol (e.g., some primates seem to enjoy eating rotten fruit that has been fermenting on the forest floor).

A photographer came to my apartment and took shots of me for the piece. I tried to keep the photos respectable. By the end of the shoot, I posed howling at the sky, wielding a frozen leg of wild boar. They arranged for a few of us to get into the American Museum of Natural History, and we got our pictures taken in front of the Cro-Magnon diorama. It was all kind of hilarious.

When the article ran in the paper, my inbox exploded. I got

inquiries from dozens of media outlets located on five different continents. I imagined every international bureau chief screaming for an article on cavemen. *"Why don't we have an article on cavemen?! Get me THE CAVEMAN!"*

The interview requests were unrelenting. Some of them were great, but many just wanted me to run around in a loincloth, climb scaffolding, and eat raw meat straight off the bone—none of which I actually did in real life. "Is it true that you only eat things that you hunt and gather in Central Park?" "Do you think we could get a shot of you hunting pigeons on the roof of your apartment?" It was the caveman jokes all over again, except presented to the world as fact.

Then *The Colbert Report* called. So what would it look like if a caveman were somehow interviewed on TV? It turns out that it would look a lot like every other interview with a bearded, hairy man.

As I got ready for the show my brain went into overdrive. My primal mind knew nothing about stage lights and TV interviews, but it knew that something big was about to go down. It was a fight-or-flight moment, and my body flooded with adrenaline.

In our primal past adrenaline was a performance-enhancing drug. Nature always tries to steal an advantage, and a well-timed dose of adrenaline allows an animal to fight harder or run faster at life-changing moments. But in front of the cameras my primal adrenaline boost was a severe *dis*advantage. It was harder for me to think and speak in a relaxed manner. I didn't want to fight or flee, nor could I.

But perhaps I could.

If my body mistakenly thought a fight was coming, then maybe I could trick my body into thinking that the fight was already over—and that I had won. Playing sports growing up, I had always been told to visualize success, so a minute before the cameras started to roll I imagined that I had gotten into a brawl with Stephen Colbert and had kicked his ass on the set of his own show.

It worked.

My anxiety dissipated, replaced by calm confidence. Athletes who have played on a championship sports team know the feeling: a confidence buzz—pure euphoria. Following a fight, victorious males experience a surge of testosterone, which is probably preparation to mate with excited cheerleaders. When I had fed the primal biology within me, my health improved—and when I tricked my primal psychology, my mindset improved.

The show started, and I explained the paleo concept to Colbert: "Say that you are a zookeeper in a zoo and your goal is to make the animals happy and healthy . . . or even reproduce in captivity, which some of them don't do. What do you do?"

"I show the animals pornography," he quipped.

"You replicate their natural habitat as closely as possible."

"Okay, yeah, yeah, sure, you fake 'em out, like some pandas, you give 'em some bamboo trees in the background."

"Yeah, and you feed raw meat to the lions. You feed rodents to the snakes. And the same principle applies to human beings. We are happiest and healthiest when we eat the types of foods that hunter-gatherers ate in the wild."

That began an adventure to understand what it means to be happy and healthy—to thrive in the modern world—which turned into a much deeper journey: to understand what it means to be human.

THIS BOOK contains three parts. Part One is a brief history of humanity through five ages of existence—Animal, Paleolithic, Agricultural, Industrial, Information—each containing lessons for how to be healthy today. Part Two applies these lessons to multiple areas of modern-day life: food, fasting, movement, bipedalism (standing, walking, running), temperature, sun, and sleep. Part Three is a more speculative vision of how those most ancient of roles—hunter and gatherer—can instruct and inspire us to build healthy and ethical relationships to other living things. In short, to understand where we come from, to make the best of where we are, and to craft a better future.

Part One

ORIGINS

KNOW THY SPECIES

ANIMAL AGE

◄ *530 million years ago to 2.6 million years ago* ►

A couple months after I appeared on *The Colbert Report* I came across a rather odd health article about a patient I'll refer to as "Michael." Michael was a medical curiosity, though his case started out commonly enough.

Born in Chicago, he moved to Cleveland when he was young. As Michael drifted into middle age he became increasingly overweight yet showed no interest in changing his habits. But after a close friend died of a heart attack, he was compelled to visit the doctor's office for a checkup. The results from a standard blood test revealed a slew of bad but unsurprising news: high blood pressure, elevated cholesterol, high triglycerides. A cardiac ultrasound showed signs of left ventricular hypertrophy, a thickening of the heart muscle and an indicator for heart disease. The doctor did what most doctors would do for someone with these symptoms: She put Michael on two blood pressure medications—carvedilol, a beta blocker, and lisinopril, an ACE inhibitor—while looking into ways to change his lifestyle.

Yet when the doctor began to probe for the typical culprits she came up short. Michael didn't smoke or drink, and he didn't eat any of the fatty foods that are widely blamed for obesity and heart disease. In fact, Michael was a vegan; red meat wasn't even on the menu. No soda either. A typical meal was a salad, some fruit, and a few fiber bars fortified with nutrients, vitamins, and minerals. If most doctors heard an overweight patient with heart disease claim to eat the way Michael did, they'd start quoting *House M.D.*: "Everybody lies."

Other common culprits included lack of exercise and bad genetics. Michael wasn't exactly an exercise buff (he never went to the gym), but, on the other hand, he walked everywhere he needed to go. Maybe Michael was just unlucky and had bad genes.

Now, if the story stopped there, it wouldn't even have garnered a brief segment on the local news. What made Michael a medical curiosity is that his actual name is Mokolo, and he is a western lowland gorilla at the Cleveland Metroparks Zoo.

In 2005 a twenty-one-year-old male gorilla in Mokolo's group died of heart failure. So the staff started to look into ways to improve the health of the remaining gorillas. At 461 pounds, Mokolo may not have been obese (for a gorilla), but he *was* overweight. His blood tests and cardiac ultrasound were worrisome.

Clearly, Mokolo didn't smoke, drink alcohol, or eat fast food. He had always been fed according to the official guidelines issued by the National Research Council, which specified the caloric density, macronutrients, and micronutrients for primates in captivity. His vegan diet consisted of "gorilla biscuits"—fortified fiber bars made by exotic pet food companies—supplemented with leafy vegetables, plant stems, and fruit.

Captive gorillas *are* less active than wild gorillas, which forage for food most of the day. Mokolo's "exercise" consisted of walking around his enclosure and, occasionally, playing around with a few ropes and artificial tree branches.

As for bad genetics, well, heart disease happens to be the number one killer of male gorillas in captivity. Heart disease is also the number one killer of male humans in civilization. Median life expectancy for male gorillas in zoos is thirty-one years, so Mokolo's age of twenty-two roughly corresponds to a man in his fifties. While heart disease may be common at this age, there's nothing inevitable about a middle-aged man—or gorilla—dying from a heart attack.

The staff at the Cleveland Metroparks Zoo decided to put Mokolo on a diet. Technically speaking, they didn't put Mokolo *on* a diet so much as they *changed* his diet. Every animal in the world—including every human being—has a diet. The question is what that diet consists of. The staff switched Mokolo to a diet that more closely resembled the diet of a wild gorilla—with stunning results: significant weight loss, unexpectedly better behavior, and improved biomarkers related to heart disease.

So were there lessons to be drawn between the gorilla in captivity and the human in civilization?

To answer that question I decided to take a field trip to the Cleveland Metroparks Zoo. My main contact was Elena Less, a PhD student at Case Western Reserve who was writing her dissertation on body fat and obesity in captive gorillas. I also spoke with Elena's dissertation adviser, Dr. Kristen Lukas, as well as Dr. Pam Dennis. Dr. Lukas is chair of the Gorilla Species Survival Plan program, an effort among fifty-two North American zoos accredited by the Association of Zoos and Aquariums to cooperatively manage the gorilla population as well as to generate and disseminate best practices regarding the health and management of gorillas in zoos. Dr. Dennis is one of the leading veterinary epidemiologists in the study of captive gorillas.

I pulled into the staff parking lot at the zoo and was met by Elena. She looked like a cross between a young Jane Goodall, the noted primatologist, and Laura Dern, the actress who played the paleobotanist in *Jurassic Park*. After she showed me around the medical facilities and introduced me to the rest of the staff, we took a walk to where the primates were housed, located on the far side of the zoo.

Dr. Lukas and the medical staff, Elena told me, were leading an effort to understand heart disease in captive gorillas. Many gorillas show no outward signs of heart disease, yet with far too much regularity a captive gorilla goes into cardiac arrest and dies.

As part of this research effort Mokolo underwent a cardiac ultrasound, which revealed the left ventricular hypertrophy. This forced the team to think about ways to slow, halt, or reverse the progression of this condition. Elena's dissertation was part of the effort to do that.

"At first we actually weren't sure the gorillas *were* overweight," Elena said, "or if so, by how much. Is a 461-pound gorilla overweight?"

It's notoriously difficult to eyeball whether an animal is overweight. Humans are pretty good at eyeballing other humans, but we aren't so good when it comes to other species. Zoo visitors often think that Mokolo and the other bachelor gorilla, Bebac, are pregnant, simply because gorillas have the disproportionately large gut that herbivores use to digest plant matter.

I had always assumed that the zoo staff would know these types of things, but there was no established "body mass index" for western lowland gorillas. There are larger differences in size between male and female gorillas than between men and women, and they can vary in size considerably based on stature and age, just like people. But the staff didn't have some chart hanging on the wall, like at the doctor's office, where they could just look up the right answer. In fact, as part of her dissertation, Elena was constructing the first body mass index for gorillas.

But in doing so Elena came upon another statistical problem. After Elena collected the data on many of the 350 or so gorillas in North American zoos, she still had no idea what it meant. If Mokolo was "average" in that pool, was that good? The average American was overweight too. Average in Elena's sample simply meant "a weight that is statistically common among gorillas in North American zoos." Furthermore, most captive gorillas have led similar lives, eating similar foods. As a result, studies conducted on zoo populations often haven't revealed large differences in outcomes.

The problem went far beyond weight. It affected every single thing that biologists measured and observed about captive animals: internal biomarkers, like cholesterol, testosterone, and blood pressure, and external behavior, like grooming, mating, and aggression.

The problem was immense. There was no standard for comparison, no benchmarks at all. What's a normal *anything* for a captive gorilla?

The best way to know whether a captive animal has normal biomarkers and behavior is to compare it to its wild counterparts. But observing animals in their natural habitat is time-consuming, difficult, expensive, politicized, and often dangerous.

To determine whether Mokolo and Bebac were, in fact, unhealthy, the staff approached the question from many different angles. Mokolo and Bebac were probably overweight. Based on past studies, they also knew that cholesterol levels tend to be higher among captive gorillas than among wild gorillas, and the same was true of Mokolo and Bebac. And they had enlarged heart muscles.

Elena pointed out that humans and gorillas have different patterns of heart disease. In humans the most common form of heart disease is coronary artery disease, where arteries narrow from a buildup of fatty deposits (atherosclerosis). This and other types of heart disease coincide with the suite of health problems known as "metabolic syndrome," indicated by obesity, insulin resistance, high blood pressure, high triglycerides, and problematic patterns of cholesterol. Zoo veterinarians suspect that many of these same indicators also define metabolic syndrome in gorillas, though they know that high cholesterol levels in gorillas do not lead to the degree of atherosclerosis that is so common in humans.

Mokolo and Bebac also had behavioral issues. After eating all their biscuits, the apes would regurgitate them and re-ingest them. They would do this every six to eight minutes once their food was gone, tapering off as it was time to go in for the night. Gorillas in the wild don't do that with their food.

Wild gorillas groom themselves, but the Cleveland gorillas plucked their own hair every day, to the point that they had several noticeable bald spots. In humans this would be categorized as a serious impulse control disorder.

Taken all together—the pattern of heart failure in other captive gorillas, the enlarged heart muscles, the excess weight, the elevated cholesterol, the chronic regurgitation, and the hair plucking—there were clear signs that something was wrong with the gorilla habitat at the zoo.

And that's when we arrived at their habitat.

"Ready to meet Mokolo and Bebac?" Elena said as we walked inside.

My eyes had to adjust to the dimly lit building. It was oval shaped, with a loop for visitors to follow. There were a few enclosures in the center, but the rest lined the exterior so that the animals could go outside when they wanted to.

The gorilla enclosure was the largest, taking up one of the long sides of the loop. It was split into two long halves connected by a short passage. Each side had its own big artificial tree and a few thick ropes. The ceilings were fairly high with a few small skylights. It was more brightly lit than the human area, making it easier for us to see the gorillas. The floor and walls were concrete, easy to clean and disinfect. A few enrichment items were scattered around the floor: large branches, more rope, and boomer balls designed for pets and wild animals.

And there they were: Mokolo and Bebac.

They were *big*. In the left half of the enclosure Bebac was awake but lying down. In the right half Mokolo was sitting and munching on some straw that had been scattered around the floor.

Then Mokolo got up and moved. His long front arms came down, and he gracefully lumbered to the front of the enclosure, looking agile and awkward at the same time. Even though gorillas aren't human, it was hard not to see human-like emotions in his eyes. It was not surprising that the staff becomes so emotionally attached to them.

"I could watch them all day," Elena said. "And I have."

"I can see why."

Mokolo had presence. His movements were slow, deliberate, confident. Without using force he still commanded respect. The mood was subdued; everyone knew who was boss.

After a few minutes of silence Elena picked back up again.

The team started by considering Mokolo's entire habitat: not just food, but the straw on the ground; the size of the outdoor area; the ropes and play toys; the concrete floor—even the presence of another bachelor like Bebac. They considered things like microorganisms, temperature, feeding times, noise level, and light. They compared Mokolo's zoo habitat with a natural gorilla habitat and looked for any differences that might explain his health problems.

Changing their diet seemed like the most likely way to address regurgitation and weight problems. The team knew that wild gorillas obviously didn't eat gorilla biscuits. So why would any responsible primatologist use them? In the past, many zoo animals weren't fed enough and were chronically malnourished. Old zoo records from the nineteenth century—even from the top zoos in the world—often included things like loaves of bread, candy, and even alcohol. Dental problems were a major problem in early zoos (and still are). In fact, many of the earliest zookeepers assumed that an animal with such fearsome teeth must surely eat meat. In the 1970s some zoos even fed items like Ovaltine and Jell-O to the gorillas.

Elena compared the nutrients in the apes' current diet to estimates of the nutrients in a wild diet. Mokolo and Bebac had never eaten meat, so the team ruled it out as a cause of the gorillas' health problems. Among other differences, the zoo diet had much more starch and simple carbohydrate, and much less fiber.

The first thing the team tried was to increase Mokolo's fiber intake. They ground up the gorilla biscuits, added a fiber substitute called resistant starch, and then made them back into biscuits. (I've since tried one—they're dry and bland, kind of like a chalky, flavorless granola bar.)

The team gradually introduced these high-fiber biscuits to the gorilla diet, but over the course of a week the gorillas developed awful diarrhea. Rather than waiting to see if the diarrhea would clear up, they decided to switch them back to the old biscuits. Since the resistant starch was wheat-based, they thought that Bebac and Mokolo's

GORILLA "DIETS"

If nutrient zoo cakes and pellets are unnatural food for gorillas, what about the conventional food items fed to those apes in captivity?
—Don Cousins, *Acta Zoologica* (1976)

Cousins collected daily feeding schedules from zoos around the world and discovered that Italian gorillas took their morning tea with milk and biscuits whereas Texan gorillas preferred horsemeat with a side of Jell-O.

Rome

8 A.M.—Mixture of tea, homogenized milk, half packet of Plasmon biscuits, 300g bread and sugar
9 A.M.—Juice of 4–5 oranges
10 A.M.—1 celery, 1 banana, or 1 artichoke
12 P.M.—200g of ground meat (cooked with salt in some oil), fresh fruit of the season (apples, pears, or 2 bananas)
3 P.M.—1 yogurt and 1 banana
6–8 P.M.—200g boiled rice, 2–3 egg yolks in homogenized milk, fruit of the season and salad (1 plant), bread and milk, sometimes 2 hard-boiled eggs.

Dallas

Morning—8 oz. milk (½ condensed, ½ water), ¼ lb. horse meat, 1 cup Jell-O
Evening—4 apples, 4 oranges, 2 bananas, 1–2 carrots, 1 head of celery, cooked yams, 5 oz. of raw spinach, kale (when available), bread, cooked rice, raisins, cooked prunes, sugar cane, 75–100 monkey chow pellets, vitamin supplement in milk.

nasty reaction was most likely due to a gluten allergy—but other gorillas eat bread without getting diarrhea, so it wasn't obvious in advance that they would have such a serious reaction.

The team knew that a handful of other zoos had experimented with removing gorilla biscuits from the diet, with positive results. The first zoo to try out the "biscuit-free diet" was Busch Gardens Tampa led by Dr. Ray Ball. Unfortunately, the team didn't collect much data about the experiment. Then Dr. Rich Bergl, the curator of conservation and research at North Carolina Zoo, made the diet switch and collected behavioral data, finding that time spent feeding doubled and that regurgitation decreased—but the positive results in North Carolina needed to be tested on a larger scale. So as part of Elena's dissertation she collaborated with Dr. Bergl to include both a health and a behavior component to the analysis, and to systematically test the biscuit-free diet at more institutions: Cleveland, Columbus, Seattle, and Toronto.

The team got rid of the gorilla biscuits altogether and replaced them with a bunch of plants, like those that gorillas would eat in the wild in Africa. Obviously flying in native African plants would be exorbitantly expensive, so they bought vegetables from the local Cleveland grocery store. Gorillas may not eat romaine lettuce in the wild, but romaine was much closer to their natural diet than gorilla biscuits were.

The team still had to follow all of the official nutritional guidelines, which increasingly looked rigid and arbitrary. Using an analysis reported by USDA, they looked at the nutrient composition of typical plants in a grocery store to figure out combinations that would satisfy the guidelines. They also continued to feed resistant starch to the gorillas as a fiber substitute, but used one that was corn-based instead of wheat-based.

This time, there was no diarrhea. But Mokolo and Bebac seemed anxious, even angry. They finally realized what was probably going on: The gorillas were cranky. There was less sugar in their new diet, and they wanted their gorilla biscuits for the sugar hit.

After about a week the gorillas adjusted and seemed perfectly happy munching on their lettuce. The hair-plucking behavior strongly receded, and the regurgitation behavior stopped completely.

The gorillas also seemed less . . . *bored*. Wild gorillas spend most of the day eating, since plant matter is so fibrous and isn't calorically dense. But at the zoo it never took them very long to eat their gorilla biscuits—and then they had nothing to do all day.

Over the next few months Mokolo lost about seventy pounds and Bebac lost about thirty-seven, about 15% of Mokolo's bodyweight and 9% of Bebac's. Then their weight stabilized, despite the fact that they were eating *twice as many calories*.

When word got out about that, the team received emails from complete strangers telling them with absolute certainty that they had to be mistaken, that their findings broke the laws of physics. Calories in and calories out is all that matters when it comes to weight gain or loss, right? But a gorilla metabolizes a hundred calories of lettuce differently than it metabolizes a hundred calories of gorilla biscuit.

For Mokolo and Bebac, all those additional calories from fresh produce weren't cheap. A year's worth of gorilla biscuits cost about $3,000 per gorilla. A year on their new diet costs about $20,000 per gorilla. The high cost of the project caused a variety of concerns. Even if it could be demonstrated that the gorillas' regurgitation, hair plucking, and signs of heart disease could be reduced with this diet, it was possible the zoo would conclude the health benefits didn't justify the additional cost. What if gorilla biscuits were deemed to be "good enough"? The team would have to watch the problems return, and they'd have to live with the knowledge that those health conditions were largely preventable.

As we walked out of the Primate House, Elena pointed to one of the other primates, a golden-bellied mangabey named Janet Lee. She had type 2 diabetes and received an insulin injection once a day. When the keeper came in for her injection, Janet Lee would stick out her arm, ready for the shot.

. . .

IN THE same way that zoo veterinarians learn from and use human medicine, perhaps it's time for humans to learn a thing or two from zoos.

Civilization isn't literally a zoo. Humans have real freedom that captive animals lack, and we receive great benefits from living in civilization. But wild animals in captivity and humans in civilization share an important quality: we are both examples of species living outside their natural habitats.

When species live inside their natural habitat they have "normal" (species-typical) health and longevity. Species are well adapted to their natural habitat, with a certain amount of balance between an organism and the challenges it faces. This doesn't mean that all wild animals are perfectly healthy—they aren't—but they are well suited to the life they lead. Wild gorillas don't brush their teeth, but they don't have to. Their two sets of teeth (baby and adult) have evolved to be functional given the types of foods that gorillas have typically eaten. Wild gorillas don't have *perfect* teeth—but they certainly don't require regular dental exams in order to avoid numerous cavities and infections, as captive gorillas do.

The history of the health of animals in captivity follows a general arc: *things got worse before they got better.*

Things got worse for wild animals living in captivity in early agricultural civilization. The earliest "zoos" were royal menageries located in city-states. Powerful rulers, like the Egyptian pharaohs, maintained a collection of exotic animals as a sign of power and a source of entertainment, and many of the fierce or "noble" animals were killed for blood sport. The inaugural games of the Roman Colosseum in A.D. 80 saw the slaughter of thousands of animals, including lions, elephants, bulls, bears, leopards, and a rhinoceros.

The Tower of London housed exotic animals for more than five hundred years, usually gifts from foreign rulers to the British Crown. According to an account from 1720, the conditions were abominable:

"The creatures have a rank smell, which hath so affected the air of the place (tho' there is a garden adjoining) that it hath much injured the health of the man that attends them, so stuffed up his head, that it affects his speech." One ostrich died from eating nails, since the public believed the birds could digest iron. An elephant was given wine to drink from April to September, because apparently the keepers believed elephants didn't drink water during that part of the year. As you might imagine, these captive animals didn't last very long. They would have been better off living in the wild.

In 1831 the remaining animals in the Tower of London were transferred to a London park under the control of the newly created Zoological Society of London. National zoos sprang up in the early nineteenth century, not long after the Industrial Revolution.

In the 1850s a gorilla could expect to live about six months in captivity, sometimes killed by a common cold. As scientists finally figured out that good hygiene kept the animals alive, cells were constructed from materials that could be easily cleaned and sterilized: concrete, steel, tile, and glass. The top zoos in the world built cells (and they did look like jail cells) that were clinical, sterile, and completely devoid of anything that might resemble an animal's natural habitat. These measures did accomplish something very important: they kept the animals from dying.

By the mid-twentieth century the top zoos had learned how to get members of most species to live beyond their typical life span in the wild: separate predators from prey; keep members of the same species from killing one another; provide sufficient food and shelter; and keep the enclosures free of infectious disease. Remove those sources of mortality, and just about anything will live longer than in the wild, including humans. Scientifically sound hygiene practices were more important than fancy medical technology.

But once captive animals matched their natural longevity in the wild and then exceeded it, chronic ailments came to the fore. Zoos had succeeded at getting animals to survive, but then they had to shift their focus to helping animals to thrive.

Some zoo animals show signs of mental problems, such as lethargy or incessant pacing. In 2005 the world-class Toledo Zoo made headlines when it acknowledged a pilot project to assess the benefits of using antidepressants to help control anxiety, aggression, and behavioral problems in zebras, wildebeest, and gorillas. Though it garnered press, the practice had been widespread in zoos for years. A 2001 survey of U.S. and Canadian zoos revealed that nearly half of them had used psychopharmaceuticals on gorillas, including Xanax, Klonopin, Valium, Prozac, Ativan, Paxil, and Zoloft. While these drugs were useful at mitigating the symptoms of mental problems, zoo personnel have increasingly attempted to address the underlying cause of the symptoms: living in a habitat that doesn't satisfy the actual physiological and psychological needs of a species.

Historically most zoos had been designed by architects who either copied designs from other zoos or created "works of art" that largely ignored the health needs of the animals. That began to change in the 1960s as landscape architects were inspired by primatologists' detailed observations of gorillas in the wild—as well as by photos in *National Geographic*. Pioneering zoos began to mimic the natural habitat of a species.

In 1978 Seattle's Woodland Park Zoo opened its new gorilla habitat. It was the first major attempt to immerse both captive animals and human observers in a naturalistic setting. The changes weren't just for show; they also had unanticipated health benefits for the apes. Previously the gorillas had chronic diarrhea, but it went away when they moved into their new habitat. The zookeepers still don't know whether it was due to a reduction in stress, a change in diet, or something else—but whatever was causing the diarrhea, it went away. The change in Mokolo and Bebac's diet at the Cleveland Metroparks Zoo was just one more step in this direction, using a habitat-based approach to address chronic health conditions.

The experience of zoos suggests a common process to understand and improve the health and well-being of any organism: *Know thy species.*

The best way to learn about a species is to study it in the wild, living in its natural habitat. This includes everything from what the species eats to how it moves, from common predators to mating behavior—*everything*. It shows the ecological niche that the species is adapted to, and gives an approximation of what kind of lifestyle will enable a member of that species to thrive.

Once a zoo understands how a species lives in its natural habitat, then it can mimic that habitat the best it can using technology. A penguin brain doesn't actually know how the Penguin House gets cold, but it cares that it *is* cold. A prairie dog brain doesn't realize that Plexiglas protects it from birds of prey; the only way it will feel safe is if it can retreat to an underground tunnel.

As with anything in life, zoos face constraints and have to make trade-offs. Mokolo's "gorilla diet" isn't actually composed of plants that a gorilla would eat in the wild, but grocery store produce was the closest, most cost-effective option available to the zoo. Furthermore, just because the zoo is taking a habitat-based approach doesn't mean it has to forgo the use of modern medical technology that isn't available in the wild, such as antibiotics.

This approach works for humans too.

In fact, the quotation "Know thy species" comes from Dr. Jonas Salk, the discoverer of the polio vaccine: "I have been trying to say that it is necessary now not only to 'know thyself,' but also to 'know thy species' and to understand the 'wisdom' of nature, and especially living nature, if we are to understand and help man develop his own wisdom in a way that will lead to life of such quality as to make living a desirable and fulfilling experience."

To understand human health we have to study our own species, the human animal. We start by looking at how we lived as hunter-gatherers on the African savannah.

3

RISE AND FALL

PALEOLITHIC AGE

◄ *2.6 million years ago to 10,000 years ago* ►

Five years after graduating, I found myself back on the Harvard campus in a familiar situation: late to meet with a professor. My destination? Harvard's Peabody Museum of Archaeology and Ethnology.

The Peabody boasts a collection of over six million ancient artifacts from around the world: a shark tooth spearhead from the South Pacific; Mayan hieroglyphics engraved on giant limestone slabs; a Native American whistle carved out of eagle bone collected by Lewis and Clark on their legendary transcontinental expedition.

The Peabody is also where Harvard stores its osteological collections: bones. *Lots* of bones. Neanderthals from Europe, mummified remains from South America, chimpanzees from Africa. The collections contain fossils famous for documenting the emergence of human beings, as well as skulls with uncommon deformities used to teach students about skeletal development. Delicate and rare, the bones in the collections are locked away in an archive, not on display to the public.

I was meeting with Dr. Daniel Lieberman, chair of the Department of Human Evolutionary Biology. Bearded and bespectacled, he looked just like a professor should; he was the ur-professor. Dr. Lieberman studies bones, both dead bones (paleoanthropology) and living bones (biomechanics). He earned tenure by studying the human head, but he earns mention in ESPN stories for his research on barefoot running.

The entire field of human evolutionary biology, Lieberman explained, is dedicated to answering a simple question: *Why are humans the way we are?*

Why are our teeth shaped the way they are—and what does that say about the human diet? Why is the foot arched—and what does that say about the biomechanics of walking and running? Why do humans sweat so much more than other mammals? Why do humans have such large and powerful brains? Embedded in the blueprint of our bodies are clues to the deep history of humanity—and many of those clues point to the Paleolithic Age.

Paleo means "old," *lithic* means "stone," and the Paleolithic begins with the first known stone tools used by hominins about 2.6 million years ago. (The term "hominins" refers to humans and our human-like ancestors such as *Homo erectus, Homo habilis,* and *Australopithecus.*) The stone tools were found in a small area of Eastern Africa in northern Tanzania, near the Serengeti, in a place known as Olduvai Gorge. Paleoanthropologists refer to the area as the "Cradle of Mankind."

The earliest stone tools were rudimentary and didn't change for long stretches of time. They might easily have remained an isolated use of technology by a specific species, the primate equivalent of beaver dams. But by the Upper Paleolithic—roughly 50,000 years ago—something important had changed: artifacts become more diverse and complex, and artistic decoration becomes easy to recognize. *Humanity* becomes easy to recognize. Scholars debate whether the Upper Paleolithic Revolution was the result of rapid changes or more gradual ones, but no one questions that those changes produced a truly revolutionary species: us.

Within a relatively short period, humans expanded into nearly every habitable land and island across the globe, from the barren Arctic tundra to remote atolls of the South Pacific. We displaced all other lineages of hominins (Neanderthals, Denisovans), domesticated another species for the first time (wolves), and hunted dozens of species to extinction. No species had ever established such widespread dominance over dry land so quickly and so thoroughly.

Humanity's explosion onto the world stage was made possible by the expansion of our most defining trait: the brain.

At the beginning of the Paleolithic, our hominin ancestors had modestly larger brains than chimpanzees. Over the next two and a half million years, brain size more than doubled. As a percentage of body mass, humans now have one of the largest brains of any species. More important than raw size is what we can do with our brains, such as communicate with complex language and learn through culture. Culture gave humans the behavioral flexibility to dramatically change how we lived, even within the span of a generation, and then pass that knowledge on to the next generation. It's what enabled hunter-gatherers to adapt to habitats across the globe with such incredible speed.

Dr. Lieberman and his colleagues are trying to figure out what factors influenced the emergence of human beings, and I got to peek into some of the experiments going on in the department.

Dr. Lieberman and his collaborator, Dr. Dennis Bramble, have proposed that bipedal humans are adapted to long-distance walking and endurance running, which our ancestors may have used for scavenging and persistence hunting (running an animal to exhaustion under the hot savannah sun). Dr. Lieberman showed me his running lab, and I got to try out one of the world's most expensive treadmills. You can't buy treadmills like this—Lieberman and his team customized it themselves. Two rubber treads—split, to record left and right feet independently—covered steel force plates, which measured the location and intensity of forces thousands of times a second. A plastic tubing contraption strapped over a runner's mouth measured oxygen consumption, enabling his team to calculate energy consumption. A series of high-speed infrared cameras tracked body movements from little reflective markers taped to the runner's body, similar to the technology used to track movements for CGI effects in movies.

In the same room I opened a freezer containing the butchered remains of a goat. They were studying the jaw forces and energy required to chew raw meat, a privilege that would be bestowed on a few lucky undergraduates. Paleoanthropologists don't agree on how our ancestors hunted before the advent of stone-tipped spears and projectile weapons, but early Paleolithic sites are often littered with bones that bear the distinct markings of an animal having been butchered. Whether by scavenging, ambush hunting, or another method they succeeded.

Changes in diet played an important role in the expansion of the human brain. A big brain is powerful, but it's also expensive. The human brain is about 2 percent of our body mass but consumes roughly 20 percent of our energy. To feed a power-hungry brain, our ancestors had to secure high-quality sources of calories and nutrients. Food sources naturally tend to fall on a spectrum from "easy to obtain, but low nutritional value" (grass, leaves) to "hard to obtain, but high nutritional value" (mammoth, tubers). Our ancestors' diet shifted away from a largely herbivorous or frugivorous diet, akin to the diets of many of the great apes, and toward an omnivorous diet—first, by adding more roots and tubers, and then by introducing more meat.

Just down the hall, scientists were in a "kitchen" heating different types of food to exact temperatures for precise periods of time. Dr. Richard Wrangham, one of Dr. Lieberman's colleagues, has been studying the role of cooking on the expansion of the brain.

Cooking acts like an external form of digestion, breaking down tough plant and muscle fibers. As a result, cooked food yields more calories than raw food—plus it kills parasites and improves the edibility of a much wider range of wild foods. The earliest evidence of cooking appears roughly a million years ago, though scholars still debate when it became a regular and widespread practice. Once hominins wielded fire, the energy constraints on brain size were relaxed even further.

It's hard to pinpoint the exact benefits of an incrementally larger

JUST-SO STORIES

The Elephant's Child sat there for three days waiting for his nose to shrink. But it never grew any shorter . . . For, O Best Beloved, you will see and understand that the Crocodile had pulled it out into a really truly trunk same as all Elephants have to-day.

—Rudyard Kipling,
Just So Stories (1902)

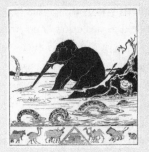

Humans are good storytellers, but not all good stories are true. The elephant didn't actually get its trunk from a tug-of-war with a crocodile. When discussing evolutionary hypotheses, it's important to keep a few things in mind.

1. **What constitutes an "adaptation" is complicated.** Most adaptations are a trade-off between multiple uses. The female pelvis must allow women to walk as well as give birth.
2. **Evolution selects for reproductive success, not necessarily health or longevity.** NFL players get lots of babes, but they get injured a lot and don't live as long.
3. **There was no single "natural habitat" for humans.** The African savannah was a very important habitat, but modern humans bear the imprint of many places and times—from the beginning of life right up to the present.
4. **Evolution hasn't stopped.** Evolution didn't stop 10,000 years ago. (In fact, it has actually accelerated.)
5. **Evolution is amoral.** Just because something is natural doesn't make it morally good ("the naturalistic fallacy"). Conversely, just because something is morally desirable doesn't make it true ("the moralistic fallacy").

Just as evolution is a continual process, so too is our knowledge of it. Evolutionary theory is great for generating hypotheses, but those hypotheses must be tested against evidence.

Source: *The Story of the Human Body: Evolution, Health, and Disease* by Daniel Lieberman

brain, but various cognitive functions must have given hominins a competitive advantage in foraging, social cooperation, language use, and sexual selection (i.e., impressing the opposite sex). However it happened, it did—and once we became big-brained hunter-gatherers, humans were hard to stop. But the most radical shift in lifestyle took place when some hunter-gatherers gradually settled down and started farming.

The Agricultural Revolution was the result of a revolutionary growth technology called domestication, a gradual form of genetic engineering. Domestication is a multigenerational process where humans breed other species to meet our needs, whether it is as a source of food (wheat), companionship (dogs), or even beauty (roses). Among animals, humans domesticated the wild ancestors of dogs, sheep, pigs, goats, cows, chickens, and horses. Among plants, humans domesticated the wild precursors of wheat, barley, rye, squash, maize, beans, millet, rice, soy, and potatoes.

Hunters of wild prey became *herders* of domesticated animals. *Gatherers* of wild plants became *farmers* of domesticated crops. "Hunter-gatherers" became "herder-farmers." Our diverse, omnivorous diet as hunter-gatherers became heavily grain-based, contributing to an overall decline in health—and I was about to hold the evidence in my own hands.

"Okay, let's go see some skulls," said Dr. Lieberman, as he led me out of the department and into the museum.

WE WALKED up to an old wooden door. Probably part of the original construction in the late nineteenth century, it had been retrofitted with an electronic security system. Dr. Lieberman swiped a key fob past it, the lock clicked open, and we walked into a brightly lit room with laboratory equipment lining one wall. It felt like moving from historic to modern, but we were actually moving from historic to *pre*historic.

The archive felt like a cross between a library and a morgue. It was lined with shelves, which were filled with boxes of bones. Handwritten

words faced outward: "Natufian—El Wad"; "Chimpanzee—Liberia."
The labels served the dual role of title and tombstone.

Dr. Lieberman handed me a pair of latex gloves.

"Here, put these on."

The gloves weren't there simply to protect the ancient remains
from me; they were also there to protect me from the ancient remains, since many had been preserved in nasty chemicals.

Dr. Lieberman pulled a box off the shelf, carried it over to a table,
and took off the lid. He gently lifted up a skull.

"This is Skhul V. This guy is famous. He was a hunter-gatherer
living more than 80,000 years ago in the Levant. That's modern-day
Israel. He's one of the earliest anatomically modern *Homo sapiens* ever
recovered. Here, you can hold his skull. There's only one rule."

Dr. Lieberman paused and looked directly at me.

"Use two hands."

It was a command, not a suggestion. This is not something you
want to drop.

With that he gingerly passed me Skhul V.

Looking at a human skull creates an optical illusion: it looks like
the skull is smiling. The brain interprets the visible teeth and up-
swept jawbone as an upturned mouth. Not only did this phenomenon
create the creepy effect that Skhul V
was somehow alive, but he seemed
downright cocky, brimming with
a confidence that even the grave
couldn't shake.

And what a grin this guy had.
What an *amazing* grin.

"Notice anything?" Dr. Lieber-
man asked. "Look at the teeth.
They're straight. And no cavities.
His wisdom teeth came in just fine.
Humans, like all animals, have
evolved teeth that are well suited to

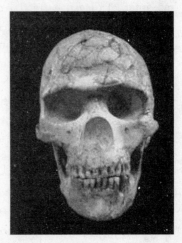

their natural diet. An infected tooth can easily kill you, and there were no dentists in the Paleolithic."

Nearly one hundred thousand years before dentists and orthodontists, this hunter-gatherer had a strong, straight set of chompers. Skhul V challenged much of what I'd been taught about the history of human health.

"Now, look," Dr. Lieberman continued, "hunter-gatherers didn't have *perfect* teeth. This guy has well-worn teeth, and he's actually missing one due to an abscess. So don't stop going to the dentist. But wait until I show you the skulls of early farmers—a lot of them would need to get fitted for dentures."

"So what's the secret? Eat less sugar?" I asked.

"Well, yes, but healthy teeth depend on a variety of factors," Dr. Lieberman explained. "First, yes, it matters what you eat. Amylase in your saliva breaks down carbohydrate into sugar in your mouth. Bacteria feed on the sugar and produce acid that wears away the enamel on teeth, giving you cavities. We'll see what happened to the early farmers who started eating a starchier diet."

To figure out what humans used to eat, teeth are a good place to start. Not only do teeth fossilize well, but they're the first point of contact between the food we eat and our body, the first part of our internal digestive tract. And if our teeth aren't well adapted to a particular food, it's unlikely the rest of our digestive tract is. But whatever Skhul V was eating, his teeth seemed to be up to the challenge.

"It also matters how tough your food is to chew," Dr. Lieberman continued. "When you put force on bones, they grow bigger and stronger. People back then ate tougher foods, they put larger forces on their jaw, and thus they had jaws large enough to actually fit all of our teeth. And those bite forces may have helped our teeth come in straight."

"And since we all eat such soft foods these days?" I asked.

"Smaller jaws."

It felt oddly insulting to hear him say that. In a sense he was pointing out that my growth had been stunted in childhood. I'm *deformed*. And not just me, but most modern people.

Dr. Lieberman took the skull and put it back in the box, then pulled out a femur and held it up.

"I don't know if you've seen many femurs, but I have, and this is quite a femur. He almost certainly has much thicker bones than either of us. Bone cross-sectional thickness increases with use, particularly before the mid-twenties. It suggests significant musculature.

"He was tall, too," Dr. Lieberman said as he held the femur up to my thigh. I'm five foot ten, and the femur was longer than mine. (Dr. Lieberman later sent me a published estimate on Skhul V: five foot ten and 150 pounds. "Yeah, I don't believe it," he said. "I suspect they estimated them wrong.") Even so, five foot ten would have been considered gigantic from the Agricultural Revolution until recently. Early farming populations lost as much as five inches of height compared with early foragers.

"So how long did this guy live?" I asked.

"Well, this guy probably fits the stereotype of dying young," Dr. Lieberman said. "Maybe thirty to forty years old. But life was dangerous back then, and it looks like he was healthy right up to the end. Plenty of ancient hunter-gatherers lived a long time. Contemporary hunter-gatherers regularly live well into their sixties and seventies."

The common misperception is that ancient people would blow out the candles at their thirty-fifth birthday party and then just drop dead. But even chimpanzees and gorillas can live that long in the wild, and there are good reasons to believe we are naturally longer lived than they are. Humans have fewer natural predators than do other primates, as well as a longer childhood before puberty. The age of the oldest documented human (122 years old) far exceeds the oldest documented chimpanzee (66 years old) and gorilla (56 years old), both of which lived in captivity with no risk of predation or starvation. The natural human life span appears to have lengthened in the late Paleolithic when humans were able to fend off external sources of mortality and bear (or support) offspring at older ages. In fact, it's likely that life expectancy initially *dropped* after the Agricultural Revolution.

The Agricultural Revolution seems like a paradox of history: if human health got worse, then why did people become farmers?

The shift to an agricultural lifestyle wasn't something that anyone consciously planned. Even so, the domestication of animals and plants appears to have taken place independently in multiple locations around the world (the Fertile Crescent, China, India, the Americas, and Africa) at about the same time, 15,000 B.C. to 5,000 B.C. It was a technology whose time had come.

In short, the Agricultural Revolution unlocked a path to more rapid growth—in population, culture, and technology—and the people who took that path left descendants as numerous as the stars in the sky. A fifty-person band of hunter-gatherers—even if they are relatively tall and healthy—will be displaced by a wealthy, technologically advanced city-state with a fast-breeding population, many of whom could be enlisted as soldiers, even if they are short and sickly.

"Shall we go look at some diseased farmers?" asked Dr. Lieberman, and he led me to another part of the archive. He pulled out a couple more boxes of bones and placed them on the counter. He lifted up another skull, holding it for me to have a look. "This is an early Neolithic farmer from Tangier, in modern-day Morocco."

Dr. Lieberman turned it over to show the dental cavity.

"These are some shitty teeth. Once you get farming, you get a lot more cavities. It's classic."

The teeth were ground flat, filled with holes, and many were missing. It looked brutally painful.

"By the way, it's not just starch that causes this. It's also the little bits of stone that get mixed into food when grinding grains. That's why the teeth are all ground flat. And see how shiny they are? They've been polished by the stone bits, like by sandpaper. A lot of starch, plus wear and tear, and a poor diet make for a lot of dental problems."

Dr. Lieberman put the Moroccan farmer away and opened another box.

"We've got lots of diseased farmers. This guy is from the fifteenth century in modern-day Montenegro."

He held up the skull. There were long gaps where teeth were missing. Based on the bones, he wasn't much more than five feet tall.

"This is a squat little person who had a horrible, nasty life," Dr. Lieberman observed. "I know you're focused on diet, but probably the biggest negative impact on the overall health of early farmers came from infectious disease: a result of living in close proximity to other people and domesticated animals for the first time."

What Dr. Lieberman said confirmed my basic take on the story of human health. It wasn't one uninterrupted improvement. *Things got worse before they got better.* Teeth got worse, stature declined, infectious disease went through the roof, and life span declined for the average person.

"Just don't forget that the Agricultural Revolution allowed more people to survive. All of us wouldn't be here without it," Dr. Lieberman said as he packed up the bones.

"Speaking of the Agricultural Revolution, who's hungry for lunch?"

JUST AS with the gorillas I visited at the zoo, understanding a species' wild origins helps make sense of its health needs in more "civilized" environments. So what did the life of a Paleolithic hunter-gatherer look like?

The answer to that question is fraught with academics, whose violent turf wars have earned themselves the name "the fierce people."

A good place to start is by asking anthropologists about contemporary hunter-gatherers. Even though they aren't actually "Paleolithic" peoples, their lifestyles provide a stark contrast with those of most people alive today and are the best living approximation of what life used to be like in the late Paleolithic. Unfortunately, few true hunter-gatherer societies exist anymore. It's down to the Inuit in the Arctic, the Aborigines in Australia, the Hadza in Tanzania, and various small tribes scattered through remote parts of the Brazilian rain forest, Papua New Guinea, the South Pacific, and Africa. They often live on marginal or remote land and have experienced fairly significant contact with the outside world, often borrowing technology or trading for nontraditional foods.

Historical accounts can provide information about "pre-contact" hunter-gatherer societies that may no longer exist. For example, a Spanish explorer named Álvar Núñez Cabeza de Vaca spent nine years (1528–1537) living with Native American tribes in the modern-day southern United States and northern Mexico. He described the indigenous people as tall and healthy: "[F]rom a distance they look like giants. They are quite handsome, very lean, very strong and light-footed." Unfortunately, few historical observations were made by scientists using hard data, and accounts can be unreliable. Even though Cabeza de Vaca was not a trained anthropologist, his report is in line with more objective sources of evidence, like indigenous skeletal remains in North America.

Archaeologists are a sadistic people who derive pleasure from forcing their grad students to dig a giant hole with a tiny paintbrush. The field is necessarily limited to parts of the body that fossilize (bones, teeth) and objects that don't disintegrate (stone tools, ashes from a fire). Height, bone density, and dental health are straightforward and reliable measurements. Hunter-gatherers from the Upper Paleolithic tended to be taller, had a thicker bone structure, had better teeth, and showed fewer signs of infectious disease than subsequent farmers. But a skeleton doesn't say much about squishy internal organs like the brain, or about important yet intangible qualities like language, culture, or social structure.

Lots of other fields have something to offer. Geneticists are unlocking a wealth of statistical inferences about our ancestors. Primatologists teach us about other closely related species, such as chimpanzees and bonobos. And paleoanthropologists put all the pieces together, grounded in a theoreotical framework based on evolutionary biology.

Combining these disciplines allows us to make an educated guess at what an ancestral human lifestyle might have looked like during the middle to late Paleolithic.

Hunter-gatherer tribes were fairly small—usually fifteen to fifty people. The tribes were nomadic and migrated with prey or sought out available plant life depending on the season. Frequently on the move, they accumulated few material possessions. In warm climates they wore minimal clothing and spent most of their time outdoors.

The primary division of labor was gender based. Men were hunters; women were gatherers. This does not mean that men only hunted animals and women only gathered plants. Women sometimes trapped small game or collected marine foods; men sometimes gathered honey, nuts, or fruit. But men pursued high risk food sources that required greater physical prowess, while women pursued low risk food sources that could be obtained while tending to small children. Food was shared (especially large game), though preference was given to those who played a role in obtaining it. There were rarely any completely specialized professions, other than perhaps a shaman.

The typical hunter-gatherer diet was very diverse. Over the course of a year a diet might have included hundreds of wild plant species and dozens of wild mammals, fish, reptiles, and insects. Almost the entire animal could be eaten or put to use, including bones, organs, and marrow. Roots and tubers were an important food source. The wild predecessors to grains—like wheat, corn, or rice—were negligible until late in the Paleolithic, though some wild grasses were consumed (we ended up domesticating them, after all). Some foods were eaten raw, but a variety of cooking techniques were used. Because of the wide variety of food available and the tribe's migrations, famine was rare to nonexistent.

Hunter-gatherers spent fewer hours procuring food than early farmers did. They walked many miles a day and engaged in more intense physical activities as life called for them: playing, tracking prey, carrying a butchered animal back to camp, digging up roots and tubers, and fighting. Nights were spent around fires, talking, eating, sleeping, or having sex. Sources of stress were acute (fight, flight) but not chronic (bad boss, credit card debt).

Mothers and other women provided most of the childcare, though mothers were not the exclusive caregiver. Mothers usually breast-fed infants for two to three years. As a result of this longer nursing period, hunter-gatherers had fewer children than did farmers, and spaced them out more. Despite narrowly prescribed gender roles, men and women were on more equitable footing than in subsequent agricultural societies.

Anthropologists have often described hunter-gatherers as optimistic and content. They experienced the full range of emotions, both positive and negative, but negative emotions were rarely chronic. Suicide was rare. They laughed a lot. They had strong personal relationships. They seemed to have a good grasp of what things in life were under their control and what things were not. Their lives appeared to be filled with the meaning that comes from the daily activities required to survive.

There were fewer chronic health problems than in modern industrial society. Obesity and diabetes were nonexistent. Cancer was less common. Dental problems were few, particularly among the young. People had good vision and didn't need eyeglasses or contacts. The human body was well suited to the lives they led.

As pleasant as this may sound, it was no paradise. There was considerable violence. There was widespread infanticide, wife-beating, adultery, rape, and cannibalism. Hunter-gatherers hunted dozens of species to extinction. There were few paths to follow in life. Experience of culture was limited to that of your own tribe and perhaps a few neighboring ones. And, of course, the small-scale nature of hunter-gatherer societies precluded most of the advances of modern civilization.

It wasn't the Garden of Eden.

But compared to the life of an early farmer—which truly was "solitary, poor, nasty, brutish, and short"—a hunter-gatherer existence probably *seemed* like the Garden of Eden.

The biblical description of the Fall of man is one of the oldest human memories. It is the origin tale that lies at the heart of the three great Abrahamic religions: Judaism, Christianity, and Islam. All three sprang from one figure: Abraham, an early herder-farmer. Abraham allegedly lived in the Fertile Crescent—just beyond the only land bridge out of Africa, where the Agricultural Revolution first took off, and where herder-farmers first displaced hunter-gatherers.

Like a dream upon awakening, we struggle to remember life before literacy, life before herding and farming, life before the Fall. But if we step back from the fine details and take in the broad contours, the biblical memory of the Fall has the following arc.

We lived in the Fertile Crescent (Genesis 2:10–14). We lived in harmony with our habitat (Genesis 2:8–25). It did not require much effort to procure food (Genesis 2:8–9). We didn't wear clothes (Genesis 2:25). Then we did something wrong (Genesis 3:6). As punishment, men had to start farming, which was hard (Genesis 3:17–19). We had to eat bread (Genesis 3:19). As punishment, women had to bear more children, childbirth became painful and dangerous, and women fell under the dominion of men (Genesis 3:16). We built the first cities (Genesis 4:17). Our nature now clashed with this new habitat (Genesis 6:5–7, 6:11–12). Agrarian civilizations struggled with famine (Genesis 41), lawlessness (Exodus 20), large-scale warfare (Numbers), and disease (Exodus 7–11). Over time, urban farmers eating plant-based diets displaced hunters and herders eating animal-based diets (Genesis 3:17–19; Genesis 4:2–17; Genesis 25:23–34).

Step even further back, and these early herder-farmers had a memory that goes something like this:

Life was good. We ate something we shouldn't have. Now life is bad.

It would be a decidedly brilliant set of cultural rules that would help a tribe of herder-farmers adapt to life in the early Agricultural Age, and its most important new habitat: the city.

4

MOSES THE MICROBIOLOGIST

AGRICULTURAL AGE

◄ *8,000 B.C. to A.D. 1769* ►

> Then the Lord spoke to Moses, saying: "You shall also make
> a laver of bronze, with its base also of bronze, for washing . . .
> And you shall put water in it . . . So they shall wash their hands
> and their feet, lest they die. And it shall be a statute forever to
> them—to him and his descendants throughout their genera-
> tions."   —*Exodus 30:17–21**

The Agricultural Age was a deeply religious era, and thus it is impossible to understand without reference to the world's great religions. Over half of the world's population adheres to an Abrahamic
religion, and they all revere one figure as a great prophet. In Judaism,
they call him Moshe—he is the great teacher, lawgiver, and most important prophet. In Islam, they call him Musa—and the Quran mentions him more than any other individual, including Muhammad.
And the Christian New Testament refers to one person from the Old
Testament more than any other: Moses.

Though the figure of Moses lies at the heart of civilization, Moses
the man is a mystery. There is nothing that points to his existence pre-
dating the biblical account. He is the putative author of the first five

---

* All Bible quotations are from the New King James Version. For looking up passages in that or other translations, visit: www.biblegateway.com.

books of the Old Testament (Genesis, Exodus, Leviticus, Numbers, and Deuteronomy), which are collectively referred to as the Pentateuch or Torah. However the books were actually written by multiple authors, include stories borrowed from neighboring cultures, sometimes diverge from the best history of the era, and weren't compiled until long after Moses allegedly lived. Seen in that light, the story of Moses is *more* than the story of one man; it's the collective memory of half the world's people.

Here's a summary: Genesis tells of the creation of the world, Adam and Eve, the Fall, and traces the ancestors and descendants of the legendary patriarch Abraham. Exodus begins with the Jews becoming enslaved by Pharaoh in Egypt—but God, acting through Moses, strikes Egypt with a series of ten devastating plagues. The Jewish people are exempt from the plagues, Pharaoh finally lets them go, and Moses leads the Jewish people out of Egypt. Leviticus, Numbers, and Deuteronomy describe the Jews' circuitous path back to Israel, the Promised Land. While wandering in the desert, Moses communes with God and gives the Jewish people laws to follow.

Collectively, these laws are known as the Law of Moses, or the Mosaic Law, which includes far more than the famous Ten Commandments. Jewish scholars count 613 commandments (248 do's and 365 don'ts), with thousands of long-standing interpretations and implications for daily life.

How curious that one of those commandments ordered Jewish priests to *wash their hands*—one of the simplest and most effective forms of hygiene ever discovered—right at the moment in history when infectious disease was exploding. And this commandment came just after the part of the story where the Jewish people distinguish themselves as being impervious to plague.

The flight from Egypt is also the moment in the story when the Jewish people transition from being pastoral herders to urban dwellers. If there is one people who not only made the transition to living in cities but also developed a reputation for thriving in cities, it is the Jewish people. Jewish culture has survived for some 3,000 years—arguably the oldest non-isolated culture with significant permanence—which suggests that it contains features that have allowed it to persist through the Agricultural Age and helped Jews adapt to life in the big city.

As EARLY agriculturalists settled down in cities, they faced very different survival challenges than did hunter-gatherers. Though agricultural diets were less nutritious, infectious disease—not diet—was the greatest health challenge of the era, the result of living in close proximity with large numbers of people and animals for the first time.

Infectious diseases like smallpox, tuberculosis ("consumption"), dysentery, bubonic plague, influenza, measles, rabies, anthrax, and gonorrhea are caused by microbes: bacteria, viruses, fungi, protozoa, and other parasites like roundworms. Pathogens are responsible for far more health conditions than is generally appreciated. Not only do bacteria cause a host of dental problems, but at least one in six cases of cancer worldwide are directly caused by infectious agents, including cervical, penile, and stomach cancers. It has been proposed that a latent or childhood infection is a major risk factor for schizophrenia. Microbes can even change an animal's behavior in odd ways: *Toxoplasma gondii* alters the brain chemistry of mice, making them unafraid of cats; a cat eats an infected mouse, *T. gondii* continues through the cat's digestive system, and gets excreted in its feces; other mice eat the infected feces, infecting themselves. Quite the circle of life.

Pathogens flourish when there are many hosts to infect and many points of contact between the hosts to spread. Growing populations of people, domesticated animals, vermin, and insects satisfied the first condition. People living in close proximity in early cities, with nonexistent public sanitation and poor personal hygiene, satisfied the second. Heaven for pathogens became hell for humans.

Many of the earliest infectious diseases were quite nasty—more deadly, in fact, than their modern-day descendants. When an infectious disease spreads via a living, robust host (e.g., influenza), it often follows the same historical pattern: it starts out virulent then becomes less dangerous over time. This pattern emerges because the most virulent strains quickly kill off their hosts and less virulent strains become more prevalent. For example, it's not in the interest of the common cold to kill off its host since a dead body doesn't walk around sneezing and turning doorknobs. (Infectious diseases like malaria, which spread via mosquitoes, do not necessarily become less virulent among humans over time. Malaria is happy to lay you out flat because mosquitoes do the work of reinoculating new victims.)

There are two and only two ways to handle infectious disease. The first way is for the population to undergo brute genetic selection, with vast numbers either dying or bearing fewer offspring than those with adaptations. The second way to foil pathogens is by using culture, such as hand washing, sewers, or antibiotics.

Whether or not early agriculturalists realized it, many ancient cultural practices were adaptations against pathogens. For example, spices have antimicrobial properties, which made them a healthy addition to food in an era before refrigeration. It's not a coincidence that equatorial ethnic cuisines are particularly spicy (food spoils faster in hot climates) and recipes for meat dishes tend to call for more spices than do vegetable dishes (meat spoils faster than plants). Water in early cities was often filthy, which helps explain the emergence of sterile alternatives such as wine (microbes can't survive in alcohol) and hot tea (boiling kills microbes). Early people didn't know that invisible bacteria were causing their cavities, but many still ended up using "toothbrushes"—wooden chewing sticks containing a natural antiseptic or treated with one.

Microbes can be beneficial too. The human body is filled with microbes—in fact, the cells of microorganisms vastly outnumber the body's own cells. Scientists are just beginning to grasp the enormous role of microorganisms in human health, including digestion (gut flora), immune function (being too clean has drawbacks), and the benefits of eating fermented foods. But back then the far greater health challenge was avoiding harmful microbes—and short of antibiotics, hygienic cultural practices had to do.

The people who adopted these beneficial cultural practices didn't have to understand how they worked. People who developed a taste for spicy food got food poisoning less often. People who drank wine instead of water were less likely to die of dysentery. Even to most modern people, the original functions of ancient cultural practices are still a mystery.

Ideas and microbes are strangely similar. Both are incredibly influential yet poorly understood. Both are (usually) invisible. Both find ingenious ways to spread: ideas use brains and books; microbes use blood and insects. Both mutate quickly, and new variants can be particularly dangerous. Both seem to have a life of their own, yet neither is viewed as fully alive. Both flourish in large, dense networks—such as cities.

We even use the same word to describe them: culture. The colloquial definition of culture refers to ideas, beliefs, traditions, practices, and technology. But culture has another definition associated with microbiology, as in a bacterial culture (as when a doctor takes a throat culture to check for an infection). Appropriately enough, both definitions of culture derive from *cultura*, which means "tillage" or "cultivation"—the same root that gave rise to the word "agriculture."

The Agricultural Revolution wasn't simply a revolution in agriculture; it was a revolution in *culture*. Agriculture led to cities, and cities led to more ideas *and* infectious disease.

Ideas flourished in early civilization in much the same way that pathogens did: more "hosts" to infect (minds) and more ways for them to spread (conquest, trade, writing). But initially pathogens spread much faster than did effective ideas on hygiene.

We know from their writings that the ancients desperately tried to understand the cause of infectious disease. Given the invisibility of germs, it's not surprising that early people blamed plague and pestilence on the will of similarly invisible gods—and looked to them for deliverance. Just as shamans played the role of "medicine men" among hunter-gatherer tribes, early priests also played the role of healers. These early healer-priests were often educated scribes, thus dealing in both forms of culture: ideas and microbes.

To learn about priestly culture from the early agricultural era, one doesn't need to study ancient bones or get access to a rare book collection. Any bookstore will do, since the bestselling book of all time—the Bible—sprang out of the Fertile Crescent thousands of years ago, where the Agricultural Revolution first took off.

In reading the Torah, one thing becomes immediately clear: life was rife with disease. Not only does the Torah describe pestilence and plague in a general sense, it also mentions dozens of distinct diseases and illnesses. Yet the Jewish people seem miraculously exempt from pestilence—when they obey God's laws.

The Torah is emphatic on this point: disobey God's rules and get hit with a huge health bill. "The Lord will strike you with consumption, with fever, with inflammation, with severe burning fever, with the sword, with scorching, and with mildew . . . with the boils of Egypt, with tumors, with the scab, and with the itch, from which you cannot be healed . . . with madness and blindness and confusion of heart" (Deuteronomy 28:22, 27–28).

There's much in the Law of Moses that remains mysterious or defies a simple explanation, but it is remarkable how much makes sense from a single point of view: infectious disease.

Some of the rules unambiguously address infectious disease, with priests explicitly playing the role of healer. For example, the laws concerning "leprosy" read like a medical text (Leviticus 13–14). Though the modern condition known as leprosy isn't itself described, the laws help healer-priests discern between multiple skin diseases and determine the appropriate treatment. The prescriptions for infected people include scientifically valid ways to halt the spread of disease: immediate quarantine, washing, and in some cases hair removal. The laws also specify how to deal with "leprous" garments or dwellings. Garments had to be quarantined and washed; if that failed to halt the spread of infection, they had to be burned. Dwellings had to be emptied, contaminated stones had to be replaced, and the walls had to be scraped down and re-plastered. If the infection persisted, the dwelling had to be destroyed.

Far beyond the laws on leprosy, it's fair to say the Mosaic Law is obsessed with cleanliness, stipulating a lengthy code of personal hygiene and public health—accounting for some 15–20% of the 613 commandments. Though many commandments applied only to priests, the practices often came to permeate Jewish culture, fulfilling the injunction: "'And you shall be to Me a kingdom of priests and a holy nation'" (Exodus 19:6). Jewish scholars have written about the importance of ritual hygiene in Judaism for a very long time (it's one of the oldest themes in written scholarship), and the tight link between physical and spiritual purity led to the religious proverb "Cleanliness is next to godliness."

The Jewish hygiene code appears to be based on four core principles.

First, certain people, animals, or things are inherently "unclean." Inorganic matter alone, such as dirt, doesn't make someone "unclean" in the literal sense of "dirty." Uncleanliness comes from *organic matter,* such as corpses, bodily fluids, insects, and certain animals. In many cases what the Jews call "unclean" we might refer to as "infected" or "diseased" (or likely to be so).

Second, this "unclean" status is *transferable* through physical contact. In the same way that germs are transmissible, "unclean" things are treated as "contaminated" or "contagious."

Third, an "unclean" person or object could become "clean" again through various *purification rituals.* It was as if these cleansing rituals were able to "decontaminate" or "disinfect" people or things.

Fourth, individual "uncleanliness" affects *the entire community.* Akin to mandatory public health measures, the Mosaic Law applies to all Jews—and the text makes clear that Jews' collective adherence to the Mosaic Law would determine the unified fate of the Jewish people.

Many sources of uncleanliness make sense given what we now know about infectious disease. The early Jews had a healthy obsession with bodily fluids, like blood, feces, saliva, pus, and semen. Pathogens love to hitch a ride in bodily fluids, and viewing all bodily fluids with suspicion would have been a prudent thing to do in that era. Eating blood was banned (Leviticus 7:26–27). Bodily discharges, including emissions of semen or menstrual blood, made a person unclean (Leviticus 15). Childbirth, entailing a great deal of bodily fluid (and potential for infection), was also a time of uncleanliness (Leviticus 12). This logic would also explain why it was prohibited to get a tattoo or to cut oneself while mourning the dead (Leviticus 19:28).

Some of the rules were clearly ineffective—touching a menstruating woman doesn't actually transmit cooties. However, ineffective rules may have been the price of a generalized obsession with potential routes of infection, and such a mindset would lead to practices that are genuinely hygienic. A general skittishness about touching people who are secreting bodily fluids would have been sensible in an era before antibiotics.

Long before modern toilets and sewer systems, the Jewish army was ordered to keep campsites clean of feces:

> Also you shall have a place outside the camp, where you may go out; and you shall have an implement among your equipment, and when you sit down outside, you shall dig with it and turn and cover your refuse. (Deuteronomy 23:12–13)

Armies, with their temporary facilities and concentration of men, are huge breeding grounds for disease—the 1918 influenza epidemic most likely bred in the trenches of World War I—and in many wars more soldiers are felled by disease than by weapons. By virtue of this rule alone, a Jewish military campsite would compare favorably to any Medieval European city—despite preceding Medieval times by more than a thousand years.

Touching any kind of corpse—man or beast—made someone unclean (Numbers 5:2; Leviticus 5:2). It was also prohibited to touch human bones and graves (Numbers 19:16). Jewish law mandated a quick burial, ideally in less than a day, an "honor" that even extended to criminals condemned to death (Deuteronomy 21:22–23). Honoring the dead benefited the living: quick burials make hygienic sense given how rapidly corpses decompose in a hot climate like that of the Middle East. Today this tradition is still important even to nonobservant Jews, who face the dilemma of interring a loved one before his or her children can return home for the funeral.

Showing a similar wariness of corpses, Jews were not allowed to eat any animal that either died of its own accord or was killed by wild beasts (Leviticus 7:24, 11:39–40). Animals weakened by disease are more likely to drop dead or be picked off by predators, and, as with humans, a corpse lying out for long enough becomes a literal breeding ground for pathogens.

When applied to humans, this same standard of edibility—avoiding anything that died of its own accord—would explain the decline of cannibalism, which had been a fairly common practice among pre-agricultural peoples. With so many people dropping dead from disease, cannibalism was a recipe for infection—thus an ancient indigenous method of honoring the dead turned into an unthinkable taboo, used in curses as a sign of the ultimate defilement (Leviticus 26:29; Deuteronomy 28:52–57). The twentieth century contains a famous example of this dynamic: kuru, the human equivalent of mad cow disease, spread among indigenous New Guineans who ate the brains of their dead ancestors.

Only healthy animals were fit for sacrificial slaughter (Leviticus 3:1), and the high standard for sacrifices to God became the minimum standard for the lowliest Jew. The result was an ancient form of food inspection: the carcass and internal organs had to be examined for defects, signs of disease, or anything that might have caused the animal to die of its own accord in the near future. Later in history, Jews even inflated the lungs and submerged them in water to look for any leaks—a telltale sign of tuberculosis.

Yet even the choicest cuts from healthy animals will quickly spoil in an era without refrigeration. When the Jews made burnt offerings, the meat had to be eaten on the first day (and in some cases, on the second). On the third day, the meat became an abomination in the eyes of God and had to be destroyed with fire (Leviticus 7:15–17, 22:30).

The Torah lays out an entire dietary code (*kashrut*), which specifies which foods are fit to eat (*kosher*). The most well-known examples are the prohibitions that rule out pork and shellfish, but they are just two of many species that are designated as "unclean" (and thus, unfit to eat) or "clean" (and thus, fit to eat).

Many of the dietary rules make a fair bit of sense in light of infectious disease. The prohibition against mice and moles (Leviticus 11:29–31) was interpreted as any type of rodent, including rats, which are notorious carriers of disease. Furthermore, nearly all insects are considered unfit to eat (Leviticus 11:20–23). Pathogens love to piggyback on biting arthropods like mosquitoes, fleas, ticks, beetles, and lice—and the insects living around a city likely would have been feeding on and hatching in refuse, feces, or corpses. Avoiding vermin and insects like the plague, as it were, would have been a simple and effective rule to avoid infectious disease.

A few insects were considered "clean," and thus edible (Leviticus 11:21–22). The Jewish philosopher Maimonides identified four types of locust, two types of cricket, and two types of grasshopper, though there is some disagreement about the number and identity of exempted species. Locusts, crickets, and grasshoppers feed primarily on plants and present little disease risk to humans. In fact, since these insects would devour crops and were themselves a good source of protein, it would have been doubly advantageous for people to consume them.

So in terms of minimizing direct contact with carriers of infectious disease, the Jewish dietary code gets it right in three important cases: vermin, insects, and corpses. But it can be hard to avoid contact with pesky vermin and insects (and corpses don't bury themselves), so it's best to have as few around as possible. Many of the remaining "unclean" species happen to feast on vermin, insects, or corpses—and thus these prohibitions protect species that provide a valuable service in the local ecology: devouring common carriers of disease.

The "unclean" lizards and amphibians (Leviticus 11:29–30) are low disease risks, but they do perform a useful function: They eat scads of insects, which carry disease. It would have been helpful having lots of them around to keep the insects at bay. Bats, also voracious insect eaters, are considered unclean and would have been far more valuable alive than dead (Leviticus 11:19). The prohibitions against eating birds of prey appear to follow a similar ecological logic (Leviticus 11:13–19). Birds of prey eat vermin and other pests. Carrion fowl, such as the forbidden vultures, conveniently dispose of corpses (Leviticus 11:13–19), as do four-pawed carnivorous mammals (Leviticus 11:27). Fewer corpses, less disease.

While this ecological explanation may seem highly speculative, the benefits of having a carnivore on the premises should come as no surprise to the one-third of American households that own a cat. House cats descend from carnivorous African wildcats, which self-domesticated by venturing into human cities to feast on vermin. Because they provided this useful ecological service, it became taboo to eat cat meat in ancient Egypt and many subsequent cultures. By excluding cats from the dinner menu, even the American diet reveals the influence of protecting a species that eats vermin.

Corpse-loving carnivores played a similar role in Zoroastrianism, another early monotheistic religion from the Middle East with a strong hygiene code. Once the dominant religion of Persia and one of the largest religions in the world, Zoroastrianism explicitly stipulated that all human corpses must be taken to a mountaintop, chained to the ground, and left to be devoured by corpse-eating wild dogs and birds (Avesta, Vendidad 6:44–51).* In fact, some of the rules in the Torah may have been borrowed from Zoroastrianism, or vice versa, during the Babylonian Exile (587–538 B.C.).

The prohibitions that rule out pork and shellfish have drawn a lot of attention from scholars, who have offered a variety of explanations. A common theory is that eating raw or undercooked pork is a good way to contract trichinosis, a parasitic disease infecting swine.

---

* References to the Vendidad are drawn from the translation accessible at: www
.avesta.org/vendidad/.

Alternatively, given the effectiveness with which food preferences separate insiders from outsiders, kashrut may simply have differentiated Jews from surrounding peoples (perhaps a pork-loving one). Without attempting to settle that debate (if that were even possible), it's worth making a few observations in relation to infectious disease and ecology. Shellfish spoil particularly quickly; as filter feeders, they are easily contaminated by polluted waters near human cities; and they clean the local water supply. Even today, shellfish can be dangerous, as in periodic red tide warnings, and the adage against eating oysters in months without an "r" (ruling out summer months). Omnivorous pigs will happily eat vermin, snakes, and refuse; plus they may carry a greater disease risk to humans due to an underlying biological similarity, the same reason that pig organs can sometimes be used as transplants for humans.

On the other hand, there may be alternative reasons, or none at all, for prohibiting the eating of pigs or other "unclean" animals (camel, horse, hare). Anthropologist Dr. Marvin Harris has proposed that swine were deemed unclean because omnivorous pigs compete with humans for food, whereas herbivorous ruminants do not. Furthermore, Harris pointed out that it would be far simpler to have a rule to thoroughly cook your meat: "flesh of swine thou shalt not eat until the pink has been cooked from it." However, if the reason that many unclean species couldn't be eaten was their role in the ecosystem, then a mandate to "cook everything" would have failed to address the underlying ecological logic. These species would have to be *alive* in order to perform their role of eating insects, vermin, and corpses—and thus each of these species would have to be specifically prohibited as a source of food. Cooked cats don't catch mice.

Finally, it is striking that the Jewish dietary code says nothing about unclean plants—even though many plant species are inedible or poisonous. This omission would make sense if one of the underlying functions of kashrut was to minimize infectious disease; plants present a much lower disease risk to humans than do animals.

The Jewish hygiene code's sophistication at identifying sources of disease is matched by its implicit understanding of how disease spreads. Germs are invisibly small and they find ingenious ways to infect new hosts: direct contact between solid objects, flowing through liquids, and even flying through the air.

Any direct contact with an unclean person (or thing) made someone (or something) unclean. For example, if a rodent carcass touched household objects or fell into food or water, it all became unclean (Leviticus 11:32–38). The idea that germs were transferable by even the slightest physical touch may seem obvious today, but it was an astonishing inference thousands of years before the formal discovery of the germ theory of disease in the late nineteenth century.

The Torah even treats liquids differently from solids. Liquids are thought to transmit uncleanliness more easily than solids (Leviticus 11:34, 37–38), yet water itself is a source of cleanliness and required in multiple purification rituals, such as bathing. Flowing water is treated as a more potent cleansing agent than sitting water (Leviticus 15:13). If a part of a carcass falls into a large body of water, such as "a spring or a cistern," the carcass is unclean, but not the entire body of water (Leviticus 11:36). The Zoroastrian hygiene code is even more specific: if a corpse lies in a pond, it defiles the water for six steps on all sides; different distances are given for wells, flowing streams, and snow. It is a grave sin for any person to come across a corpse in a body of water and not immediately remove it (Avesta, Vendidad 6:26–41). As a result of water's dual nature (easily transmitting uncleanliness, yet itself a source of purification), Jews became fixated on ensuring the purity of their water supply. A clean water supply would have resulted in less exposure to deadly waterborne illnesses, such as cholera.

The Torah views uncleanliness as airborne only under certain conditions. If a person dies in an enclosed area, like a tent, then others become unclean through their mere presence. This sensitivity to open and closed spaces also extends to open and closed containers:

> This is the law when a man dies in a tent: All who come into
> the tent and all who are in the tent shall be unclean seven days;

and every open vessel, which has no cover fastened on it, is unclean. (Numbers 19:14–15)

Given the many sources of uncleanliness and the ease of transmission, it's a wonder the early Jews could get clean at all. Thankfully, they could turn to a set of religious rituals to purify themselves in the eyes of God.

One of those purification rituals requires an unclean person to take both hands and rinse them in clean water (Exodus 30:17–21; Leviticus 15:11; Deuteronomy 21:6). The Nobel-worthy commandment to wash your hands is called for in a few specific circumstances, but it was subsequently extended to mean that Jews should wash their hands after waking up, after going to the bathroom, before meals (eating bread), before worship, after being in a cemetery, after coming within a certain distance of a corpse, after touching private parts, and a Talmudic list of other situations. Today, hand washing is known to be one of the simplest and most effective ways to avoid infectious disease—and even washing without soap is better than nothing. Islam mandates hand washing at least five times a day (before prayer), and if clean water is unavailable, scrubbing the hands with clean earth or sand will do (Quran 5:6).

Another form of "ritual" purification required Jews to immerse themselves in a pool of water—also known as taking a bath. For example, on the Day of Atonement (Yom Kippur), the holiest day of the year, the high priest had to bathe before making the burnt offering, emphasizing the importance of cleanliness in the eyes of God (Leviticus 16:24). While it might seem obvious to modern readers, the hygienic benefits of bathing went unappreciated for long stretches of history. But the Jews have been avid bathers for millennia, finding an opportunity at nearly every turn.

One of those opportunities recurred every seven days: the Sabbath.

Keeping the Sabbath holy—one of the Ten Commandments—may have functioned as a way to enforce minimum standards of personal hygiene throughout the community. Similar to how modern parents have to force children to brush their teeth twice a day—a secular hygiene ritual—early herder-farmers probably had to be forced to bathe on a regular basis. Observing the Sabbath was very important: the penalty for not observing a day of rest—taking a vacation day— was death (Exodus 31:12–17). In preparation, Jews had to undergo multiple purification rituals: take a bath, wash their hands, launder their clothes, and clean their home. All Jews had to come clean, so to speak, on the Sabbath.

The Jewish people also knew about at least one form of sterilization: fire. After the Bible says they conquered the Midianites, the priests instructed the soldiers to sterilize their plunder:

> Only the gold, the silver, the bronze, the iron, the tin, and the lead, everything that can endure fire, you shall put through the fire, and it shall be clean; and it shall be purified with the water of purification. But all that cannot endure fire you shall put through water. (Numbers 31:22–23)

Here's how to make that "water of purification": slaughter a cow, burn it whole, and throw some "cedar wood and hyssop and scarlet" into the fire. Then take the ashes and add water (Numbers 19). Water, ash, and animal fat are ingredients for soap. This might explain why the Jewish people seem to use purification water as a potent cleansing agent in rituals throughout the Torah. Simple soap-like substances were known in Babylon as far back as 2800 B.C., as well as in ancient Egypt.

Even though Jews stopped sacrificial slaughter thousands of years ago, Jewish rabbis offered a different interpretation of "water of purification": scalding hot water (Talmud, Avodah Zarah 75b). As a result, Jews sterilized their dishes and eating utensils by submerging them in water that had been brought to a boil.

The purification laws also distinguish between objects made from different materials. Earthenware pots, which are porous and difficult to sterilize, had to be broken and could never be used again if they became unclean (Leviticus 6:28, 11:33). In contrast, bronze pots could be scoured and washed (Leviticus 6:28). Items made from wool, linen, leather, and wood could usually be washed (Leviticus 11:32, 13:53–59, 15:12; Numbers 31:20), though sometimes they had to be destroyed with fire (Leviticus 13:47–52).

The Torah also recognizes that the passage of time has the power to purify, such as during quarantine. Clearly, the body is capable of fighting off infection on its own.

All these purification rituals were brought to bear after the Jewish military conquered filthy, infected foreigners (Numbers 31:19–24). Oddly for a victorious army, the rules for soldiers and captives were largely the same: a weeklong quarantine; two bouts of washing for anyone who killed someone or touched a corpse; two bouts of additional washing for the captives; washing all garments, leather goods, and wooden implements; sterilization of metal plunder with fire; then either washing plunder with soapy water or by submersion in boiling water.

(In fact, this passage in Numbers became the basis for many rules governing any type of contact with Gentiles and their possessions, which were assumed to be unclean. This wariness of contact with filthy foreigners, plus an obsession with hand washing, would have given Jews an advantage in commerce, both as middlemen—as hubs in trade networks—and long-distance merchants visiting lands with novel pathogens—key edges in trade networks. Another people similarly distinguished are the Parsis of India; curiously, they are some of the last remaining followers of Zoroastrianism.)

Not only did the physical plunder have to be cleaned of infection, so did the captive women (all the men were killed). Female captives were forced to shave their heads and trim their fingernails (Deuteronomy 21:10–12), which has typically been interpreted as a mourning ritual. Oddly, the Zoroastrian holy book devotes an entire chapter to the evils of hair and fingernail clippings, explicitly associating them with lice and other insects (Avesta, Vendidad 17). Pathogens are now

known to hide in hair and under fingernails, which is why nurses
with long hair have to wear it up and the Centers for Disease Control
instructs them to keep their fingernails trimmed to less than a quarter of an inch.

Only virgin women could be captured; all other women had
to be killed (Numbers 31:15–18). This was a direct result of past
experience—see "the Peor incident" (Numbers 25)—when the Jewish soldiers kept all the conquered women alive, had sex with them,
and brought a plague upon themselves. Keeping only the virgins
would have largely eliminated the likelihood of contracting a sexually
transmitted disease (STD).

STDs certainly existed before the Agricultural Revolution, but
after it they became more numerous and widespread—just like other
types of infectious disease. Leviticus describes an STD that scholars
believe was gonorrhea (Leviticus 15:1–15). Left untreated, gonorrhea
can cause infertility in women and blindness in children at birth.
Both conditions are referenced in the Bible (Exodus 23:26; John
9:1–2), barren women with some frequency. Exposure to infertility-
inducing STDs would have been a heavy cost of any type of sexual
behavior, but particularly behaviors that increased the risk of infection and did not bring a reproductive benefit.

The more promiscuous instincts of our forager ancestors (relative
to lifelong monogamy) would have exposed them to disease in this
new habitat. Early agricultural sex cults—of which there were more
than a few—tended to die out. Religions that placed restrictions on
our sexual impulses did not. Untreatable, virulent STDs were clearly
a reason. It's no coincidence that more permissive sexual practices
began to emerge in the late 1950s, soon after the discovery of penicillin in 1943. Antibiotics allowed people to treat previously untreatable
STDs, like syphilis, gonorrhea, and chlamydia.

The early Jews didn't have antibiotics or latex condoms, but the
Torah imposes other measures to minimize the spread of STDs. Prostitutes often carry a high number of STDs—and not only were parents ordered to prevent their daughters from becoming prostitutes

(Leviticus 19:29), but high status priests were also prohibited from marrying "harlots" (Leviticus 21:7). In addition to prostitution, forms of sex outside of a monogamous (or polygamous) relationship were frowned upon or explicitly prohibited, including premarital sex, adultery (Leviticus 20:10), sex between men (Leviticus 18:22), and bestiality (Exodus 22:19; Leviticus 18:23).

Since women bear more of the health burdens from STDs than men do, the average Jewish woman would have benefited considerably from these measures. For example, for over a century doctors have noticed that Jewish women have particularly low rates of cervical cancer, the second most common cancer in women worldwide. Cervical cancer is caused by an STD called the human papillomavirus (HPV). The connection between cervical cancer and sexual activity was discovered by observing that celibate nuns were unafflicted by cervical cancer, whereas the affliction was relatively common among prostitutes. In all likelihood, Jewish women throughout history can thank some aspect of Jewish sexual practices for their low rate of cervical cancer.

In light of all this, it seems fitting that one of God's great covenants with the Jewish people was a medical procedure that helped combat infection: circumcision (Genesis 17:9–14). In 2012, a task force on circumcision organized by the American Academy of Pediatrics published a review of the costs and benefits of male circumcision. In their estimation the primary benefits are a reduction in urinary tract infections among infants; lower transmission of some STDs, such as HIV and HPV; and fewer cases of penile cancer (often caused by HPV infections). To be sure, circumcision does not appear to reduce transmission of all kinds of STDs; the surgical procedure itself carries a small, non-negligible risk of complications; and some people have raised ethical issues with removing a sensitive part of an infant male's penis. However, in an era when infectious disease was the number one cause of mortality and incurable STDs could easily cause sterility, male circumcision was probably a wise decision.

Without question, hygiene is not the only explanation for these

biblical rules—and in practice, individual rules may have had no hygienic impact at all (or a negative one). Even though a unified explanation for rules covering such disparate domains of life may seem like
the product of a Bible-code conspiracy theorist, germs *are* pervasive.
Any hygiene code that didn't address such widely disparate domains
would be a poor one. God works in mysterious ways; so do germs.

Taken as a whole, the knowledge of hygiene contained in the
Mosaic Law is nothing short of stunning. It correctly identifies the
main sources of infection as vermin, insects, corpses, bodily fluids,
food (especially meat), sexual behaviors, sick people, and other contaminated people or things. It implies that the underlying source of
infection is usually invisible and can spread by the slightest physical
contact—while taking into account the different physical properties
of solids, liquids, and gases; the passage of time; open and closed
spaces; and different types of materials. And it prescribes effective
methods of disinfection, such as hand washing, bathing, sterilization
by fire, boiling, soap, quarantine, hair removal, and even nail care.

Yet even when health rules are scientifically sound, it can be exceedingly difficult to get people to actually comply with them. Effective public health measures require the coordination of the entire
population, as modern efforts have demonstrated. If enough people
don't get vaccinated, viruses persist. A small number of people abus-
ing antibiotics can breed antibiotic-resistant strains of bacteria that
can harm everyone else. Just a few transgressors can introduce disease into a population. Nearly everyone has to be on board for public
health measures to work.

Impressively, the Mosaic Law treats infectious disease as a public
health issue affecting the entire community. It enforces mandatory
measures to prevent the spread of disease: clean water, toilets, food
inspection, pest control, hygienic burial practices, STD awareness,
circumcision, and codes of sexual conduct—as well as regular house-
cleaning, dishwashing, laundry, and bathing in preparation for the
Sabbath and other holy days. These were matters of life and death
for the entire community, and transgressors were punished severely.

In light of the scientific nature of the Jewish hygiene code and the need for community-wide enforcement, the Jewish God's threats start to make sense. Follow God's hygiene rules and emerge unscathed from the great plagues that destroy rival peoples: a sign of God's favor. Disobey God's hygiene rules and be struck down by pestilence: a sign of God's displeasure.

I propose that a scientifically sound set of hygiene rules could explain why the Jewish God was a jealous, monotheistic God: He could brook no compromise with the filthy practices of rival gods. Famously faceless, abstract, and unsuperstitious, the Jewish God was *science*.

God was exceedingly clear about the consequences should Jews ever abandon the Mosaic Law: plague and disease. Fatefully, an influential Jew—Jesus of Nazareth—formed a splinter sect and instructed his followers that it was all right to abandon these ancient Jewish customs. In an underappreciated moment in human history, Jesus and his disciples didn't bother to wash their hands before meals (Matthew 15:1–20; Mark 7:1–23; Luke 11:37–41).

The Pharisees were aghast: how could a Jew not wash his hands before eating? Jesus argued that defilement came not from external sources but from within. Jesus had a valid point about moral conduct, but with respect to the hygienic value of hand washing, it's fair to say the Pharisees were right and Jesus was wrong.

The deadly consequences of this schism would not be felt immediately. Christianity rose to prominence during the relatively hygienic Roman Empire, which mitigated infectious disease through sewers, aqueducts, and a civic religion of public baths. But when the Roman Empire fell and Europe entered the Dark Ages, Christendom became a filthy place ("a *filthier* place" might be a more accurate description, since the Roman Empire was still quite filthy by today's standards). The decay of Roman sewers and aqueducts meant more feces, refuse, and rats. Bathing was no longer a daily activity for most Medieval Christians—and sometimes not even a weekly or monthly one. While Medieval books on manners encouraged hand washing, Christian doctrine did not mandate the practice as a daily, central, universal feature of religious observance in the way it was by Jewish (and Islamic) doctrine.

Christendom would pay a high price for abandoning the Mosaic Law: the Black Death.

In 1348 bubonic plague broke out across much of Europe, killing a third or more of Europe's population within just a few years. People had no idea what caused it—some thought it could be transmitted "by look alone." The two most common explanations were bad air, vapors, and stench; or divine retribution and acts of God. While the idea of divine retribution may seem medieval, Medieval Christians would have been wise to take that idea a little more seriously—their own holy book explained how to avoid God's wrath. Modern researchers have determined that bubonic plague was caused by *Yersinia pestis,* a bacterium transmitted by two "unclean" species: the fleas on rats.

In a tragic historical turn, Christians in some cities claimed that fewer Jews were dying from the plague. They tortured prominent Jews and extracted forced confessions that Jews had conspired to poison the water supply; the fact that Jews (sensibly) covered their own wells was offered as "proof." Across Europe, violent rioters killed tens of thousands of Jews and caused many more Jews to flee to Eastern Europe. Pope Clement VI tried to quell the massacres by issuing a papal bull stating that just as many Jews were dying from plague as were Christians. Subsequent historians have asserted the same belief, perhaps not wanting to validate claims that were used to persecute the Jewish people.

But what if the Jewish people actually *were* less afflicted by the Black Death?

Not because of a global Jewish cabal, but because of their adherence to a stunningly brilliant, scientifically sound set of hygiene rules called the Law of Moses. They protected their water supply from contamination; bathed regularly; washed their clothes; inspected their food; avoided vermin, insects, and corpses—and they washed their hands.

It took a few thousand years for scientists to catch up with the book of Leviticus.

In the mid-nineteenth century, the hygienic value of hand washing was "discovered" by a Hungarian physician, Dr. Ignaz Semmelweis, who noticed particularly high mortality rates in one of two maternity wards at Vienna General Hospital. Adjoining that maternity ward was a morgue, and doctors would perform autopsies then proceed to deliver a baby without washing their hands. (Midwives delivered the babies in the ward with lower mortality rates.) Semmelweis hypothesized that doctors' hands picked up "cadaverous particles" from the dead and transferred them to the living. Ignored at the time, Semmelweis now receives credit for discovering the hygienic value of hand washing—even though he lived more than two millennia after Jews not only adopted the practices of washing their hands, avoiding corpses, and isolating women during childbirth, but also had their "findings" published in the most accessible and well-known text in Western civilization.

The relationship between Judaism and hygiene did not go unnoticed by the scientific world. Jewish scholars had long written about the hygienic value of Jewish purity laws, but scientific proof of their effectiveness was scant. It was still just a good story.

At the end of the nineteenth century, Dr. Maurice Fishberg, a Jewish physician living in New York City, began to gather statistics on Jewish mortality rates to see if there was anything to the Jewish reputation for "unprecedented tenacity of life." In Europe, from the Black Death onward, Fishberg uncovered reports of Jewish people dying at lower rates than Christians during major epidemics: a typhus epidemic in 1505; fevers in Rome in 1691; dysentery in Nimègue in 1736; and typhus in Langeons in 1824. By the nineteenth century, public health statistics revealed not only that the effect was real, but that it was enormous: a ten-year advantage in life expectancy in many European cities. This disparity was even more remarkable considering that Jews were often forced to live in crowded and damp urban ghettos—places conducive to the spread of disease.

In the United States, the story was the same. Fishberg noted that a Jewish five-year-old could expect to live to the age of sixty-seven, whereas the average non-Jewish five-year-old (from Massachusetts) could expect to live to fifty-eight—a stunning nine-year gap. As in Europe, the Jewish population was overwhelmingly concentrated in the densest parts of the biggest cities, especially New York City's Lower East Side. The Tenth Ward was crowded, filthy, overwhelmingly Jewish—and had the lowest mortality of any ward in the entire city. Fishberg noted that this lower mortality was driven by lower rates of infectious disease: "tuberculosis, pneumonia, nephritis, typhoid, malaria, etc." He even observed that the Jewish population's "unprecedented tenacity of life" did not extend to some noncontagious conditions, including diabetes. (Fishberg skeptically noted, "Some have even gone so far as to say that the Jews consume very many sweets, and that on this account they are more liable to diabetes than Christians.")

In an era when racial theories were prominent, Fishberg ruled them out. In Europe the differential resistance to infectious disease "diminish[es] gradually as we proceed from East to West, from the countries where the Jew lives isolated, pursuing his life in his own fashion, adhering to the customs of his forefathers, to those countries where the Jew commingles and assimilates with the non-Jewish inhabitants, adopting their modes of life and habits. This has been observed in the United States." In other words, when Jews started to live like Gentiles, they fell prey to the same illnesses.

But what about the reverse? What about Christians living like Jews?

A 2012 study published in *Economics and Human Biology* examined late-nineteenth-century mortality in the Jewish and Catholic population of Gibraltar, the small British territory at the southern tip of Spain at the entrance to the Mediterranean. The authors combined census records from 1878 with cause of death statistics over a seven-year period. They found that the Jewish population could expect to live eight years longer than the Catholic population. Perhaps the most striking finding was that Catholics living in Jewish tenements had greater longevity than Catholics living among themselves. The authors attributed the effect to more hygienic conditions because the Catholics were living among Jews.

Today many of these ancient traditions are either ignored or held up to ridicule—by the same people who wash their hands multiple times a day, use soap, bathe regularly, launder their clothes, own a dishwasher that uses scalding hot water, think it's wise to wear a condom, depend on a clean water supply, flush human waste to a distant location, eat meat that has passed inspection, and dare not touch corpses—and even though they can't see germs, they have an unshakable faith in the germ theory of disease.

We *all* follow the Law of Moses.

It is probably no coincidence that the most urban people in history—across eras and empires—foiled bacterial culture with another type of culture: ideas. But by the dawn of the Industrial Age, humans would be traveling into new habitats faster than even culture would allow them to adapt.

5

HOMO INVICTUS

INDUSTRIAL AGE

◀ *1769 to 1946* ▶

On September 5, 1862, two British gentlemen waved to an assembled crowd, stepped into the gondola of a hot air balloon, and took an extraordinary journey into a habitat no human had ever experienced before: earth's upper atmosphere.

Over the next hour James Glaisher and Henry Coxwell broke the prior altitude record of 26,000 feet, rising to somewhere between 35,000 and 39,000 feet. The exact altitude is unknown, since Glaisher stopped taking measurements when his vision failed—just before he passed out. Thirty-nine thousand feet is more than seven miles, higher than the typical cruising altitude of 747s. It is higher than Mount Everest, the highest point on earth, by about a third.

As the balloon began to rise, Coxwell, the pilot, paid attention to flight dynamics. Glaisher, the meteorologist, took scientific measurements such as temperature, humidity, and pressure. As they approached 26,000 feet, the prior record, the men began to feel light-headed. They had traveled from sea level to the equivalent of 3,000 feet short of the peak of Mount Everest, and had done so in under an hour.

Glaisher's account of the journey demonstrated that the men were ignorant of the physiological effects of extreme high altitude and, in retrospect, thoroughly unprepared for their journey. When Glaisher began to lose his vision, he believed it to be only a "temporary inconvenience." Next he lost control of his arms. He tried to shake his body and realized he could no longer control his legs. Glaisher tried to call out to Coxwell. To his dismay, he had already lost power over his voice. After incrementally losing control over the rest of his body and all his senses, Glaisher remained conscious for long enough to realize that he was probably about to die.

As Glaisher slumped unconscious in the basket of the balloon, Coxwell was above the gondola, untwisting a rope that had gotten tangled. He saw Glaisher passed out. Unaware of the rapidly diminishing oxygen level, he believed his colleague was resting. Suddenly realizing that he himself was growing light-headed, Coxwell attempted to open the appropriate valve to initiate the descent. To his surprise, his hands were completely frostbitten and useless. Desperate, he used his teeth to open the valve—narrowly avoiding certain death for him and his companion.

As the balloon descended to a more heavily oxygenated altitude, Glaisher came to. In a classic display of British stoicism and understatement, Glaisher observed to Coxwell, "I have been insensible." Then he picked up his pencil and noted what it felt like to nearly die from asphyxiation. The men then poured brandy over Coxwell's still black hands. The balloon landed in a rural area, and they concluded their journey with a civilized eight-mile stroll through the English countryside.

From a modern perspective, it seems strange how woefully unprepared Coxwell and Glaisher were for high altitude. Incredibly, they were the most knowledgeable people of their era: Glaisher was a founding member of the Royal Meteorological Society, and Coxwell was the premier hot air balloon pilot in the world, having engaged in over four hundred prior ascents.

But how were they supposed to know? No human had ever traveled nearly so high in the atmosphere. They had traveled to a habitat that was completely inhospitable to human life.

It happened so fast, they were unprepared both genetically *and* culturally.

What made Coxwell and Glaisher's hot air balloon possible was the Industrial Revolution. Originating in Britain in the eighteenth century, the Industrial Revolution was marked by accelerating economic growth and technological change in a variety of fields: transportation, mining, metallurgy, chemistry.

Coxwell and Glaisher's journey depended on these new technologies. They had chosen Wolverhampton, their point of departure, due to the presence of a gas works, which could provide the coal gas in their balloon. The gas works itself needed to be located near the vast coal deposits outside the manufacturing mecca of Birmingham. Not only was Britain the epicenter of the Industrial Revolution, but the area around Birmingham was the industrial center of Britain. That's where the Industrial Revolution took off—and it's no coincidence that's also where Coxwell and Glaisher took off.

Industrial technology propelled humans into completely novel habitats, ones that our ancestors had never experienced during eons of genetic and cultural evolution.

Advances in long-distance seafaring revealed the bitter colds of Antarctica. Hot air balloons, dirigibles, and fixed-wing aircraft opened up the skies. Diving bells and submarines took us far beneath the sea. Supplemental oxygen systems allowed mountain climbers to reach the highest peaks on the planet. Rocket and shuttle technology took humans into the vacuum of outer space. These "famous firsts" start with advances in sailing in the sixteenth century, pick up with the Industrial Revolution in the eighteenth and nineteenth centuries, and culminate in the mid-twentieth century with space, "the final frontier."

During the Industrial Age, explorers pushed the human body in ways it had never been pushed before—many dying as a result. Extreme deaths in harsh habitats show the limits of the human organism. But by venturing into uninhabitable places, explorers also reveal which features make a habitat *habitable*. By demonstrating what kills us, they reveal necessary conditions for human life.

In the centuries leading up to the Industrial Revolution, millions

FAMOUS FIRSTS IN EXPLORATION

1522—Circumnavigation of the globe *(Magellan)*

1620—Navigable submarine test *(Drebbel)*

1783—Untethered hot air balloon flight *(Montgolfier Brothers)*

1783—Parachute jump *(Lenormand)*

1820—Landing on Antarctica *(Davis)*

1862—Hot air balloon to 39,000 feet *(Glaisher and Coxwell)*

1863—Mechanically powered submarine *(Bourgeois and Brun)*

1889—Ascent of Mount Kilimanjaro *(Meyer and Purtscheller)*

1903—Airplane flight at Kitty Hawk *(Wright Brothers)*

1911—Reaching the South Pole *(Amundsen)*

1911—Parachute jump from an airplane *(Morton)*

1927—Nonstop flight from New York to Paris *(Lindbergh)*

1953—Ascent of Mount Everest *(Hillary and Norgay)*

1957—Animal in space *(Laika, a dog)*

1960—Submarine to the Mariana Trench *(Piccard and Walsh)*

1961—Human in space *(Gagarin)*

1969—Human on the Moon *(Armstrong and Aldrin)*

of sailors became unwitting subjects in grisly diet experiments. Advances in seafaring technology, such as the compass, allowed for longer voyages. Ships were stocked with foods based on how slowly they would spoil, not on whether they provided essential micronutrients. The result was a host of gruesome health conditions.

For centuries *scurvy* was the scourge of sailors—killing millions. Early signs of scurvy are extreme lethargy, depression, mottled skin, bleeding from mucous membranes, and spongy gums before advancing to loss of teeth, jaundice, fever, and death. According to historian Jonathan Lamb, Ferdinand Magellan lost 90% of his crew (208 out of 230), principally to scurvy. In the eighteenth century, British sailors had a greater chance of dying from scurvy than in combat. During the Seven Years' War (1756–1763), records from the British Royal Navy show that 1,512 sailors died in battle, whereas 133,708 died from disease or went missing—the bulk of which historians attribute to scurvy. Just a few years earlier, Scottish physician Dr. James Lind had discovered that citrus fruit cured sailors of scurvy in what was perhaps the world's first clinical trial. Scurvy, as we now know, is a condition caused by a vitamin C deficiency. Humans are not adapted to a prolonged diet of salt pork, hardtack (a long-lasting biscuit), and alcohol. Unlike many other mammals, we cannot synthesize vitamin C. We need to get it directly from fresh food—fruits, vegetables, raw animal foods—since cooking destroys vitamin C.

Another scourge of sailors was *beriberi*, which is characterized by severe lethargy, impaired senses, swelling, and death. It became widespread in nineteenth-century Japan after the introduction of polished white rice—a novel industrial food that spoiled less quickly than brown rice. The dietary cause of beriberi was discovered in 1884 by a Japanese naval doctor who observed that low-ranking sailors who ate little else than white rice suffered and died, while officers and Western crews who had a more varied diet did not. The cause of beriberi? A vitamin B1 deficiency.

Long-distance seafaring was indirectly responsible for another nasty condition called *pellagra,* caused by a vitamin B3 deficiency and characterized by "the Four Ds": diarrhea, dermatitis, dementia, and death. When European explorers brought back corn from the New World soon after 1492, they neglected to bring the traditional Mesoamerican food processing methods with them. In a process called nixtamalization, Mesoamericans prepared corn with lime, making vitamin B3 available in the process. In the following centuries pellagra afflicted people all over the world who ate heavily corn-based diets—except for Mesoamericans eating corn in traditional ways.

Vitamin C (scurvy), vitamin B1 (beriberi), and vitamin B3 (pellagra) are not the only nutrients with a long trail of dead leading to their discovery. Essential nutrients have largely been "discovered" by their absence.

A few decades after essential nutrients were discovered, industrial food manufacturers began to fortify foods with them. In 1941

Wonder Bread released a new line of enriched white bread, fortified with B vitamins designed to combat beriberi and pellagra. These advances in food fortification were improvements on what existed at the time, but it's not as if the human diet had always been chronically deficient in certain nutrients. Chronic nutrient deficiencies were a problem of our own creation, caused by inadvertently changing the human diet long ago—primarily during the Agricultural Revolution, and then during the Industrial Revolution.

Science discovered the bare essentials required for human survival, and the industrial food system found ways to provide all the essential nutrients as inexpensively as possible to as many people as possible. It was a magnificent success that alleviated enormous human suffering. It was a great victory against death—we learned how to *not die*—but it didn't show the optimal way to thrive.

Even as sailors were venturing across the sea, inventors were trying to dive underneath it.

In 1620 Cornelis Drebbel built the first crude "submarine" for the English Navy and tested it in the Thames. Fifty years later the British scientist Robert Boyle would demonstrate a danger of undersea exploration: *decompression sickness*. High air pressure forces more gases to dissolve in the bloodstream, but a quick drop in pressure causes those gases to bubble out of the blood—not a pleasant sensation. It is characterized by localized joint pain, dizziness, neurological problems, and sometimes even death.

Decompression sickness, more commonly known as "the bends," afflicts scuba divers if they move too quickly from high to low air pressure. In 1840 the symptoms of the bends were first described in humans after the undersea removal of a sunken British warship: "of the seasoned divers, not a man escaped the repeated attacks of rheumatism and cold." Though frequently associated with modern scuba diving, decompression sickness was common among nineteenth-century industrial workers. Miners and bridge builders sometimes worked in chambers filled with compressed air in order to keep the space from flooding. The term "the bends" originated during the construction of the Brooklyn Bridge in the early 1870s. Hundreds of workers who worked in compressed air environments faced health problems associated with decompression sickness for the remainders of their lives.

Humans are adapted to only certain levels of atmospheric pressure, and slow changes to it. In the ancestral human habitat, humans did not experience fast changes to air pressure.

Not only did industrial technology make it possible for explorers to push into new habitats, but it also revolutionized how ordinary people lived. Since Britain was at the forefront of the Industrial Revolution, the British people were often the first to face these challenges—earning their reputation for having a stiff upper lip.

The British were one of the first people to have large amounts of refined sugar in their diet—and they had the *cavities* to prove it. In the seventeenth and eighteenth centuries, sugar was still a luxury good. From there onward, it increasingly became a staple of British society—consumed whenever tea was (i.e., often). The diet of working-class Brits became heavily concentrated in bread, potatoes, sugar, tea, and alcohol. According to bioarchaeologist Dr. Simon Hillson, "In London, mostly 1800 onwards, they have absolutely dreadful teeth." That is to say, the British reputation for poor teeth began after they first developed a sweet tooth—over two hundred years ago.

Given the rise of sweet and starchy foods in the British diet, it should come as no surprise that around this time, *obesity* started appearing with greater frequency among the British people. In 1863 a formerly obese Englishman named William Banting published the first popular "diet book," called *Letter on Corpulence, Addressed to the Public*. The Banting Diet restricted the sweet and starchy foods that had recently come to dominate the industrial British diet.

Ordinary British citizens were unwitting pioneers of another novel habitat: the great indoors. The indoors may not sound like a harsh habitat, but a sunless environment is quite inhospitable to a savannah species.

In 1651 a British physician named Francis Glisson published the world's first comprehensive treatise on *rickets,* an "absolutely new disease . . . never described by any ancient or modern writers." Now seen the world over, it was dubbed "the British Disease." Rickets is a childhood condition characterized by skeletal deformities, twisted bones, bone pain, dental problems, and muscle weakness. Left untreated it will disable a child for life. Rickets is caused by a vitamin D deficiency, resulting from a lack of sun and a poor diet—two things for which Britain has long been known.

Though most people associate rickets with the urban industrial poor, holed up in windowless tenements, rickets started out as a disease of the proto-industrial rich. The rich were wealthy enough to avoid the most widely available cure for rickets—sunlight—because they didn't have to work in the fields. Pale skin even became fashionable. Rickets emerged just decades after the reign of Queen Elizabeth I, who was famously pale; the aspirational merchant class mimicked the high status behaviors of the hereditary elite. The very term "blue blood" is a reference to paleness so extreme that a person's veins are visible through the translucent skin.

In 1919 British doctor Edward Mellanby, suspecting there was a dietary cause for rickets, re-created it in dogs by feeding them a diet of oats and keeping them indoors; dogs that were fed cod-liver oil (which is rich in vitamin D) were unaffected. Just a few years later American researcher Dr. Alfred Hess showed that exposure to ultraviolet light helped synthesize vitamin D in the body. Clearly, the ancestral habitats of humans had plentiful sources of vitamin D— from sun, diet, or both. In 1933 the U.S. government began an effort to fortify milk with vitamin D in order to combat rickets. This was another great advance in public health, but it was solving a problem of our own creation: lives increasingly spent indoors, consuming a nutrient-poor diet. Again, we learned how to *not die.*

In the early twentieth century, industrial production of compressed air led to the creation of supplemental oxygen systems, which allowed pilots and mountain climbers to ascend to higher altitudes without dying. In 1953 Sir Edmund Hillary—a New Zealander of recent British descent—and his Nepalese climbing partner, Tenzing Norgay, became the first humans to reach the tallest point on the planet: the peak of Mount Everest. On their backs each carried supplemental oxygen systems weighing twenty-two pounds.

As altitude increases, atmospheric pressure drops—and with it the concentration of oxygen in the air. Mountain climbers without access to supplemental oxygen can suffer from *altitude sickness*. Also called acute mountain sickness (AMS), it has been described as feeling like "flu, carbon monoxide poisoning, or a hangover." It can progress to fatal forms, including high altitude cerebral edema (HACE) and high altitude pulmonary edema (HAPE), where fluids leak into the brain and lungs, respectively. Permanent human settlements have not been found at altitudes over 18,000 feet, and altitude sickness can start much lower, as can declines in physical performance. Many competitive athletes—including mountain climbers—will often go early to high altitude locations in order to acclimate.

Just a few years after Hillary and Norgay reached the highest point on Earth, the Soviets left Earth altogether. In 1957 the Soviet Union launched the first satellite, *Sputnik,* into orbit. Later that same year the Soviets launched *Sputnik 2,* this time with a passenger: a dog named Laika. She holds the dual distinction of being the first animal to go to space and the first animal to die there.

Preventing living creatures from dying in outer space was a huge technological challenge for the Americans and the Soviets. Though some of the technology already had been developed due to high altitude flights, new innovations were needed to protect astronauts from being bombarded by the cosmic rays and solar radiation typically absorbed by Earth's atmosphere. The engineers had to address the effects of a zero gravity environment, and to insulate the astronauts from the heat generated by reentry into the atmosphere.

Only twelve short years after the Soviets sent Laika on a suicide mission, Neil Armstrong and Buzz Aldrin became the first humans to set foot on the Moon. The culmination of roughly a hundred thousand years of human exploration since leaving Africa, the Apollo 11 mission demonstrated that we were technologically capable of sending astronauts to the Moon and returning them safely to Earth.

OVER THE next half century, NASA and the Soviet space program assessed the feasibility of more challenging manned missions: building a space station, establishing a lunar colony, or even sending a man to Mars. Long-duration spaceflight presents an entirely different set of problems than short missions like Apollo 11, which lasted only eight days. The challenge of lengthy missions isn't keeping astronauts alive as much as keeping them sane. Worries include "low sensory input, lack of motivation, confinement, isolation, monotony, long-term dangers and sudden emergencies, and personality conflicts with other crew members."

Only ten astronauts have spent more than 200 continuous days in space. The record for the longest continuous time spent in space is 437 days. Given the current technology and the orbits of Earth and Mars, a round-trip mission to Mars would take an absolute minimum of 500 days. The longer the mission, the more the astronauts' performance and health deteriorate. Basic survival isn't sufficient—astronauts would have to function at a high level over a long period of time. In other words, they'd have to thrive, not simply survive.

At a fundamental level, a space station, lunar colony, or spaceship to Mars would have to be engineered for humans, based on a deep understanding of how humans themselves are "engineered." The technology used to build such a habitat would have to match the "technology" inside a human being. The consistent lesson from the history of exploration is that there's a mismatch between human biology and a small box, whether that box is a ship sailing across the Atlantic, a research station in the Antarctic, a nuclear submarine deep below the sea, or a space shuttle orbiting Earth. The same concept applies to gorillas in a zoo enclosure and modern humans in a New York City apartment—the habitat doesn't match the organism's built-in needs.

Since outer space is mostly just a giant vacuum—the absence of a habitat—long-duration spaceflight presents a novel challenge: *How would one build a human habitat from scratch?*

One way to think about potential habitat features is to start big and narrow it down.

Mankind evolved in a specific universe. Our universe operates according to certain laws of physics, such as motion, electromagnetism, gravity, energy, and relativity.

We evolved in a specific solar system. Our solar system contains a star of a particular size and intensity, as well as Earth, the Moon, and other planets. The Sun gives off a certain amount of radiation. Earth has a particular orbit around the Sun, and the Moon has a particular orbit around Earth.

We evolved on a specific planet. Our planet—Earth—has a particular set of characteristics: strength of gravity, atmospheric composition, and a magnetic field.

We evolved in a specific set of habitats on Earth. This set had particular characteristics relevant to human evolution. It was near the equator, and thus we evolved under a fairly regular transition between night and day. It was on dry land. It was in the presence of other human beings. And it had many more features that varied substantially at any given moment, such as temperature or energy intake. Our day-to-day existence is a mash-up of all these different forces and features, and somehow the body makes sense of it all.

If one had to categorize all these habitat features based on how our species experienced them over the course of our evolution, they would fall into three broad categories: (1) features that were *constant* at a certain level (e.g., gravity), (2) features that were *cyclical* over a certain period (e.g., day and night), and (3) features that were *varied* within certain bounds (e.g., temperature).

THE CONSTANT category includes:

- Universal laws of physics (gravity, electromagnetism, energy)
- Earth's gravity
- Earth's atmospheric pressure and composition

Most of these habitat features are so pervasive and unchanging that most people never even register them. They are the ultimate white noise, fading to the background of our consciousness. Only a few explorers have ventured to places where these forces change, such as at high altitudes, deep underwater, or outer space. Humans can survive limited, gradual, or temporary changes in a few constants of Earth, such as atmospheric pressure or composition. In contrast, pressure changes are a fact of life in the air or underwater, and many aerial and aquatic species are very well adapted to extreme changes in atmospheric pressure. But overall, most species are not well adapted to changes in fundamental forces that have always been constant.

THE CYCLICAL category includes:

- Day and night
- Seasons
- Tides

These habitat features repeat in cyclical, regular patterns—the product of spinning spheres moving in cyclical orbits (Earth, Moon, Sun). They are extremely predictable: sunset/sunrise charts, equinox calendars, and tidal tables.

They change at different locations on the planet. Humans spent much of our recent evolution in equatorial regions and are thus adapted to a fairly regular twenty-four-hour cycle between night and day. We adjust easily to moderate changes in the length of night and day, but if this cycle does not occur at all—as for Arctic explorers or submarine personnel—circadian rhythm dysregulation can cause depression, anxiety, insomnia (too little sleep), and hypersomnia (too much sleep).

Seasons matter, too. The more distinctive the seasons in a given geography (e.g., big changes in temperature, precipitation), the more that species have life cycles well-adapted to them. For example, the reproductive cycles of North American white-tailed deer are based on the seasons: does give birth in spring in order to give their offspring the maximum time to grow before winter comes.

THE VARIED category includes:

- Energy (intake, expenditure)
- Food (type, availability, amount, eating times)
- Water (availability, intake, expenditure)
- Movement (type, intensity, duration, conditions)
- Temperature (external, internal)
- Sun (intensity, duration)
- Social interactions (type, intensity, duration)

These habitat features vary in somewhat unpredictable ways. A physicist can draw up a precise calculation of Earth's orbit around the Sun, but not of a young boy's orbit around his mother. In contrast to physics, biological systems tend to be complex and unpredictable, vary in semi-random ways, and contain feedback loops that interact in unanticipated ways. This is why planned interventions often produce unintended consequences in fields as disparate as pharmaceuticals (prescription drugs), economics (central planning), and wildlife conservation (invasive species).

Living organisms do not take in or expend the exact same number of calories each day, each hour, or each minute—there's natural variation. Natural surfaces are rarely flat and predictable like a treadmill or running track—they incline and decline, are uneven and rough, and are made of materials with different properties (dirt, wood, stone). Living creatures are not industrial robots made to do the exact same thing over and over.

So to design a habitat from scratch, some good guidelines become apparent:

1. If a species evolved with a *constant* habitat feature at a certain level, members of that species are likely heavily dependent on that feature *remaining constant* at that level. (Don't mess with gravity.)

2. If a species evolved with a *cyclical* habitat feature with a certain period, members of that species are likely dependent on that feature *remaining cyclical* with the same period. (Don't mess with day and night too much.)

3. If a species evolved with a habitat feature that *varied* within certain bounds, members of that species probably thrive when that feature *remains varied* within similar bounds. (Variation can be healthy.)

Or to put it simply: *An organism is likely to thrive in a habitat that resembles its ancestral habitat.**

The history of exploration (and zoos and civilization) demonstrates that problems seem to occur when this guideline isn't followed. Either constant habitat features are set at the wrong level (zero gravity) or change too quickly (decompression sickness); cyclical habitat features get out of cycle (circadian rhythm dysregulation); or varied habitat features become too monotonous (boredom, confined spaces) or vary beyond the tolerated bounds (rickets, sunburn).

---

* In this context, I am using the word "thrive" to mean individual health and well-being, not reproductive success. Many species enter novel habitats and thrive in the Darwinian sense, such as pigeons in New York City.

Even so, it is a testament to human ingenuity that we have been able to transform harsh environments to make them habitable. More amazing than the unforgiving conditions where humans haven't survived are the inhospitable conditions where humans have. Our resilience is not simply a function of "physical" attributes—it is psychological resiliency too.

Dr. Peter Suedfeld is a scholar who studies the survivors of traumatic events: failed expeditions, industrial and environmental disasters, and imprisonment. Though many psychologists focus on frailty and exalt victimhood, Dr. Suedfeld consistently found stories of incredible resiliency among ordinary people. He described individuals who prevail over extreme stress as having "the ability to perceive meaning in seemingly random events, dedicating oneself to an ideal or a future plan, believing in one's ability to meet challenges, and exerting whatever control is possible over the environment and oneself." In other words, survivors had a sense of purpose to their life and took steps to achieve that purpose.

Dr. Suedfeld concludes that humans can survive almost anything, dubbing us "Homo Invictus." *Invictus* is the Latin word for "unconquerable," "undefeated," or "indomitable," a word that Suedfeld borrowed from the poem of the same name by Victorian poet William Ernest Henley. Published in 1875, it captures not only the intrepid spirit of the Industrial Age, but also the stoicism of its exemplars, the British people: the millions of sailors who died of scurvy; the polar explorers, mountain climbers, and deep-sea divers who braved hypothermia, asphyxiation, and the bends; the commoners who labored in coal mines and factories; and the entire British people who suffered from lousy weather, dreadful food, and rotten teeth.

As the Industrial Age came to a close, so too did the frontiers of physical space. But the rise of computers and the dawn of the Information Age opened up a new frontier: cyberspace. The pioneering, risk-loving, rule-breaking philosophy of exploration was passed from jocks to geeks.

INVICTUS

Out of the night that covers me,
Black as the Pit from pole to pole,
I thank whatever gods may be
For my unconquerable soul.

In the fell clutch of circumstance
I have not winced nor cried aloud.
Under the bludgeonings of chance
My head is bloody, but unbowed.

Beyond this place of wrath and tears
Looms but the Horror of the shade,
And yet the menace of the years
Finds, and shall find, me unafraid.

It matters not how strait the gate,
How charged with punishments the scroll.
I am the master of my fate:
I am the captain of my soul.

—*William Ernest Henley*

6

BIOHACKERS

INFORMATION AGE

◄ *1946 to present* ►

"**W**e have found the secret of life."

It was February 28, 1953, and the man uttering those words had just burst into the Eagle Pub near England's Cambridge University. The patrons must have thought it was the ravings of a madman, but it wasn't: "we" was Francis Crick and his collaborator, James Watson—and "the secret of life" was the double-helix structure of DNA.

DNA (deoxyribonucleic acid) is the structural medium of genetic code, the programming language of life. Its existence had been discovered nearly a century prior, and its constituent parts had been subsequently identified. What hadn't been clear was the precise mechanism by which hereditary information is encoded in the genome and replicated throughout successive generations. It was this discovery—the double helix—that led Francis, Crick, and Maurice Wilkins to receive the Nobel Prize in 1962.

DNA has an elegant simplicity. Two mirror-image strands spiral around each other like dance partners in perfect synchronization. The strands are bonded in such a way that they can be easily separated and replicated. Just four repeating molecules—adenine (A), guanine (G), thymine (T), cytosine (C)—form the basis of the code itself, each bonding with only one of the others (A with T, G with C). These base pairs form various functional units (codons, genes), which govern everything from protein synthesis to hormone signaling. Its beauty is undeniable: at the heart of all complex life, from mosquitoes to mankind, sits the same simple code.

But before the genome could be decoded it had to be sequenced. In 1977 researchers sequenced the entire DNA-based genome of a living organism for the first time. Phi X 174, a tiny bacteriophage, had a genome that only contained 5,386 base pairs. Over the decades that followed, advances in laboratory techniques grew alongside the computing power and software required to store and analyze genomic data. At roughly 3.3 billion base pairs, the human genome is more than 600,000 times larger than that of phi X 174. When two teams of scientists announced maps of the human genome in 2000, they were years ahead of schedule. The effort would have been impossible without the technology that came to define the Information Age, the digital computer, and the exponential growth of its power.

That advances in genomics depended on advances in computing was not lost on people in either field—nor were other similarities between biology and computers. Organisms are built on a base of genetic code, while computer programs are ultimately based on binary code. Both types of code are digital, encoding information in discrete bits (ATGC; 1s and 0s). Biological viruses infect living organisms, while computer viruses "infect" electronic devices. As Bill Gates observed, "Human DNA is like a computer program but far, far more advanced than any software ever created." The rise of computers led to a profound idea: biology is an information technology. In fact, biology was the original information technology, humming along for eons before computers ever came around.

But what did that actually *mean*? To most people, genetic code was as foreign as software code. However, there was one group of people who thrived in this new cyber-habitat, a new breed of net denizens who finally felt at home in the Information Age: hackers.

HACKERS HAVE an image problem, particularly with nontechnical people. A "hacker" may summon the image of a rogue programmer;

a "hack" may refer to an unwieldy fix (a kluge); and "hacking" sure
sounds illegal. However, the true and original meanings were quite
different. The term "hacker" originated at the Massachusetts Institute of Technology in the mid-twentieth century. Initially the word
"hack" referred to the infamous pranks pulled by students, such as
putting a fire truck on top of the MIT dome. As tech journalist Steven
Levy writes in *Hackers*, "To qualify as a hack, the feat must be imbued
with innovation, style, and technical virtuosity," and this ethos carried over to computer hackers in the 1950s and '60s. At MIT, hackers
were respected as hands-on virtuosos—even if they pulled all-night-
ers, slept through class, and received poor grades. The students who
always went to class, never left the library, and got straight As? They
were called "tools."

Early hacker culture took root at a few large universities and
corporations (MIT, Xerox PARC), but it blossomed with the release
of the personal computer and the rise of the Internet. In 1986 an
online magazine for hackers called *Phrack* published Hacker's Manifesto by The Mentor. The piece famously describes the feeling when
a "damn underachiever" discovers computers: "a door opened to a
world . . . rushing through the phone line like heroin through an
addict's veins, an electronic pulse is sent out, a refuge from the day-
to-day incompetencies is sought . . . a board is found. 'This is it . . .
this is where I belong.'"

From the beautiful minds of these misfits emerged the new ethos
of the Information Age. This hacker philosophy favored hands-on
learning over book smarts; trial-and-error over theorizing; speedy
solutions that were "good enough" over the endless pursuit of perfection; resourcefulness, simplicity, decentralization, and openness.

The starting point for a hacker is acknowledging his own ignorance: *How does it work?* "It" might be anything from a ham radio to
word-processing software. Rather than looking for the answer in an
instruction manual or a classroom (like the tools at MIT), hackers got
their hands dirty through what they described as the Hands-On Imperative. This approach is also called learning by doing, do-it-yourself

(DIY), self-experimentation ($n=1$), and trial-and-error. Hackers don't try to avoid failure; they embrace it. Facebook founder Mark Zuckerberg adopted a company slogan rooted in hacker culture: "Move fast and break things." The faster you fail, the faster you learn from your failures—and the sooner you succeed.

One benefit of speed is that it preempts the pursuit of perfection. Hackers live by the proverb, "Perfect is the enemy of the good." During all-night "hackathons"—whether alone in a dorm room or at Facebook HQ—perfection is impossible, so it's pointless to try. The same concept is articulated by the 80/20 rule or the Pareto principle—20% of the input produces 80% of the outcome—and trying to achieve 100% perfection is a waste of time and resources.

Time pressure also forces hackers to repurpose existing things to completely new uses. One of the most famous examples of hacking took place on Apollo 13 when endangered astronauts had to jerry-rig a square carbon-dioxide scrubber to fit into a round container. In fact repurposing existing inventions to new uses is a recurring theme throughout history. Coca-Cola was originally concocted as a medicine, Play-Doh was devised as wallpaper cleaner, and Viagra was developed to treat hypertension. Many major scientific breakthroughs were either discovered accidentally by hands-on experimenters (penicillin) or were first demonstrated through self-experimentation (the bacterial cause of ulcers).

Hackers also place aesthetic value on simplicity and elegance. The early hackers at MIT had to share computer time, so there was an incentive to write code as succinctly as possible. Today "Keep It Simple Stupid" remains a mantra among programmers. Simple isn't just efficient, it's also beautiful.

Hackers aren't fond of authority figures, particularly tools who "earned" their authority while safely within the confines of academia, big business, or government. Two hacker principles speak to their fondness for open systems: "Mistrust authority—promote decentralization" and "Information wants to be free." Open-source systems (Linux) stand in contrast to closed, proprietary systems governed by "authorities" (such as Microsoft Windows or Mac OS). Programmer Eric Raymond described these two approaches as "the Cathedral" (top-down, centralized authority enforcing a closed system) versus "the Bazaar" (bottom-up, decentralized equals collaborating in an open system).

These hacker principles aren't just useful for understanding computers; they're also applicable to understanding just about any complex system. Noted programmer, essayist, and venture capitalist Paul Graham likes to invest in "world hackers . . . who not only understand how to mess with computers, but mess with everything." Kevin Kelly, founding editor of *Wired*, is also co-creator of Quantified Self, a movement of (mostly) techies who are applying the principles of hacking to improve their own personal health. Appropriately, they are referred to as *bio*hackers.

If there are two things hackers love, they're gadgets and data—and biohackers are no different. An increasing number of devices allow people to collect data about themselves: blood sugar levels, the number of steps taken each day, and sleep cycles. It won't be long before checking blood work will only require a relatively inexpensive device that plugs into a smartphone, not a visit to the doctor's office. The cost of sequencing the genome continues to drop, and soon it will be as unremarkable as taking a fingerprint. The marriage of big data and human health will give birth to personalized medicine, gene therapy, and countless treatments yet unknown.

But one doesn't have to love gadgets or data in order to be a biohacker. The only requirement is taking responsibility for one's own health. There's no one else who can make the daily decisions—eating well, exercising regularly—that deliver lifelong health. In other words, being healthy *is* a "do-it-yourself" project. Seen in that light, we are all biohackers. Yet too many people entrust their day-to-day decisions to authority figures—the tools, as it were—on the assumption that the experts actually know what they're talking about. In contrast, biohackers begin by acknowledging their own ignorance: *How does the body work?* The simple truth is that no one has a very precise idea. Not doctors, not molecular biologists, and not the average Joe.

Rather than looking for the answer in a scientific journal, molecular biology textbook, or classroom (like tools would), biohackers get their hands dirty. They, too, follow the Hands-On Imperative. Biohackers experiment on themselves: trying new foods, removing others, and tracking how their body responds. This trial-and-error approach has a number of virtues: it's fast and cheap; the results are customized to unique persons or circumstances; and it doesn't require a PhD in molecular biology.

Biohackers also understand that "Perfect is the enemy of the good." Nobel laureate Max Planck pointed out the slow and halting progression of science, giving rise to the adage, "Science advances one funeral at a time." Waiting for scientists to reach a consensus is waiting for your own funeral. There's no such thing as perfect— no perfect diet, no perfect exercise, no perfect lifestyle. Unconcerned with perfection, biohackers adopt smart rules of thumb that stand a decent chance of being more or less right (the 80/20 rule).

Here's how a smart biohacker would quickly get a handle on an aspect of health—say, diet. She would begin by looking at how diets vary across species (Animal). Then, she would learn about the human diet over the course of our formative years as hunter-gatherers (Paleolithic). Next, she would take into account cultural rules and possible recent adaptations among herder-farmers (Agricultural). Then, she would learn from the mistakes of explorers and producer-consumers eating industrial diets (Industrial). Finally, she would use self-experimentation to devise customized solutions that work for *her* (Information). She would be unconcerned with temporary failures— there's no such thing as perfection—and eventually stumble on long-term success: a diet that allows her to thrive.

Nothing could be more appropriate than applying the hacker philosophy to biology. After all, that's how evolution by natural selection works: "amateurish" trial-and-error, repurposing existing bits to new uses, and acceptance of "good enough" solutions. Nobel laureate Max

Delbruck observed, "Any living cell carries with it the experiences of a billion years of experimentation by its ancestors." The most brilliantly "engineered" organisms are actually the result of trial-and-error by countless generations of organisms. Another Nobel laureate, geneticist François Jacob, made the point that "Nature is a tinkerer, not an engineer." In other words, nature is a hacker, the best there ever was. Trial-and-error, self-experimentation, tinkering, and hacking do not just contribute to the progress of science; they lie at the very core of evolution itself.

IF THINKING like a hacker is useful, then it may also be useful to think of the human body as an information technology—and it may be possible to borrow wisdom from the world of computer programming to make smarter health decisions.

There's a saying among software developers: "It's not a bug, it's a feature." It's said in situations when a user *thinks* the software is malfunctioning, when it's actually working as designed. A nontechnical example is when airlines overbook flights, selling more tickets than there are seats on the plane. The first time a person gets bumped he usually thinks there must be some mistake—that is, a bug. But airlines overbook on purpose because they know that, on average, a few people miss flights, which means empty seats and forfeited revenue. Overbooking isn't a bug; it's a feature.

Similarly, many people view the human body as "buggy." But the human body is stunningly sophisticated, and more often than not we simply don't understand it or misuse its features. For example, morning sickness in pregnant women has often been thought an unfortunate side effect of pregnancy. But morning sickness has a biological function: it makes a mother sensitive to unfamiliar and strong-tasting foods that are (or were) more likely to contain pathogens or toxins. Morning sickness is not a bug, but a feature of the human body.

Software developers have another phrase: "garbage in, garbage out"—or GIGO, for short. GIGO refers to how computers unquestioningly accept bad inputs ("garbage in"), process them, and spit out an incorrect "answer" ("garbage out"). If a fat-fingered accountant enters wrong numbers into accounting software, the software isn't going to magically spit out an accurate set of books. Yet many people have too much faith in computers to correct for user error.

If the lesson of "It's not a bug, it's a feature" is to trust our evolved biology, the lesson of "garbage in, garbage out" is to not trust it too much. There are limits to computer technology, and there are also limits to our own biological technology. Send the wrong inputs to the body, and the body will still start to malfunction. Send the right inputs to the body, and everything works smoothly again. For example, many people struggle to get to sleep at night, relying on sleeping pills, alcohol, or other sedatives; they then struggle to wake up in the morning, relying on coffee, sugar, and other stimulants. This is often due to a circadian rhythm dysregulation caused, in part, by being exposed to indoor lights at night (It's day!) and waking up to a dark room (It's night!). It's no wonder that the body becomes confused. Garbage in, garbage out.

Conceiving of the human body as an information technology is a recent phenomenon. Throughout history most people used other metaphors to try to understand how the body worked, many of them based on the technology of the age: fluid dynamics, hydraulic pumps, engines, and energy. The metaphors are worth understanding since many of them still creep into modern debates over health.

A fluid-based philosophy of health, humorism, was popular among Greek and Roman physicians and persisted all the way into the nineteenth century. Humorists (no pun intended) believed that the body contained four fluids, or humors: blood, yellow bile (urine), black bile, and phlegm. When the humors were out of balance, the result was disease. Humorism led to an unhealthy obsession with bodily fluids. Its prescriptions—bloodletting, purges, vomiting, and cupping—often had disastrous consequences. As George Washington fought the infection that would take his life, his doctors bled him of several pints of blood—most likely contributing to his demise.

Fluid-based metaphors for life underwent a renewal with the

advent of industrial hydraulic technology: pumps and pressure. In psychology, no less a figure than Sigmund Freud popularized a fluid-based, hydraulic metaphor for the mind. As cognitive psychologist Steven Pinker writes in *How the Mind Works,* "The hydraulic model, with its psychic pressure building up, bursting out, or being diverted through alternative channels, lay at the center of Freud's theory and can be found in dozens of everyday metaphors: anger welling up, letting off steam, exploding under the pressure, blowing one's stack, venting one's feelings, bottling up rage." As it turns out, thoughts and emotions aren't actually determined by hydraulic pressures in the brain. The brain can't be understood without reference to the information content of cognition, and cognition can't be fully understood without reference to the challenges humans regularly faced over the course of our evolution.

Combustion and energy are two additional metaphors borrowed from physics. Human metabolism has been variously described as a fire, furnace, or factory that produces energy. These days everyone wants more energy, as demonstrated by the popularity of energy drinks and countless energy bars. It's also common to hear people cite the first law of thermodynamics—"Energy cannot be created or destroyed, simply transferred or transformed"—in support of the notion that "calories in" must equal "calories out." While the laws of physics do apply to biological processes, biology is not physics, and metabolism isn't actually a simple mechanical system. Bacon is not grass, and grass is not gasoline; humans are not cows, and cows are not cars. Energy is real, of course, and vitally important to life. But the average person already carries around enormous stores of energy in the form of body fat. People don't actually want more energy; what they want is to *feel energetic*. Two of the most well-known factors that influence feeling energetic have nothing to do with energy intake: the perception of a serious threat causes the release of adrenaline, and morning sunlight causes us to wake up.

Of course, the human organism does contain fluids (blood), circulates them with a hydraulic pump (the heart), uses energy (food), and obeys the laws of physics (calories), but all of these systems are influenced by information. In a sense, information must be essential to life. Any system as improbably complex and self-sustaining as a human body could persist only if it were governed by intricate internal feedback loops that preserve functionality in the face of the relentless forces of decay: parasites, pathogens, predators, human enemies, and heat loss.

So when Watson and Crick exclaimed that they had found the secret of life, they weren't just talking about some obscure aspect of molecular biology. The citation accompanying their Nobel Prize captured the true significance of their work: "for their discoveries concerning the molecular structure of nucleic acids and its significance for *information transfer* in living material [emphasis added]." Their discovery unlocked the source code that lies at the heart of heredity, how so much information about the world gets transferred from one generation to the next.

That's why it's so important to understand the path our species has trodden: primates, hunter-gatherers, herder-farmers, and industrial producer-consumers. And now, biohackers.

Part Two

HERE AND NOW

7

FOOD:

THE CONVENTIONAL WISDOM

What is a healthy diet?

Advice comes from all directions: doctors, newscasters, the trainer at the gym, government officials, corporate advertising, celebrity tabloids, late-night infomercials, and nagging spouses.

The advice on animal protein, in particular, ranges from "eat as much meat as you want" (Atkins) to "don't eat animals at all" (veganism). The mainstream compromise is boring and bland, cooking by committee: skinless chicken breast as far as the eye can see.

When it comes to carbs, the competing schemes also range the spectrum, even while managing to rhyme: no carb, low carb, and slow carb. There's even "mo' carb," as in the high-carb diet recommended by the USDA.

As for fat, we all know from decades of stern admonishments from health authorities that all fats are bad for us—except the good ones.

The only things that health authorities seem to agree on are that fish is healthy and Twinkies are not. Yet even that came into question after a Kansas State University professor went on a "Convenience Store Diet." Eating mostly junk food—but strictly controlling his caloric intake—he lost twenty-seven pounds in two months while registering an improvement in his blood work (triglycerides and LDL down, HDL up). The media speculated that perhaps we can have our health and eat our cupcakes too.

Our national schizophrenia on healthy eating explains the grow-ing popularity of the adage "Everything in moderation." It isn't a pre-scription to stay slim so much as a way to stay sane. It helps us keep our sanity under the alternating onslaught of junk food on the one hand and guilt-inducing health guidelines on the other.

Yet as scientifically sound health advice, "Everything in modera-tion" is as nourishing as white bread. The very people who need to eat more moderately are also the ones who seem to have the most difficulty actually doing so. The Convenience Store Diet requires people to strictly control their caloric intake, which very few people actually seem able to do over the long run. As science journalist Gary Taubes has written, at a certain point telling the obese to eat more moderately just restates the problem; it doesn't provide a solution.

Some people expect science will settle everything. If nerds in white lab coats just run some big studies, the thinking goes, they could tell everyone what's healthy. Case closed!

Unfortunately, it's not that easy. Science is hard. Good science? Really hard. Controlled, double-blind, long-term, large sample clini-cal experiments on diet? Damn near impossible. They're expensive, politicized, time-consuming, difficult to structure properly, and, in some cases, unethical.

Bad science, on the other hand, is easy—and bad science makes for good press. Most news commentators draw the wrong conclusions from unreliable and unreplicated studies yet parade them around as newfound scientific truths. The scientific establishment's dirty secret is that lots of studies never get replicated, and journals often don't publish studies that didn't find effects—even if they contradict prior findings.

Is there no solid ground? No place to start?

As it turns out, there is: everyone's very first meal.

Inmates on death row may get to choose their last meal, but no one gets to choose their first meal. It wasn't a grilled cheese sand-wich or a hot dog. It wasn't even breast milk or infant formula. It was whatever their mother's body fed them in the womb.

The womb is the original cave—tricked out with central heating, an all-you-can-eat buffet, and all the free drinks a growing cavebaby could ever want. The embryo and then the fetus ingests an all-liquid diet and hardly exercises at all, apparently a great way to gain weight. Nine months later that baby weighs 7.5 pounds on average. This is a nearly infinite percentage gain in weight relative to the negligible weight at conception. The human metabolism is so sophisticated that it can reliably govern the growth of a few microscopic cells into a full-grown adult—but health experts think that very same metabolism is too crude to maintain a healthy body weight without, say, consciously counting calories at every meal.

Experts may debate what mothers should eat during pregnancy, but nobody debates the optimal mechanism for a fetus to receive nutrition: from the womb. The womb is a far more sophisticated piece of biological technology than its synthetic imitator, the incubator. The earlier a baby is born before term, the more he is likely to face health complications, even well into adulthood. Not only do the earliest preemies have extremely high rates of birth defects and mental retardation, but even babies born on the early side of normal, thirty-seven weeks, are more likely to have moderate reading or math impairment in elementary school.

For the first nine months of a developing child's existence, everyone respects the nutritional wisdom that is embedded in a mother's body. Food cravings and aversions are respected. Mothers can mess it up by eating an awful diet, smoking, or using narcotics, but there's not a whole lot anyone can do to improve upon the process—and incubator technology still hasn't come close to matching it.

During the most important developmental period in any of our lives, we trust in our evolved human biology.

After birth? There's hardly any disagreement that human breast milk is preferable to infant formula. Breast-fed children are significantly more likely to survive infancy, particularly in developing countries. They have fewer infections, allergies, and incidences of asthma, and are less likely to become diabetic or obese later on. Mothers benefit too: breast-feeding is inexpensive, accelerates weight loss, releases bonding hormones, and reduces rates of breast and ovarian cancers. It even acts as a reliable form of birth control, as long as the infant is breast-fed on demand (day and night)—it's nature's way to space out pregnancies.

There is no longer much of a debate on whether to breast-feed, but rather on how long to breast-feed, how often, and the nature of the mother's diet while breast-feeding. Yet it wasn't that long ago that infant formula was seen as comparable to breast-feeding—even superior to it. Industrial food producers thought they could simply extract the whey and casein protein from cow's milk, mix it up with some fat from vegetable oils, dose it with some carbohydrate from lactose, swirl in some vitamins and nutrients—and just add water. But real human breast milk is a bit more complicated and contains hormones, digestive enzymes, and antiviral agents. Some of the mother's own gut bacteria is transferred to the baby, and breast milk contains molecules that feed beneficial bacteria in the baby's stomach, seeding and strengthening his immune system.

Prior to the rise of infant formula during the Industrial Age, infants had always been breast-fed by their mother (or, in some cases, a wet nurse). Breast-feeding isn't something that herder-farmers started doing a few thousand years ago during the Agricultural Age or hunter-gatherers started doing a couple million years ago during the Paleolithic Age. Breast-feeding is how mammals have fed their young going back hundreds of millions of years. Breast-feeding (via mammary glands) is more essential to being a mammal than bearing live young. Even the five "primitive" mammals that lay eggs—the platypus and four species of echidna—all breast-feed their newborn.

The advice to breast-feed—the least controversial health advice in the entire diet world—boils down to this: "Eat like a mammal."

Breast milk isn't healthy because it's "low-calorie" or "low-fat" (it's not). Breast milk isn't healthy because it's artificially fortified with vitamins (it's not). Breast milk isn't healthy because it's "certified organic" or "Fair Trade" (it's not). And breast milk definitely isn't healthy because it's vegan (it's not).

Breast milk is healthy because it is a biologically appropriate food, one that human infants are well adapted to eating. Babies don't count calories, read ingredient labels, fear fat, understand biochemistry, or insist on organic certification. They just eat the right stuff. As long as the mother is healthy, everything takes care of itself.

When it comes to the womb and breast-feeding, everyone uses an evolutionary standard for what's healthy. It's only after breast-feeding when opinions really start to diverge, food corporations profit from the confusion, and nanny state bureaucrats stumble to the rescue.

Some of our dietary confusion stems from the nature of human development in the two decades after infancy. Humans move from infancy, a phase where there are few options of what to eat (and the optimal option is fairly clear), to a phase when growing children seem to be able to eat just about anything and still remain relatively healthy (though with the rise of childhood obesity and diabetes, that is less true than it used to be).

The problem is that many people emerge from this long stretch of seeming invincibility with poor eating habits and little idea of what healthy eating even means. They grow up thoroughly unprepared to address more serious health conditions that afflict them as they age. It's hardly inevitable that so many people look so much worse at their ten-year high school reunion. At that point, if they decide to get healthy, they turn to one of many popular health standards—low-calorie, low-fat, organic, vegetarian—having forgotten the evolutionary standard of that first meal.

DESPITE THE various standards for what makes food healthy, mainstream health authorities from Dr. Oz to the Mayo Clinic actually make fairly similar dietary recommendations. They boil down to the following guidelines:

1. *Eat fewer processed foods* (soda, white flour, pizza).
2. *Eat more whole foods* (grains, fruits, vegetables).

Among "whole foods," many conventional health authorities also emphasize avoiding high-calorie, high-fat animal products (such as red meat and eggs) and eating organic (if one can afford it). The overall set of dietary recommendations, according to the conventional wisdom, becomes something like this:

1. *Eat fewer processed foods* (soda, white flour, pizza).
2. *Eat more whole foods* (grains, fruits, vegetables).
   a. *Eat organic* (no chemical pesticides, hormones).
   b. *Eat low calorie/low fat* (lean meats, vegetarian).

But there's a language problem here. Many of these terms (processed, whole, organic) are inaccurate at best. Once the conventional advice is decoded into clearer and more accurate language, it's actually easy to understand what's right with it, what's wrong with it, and why.

1. "Eat Fewer Processed Foods"

The colloquial understanding of "processed food" is defined by two qualities: (1) it appeared relatively recently, and (2) it is particularly unhealthy.

But strictly speaking, humans have been processing food for a very long time. A loaf of bread requires an enormous amount of "processing": threshing, grinding, mixing, kneading, leavening, baking. Yet most people don't consider a loaf of whole grain bread to be a "processed" food. Not only is the practice of baking bread thousands of years old, but using fire to cook is a million years old. Tenderizing meat—pounding it to break muscle fibers—is even more ancient than cooking. Even chewing is a form of processing.

Clearly, not all methods of processing food are unhealthy. Cooking kills harmful bacteria. Fermentation harnesses the processing power of healthy bacteria to transform milk into yogurt. Processing is just a way to transform food, and whether a transformation is healthy or not depends on how the food has been transformed.

When people use the phrase "processed food," they are actually referring to foods that our great-grandparents wouldn't recognize as food. What they really mean is industrial food.

The advice to "Eat fewer processed foods" actually means "Eat fewer industrial foods."

Industrial foods are ones that couldn't be made without the novel technologies of the Industrial Age, those made with industrial methods or ingredients. They are developed in laboratories and made in factories (or factory farms). In contrast, foods from the Agricultural Age are grown on a farm or herded on a ranch, and foods from the Paleolithic Age are hunted or gathered in the wild.

Consider Cheez Whiz. Before Kraft introduced Cheez Whiz in 1953, there had never been anything quite like it in the history of life on this planet. (There's still nothing quite like it.) It was developed in a laboratory, produced in a factory, and was made with industrial ingredients and methods—a "miracle" of industrial food science. Other notable "processed" foods were invented or released as the Industrial Revolution spread to food: margarine (1869), Coca-Cola (1886), Crisco (1911), Twinkies (1930), SPAM (1937), the Big Mac (1967), Pop-Tarts (1967), and canola oil (1978).

There is overwhelming evidence showing that an industrial diet is unhealthy. In 2010 the CDC found that 35.7% of adult Americans were obese, as well as 17% of children. Needless to say, obesity is a risk factor for pretty much every negative health condition that Americans worry about. Although many Americans had been overweight after World War II, the obesity rate noticeably accelerated in the late 1970s. The obesity epidemic has also taken off in other parts of the world—Brazil, India, China, the Middle East—as they have taken to eating an industrial diet.

Not all industrial processing methods or industrial foods are unhealthy. Soon after the discovery of vitamins in the early twentieth century, the fortification of foods with vitamins began to help people avoid conditions like rickets, beriberi, and pellagra (though these were problems of our own creation: eating a heavily grain-based diet). The availability of cheaper food also enabled more people to simply survive, just as the grains from the Agricultural Revolution did. Of course, thriving is another question entirely. Industrial foods appeared so recently in the human diet that the human metabolism hasn't had the time to adapt to them. (Note that most health authorities accept this evolutionary shorthand when applied to industrial food but often fail to apply it to agricultural food.)

As a result, almost any change in diet that results in eating less industrial food will improve one's health. It doesn't matter whether it's due to veganism or Atkins—people who stop drinking soda will get healthier. This is a major reason that so many wacky diet programs work initially: they get people to avoid a similar set of industrial foods, such as white flour, refined sugar, and vegetable oils.

2. "Eat More Whole Foods"

The word "whole" stands in contrast to "processed"—and since it was chosen in direct opposition to a misnomer, it is a misnomer itself. A walk through Whole Foods reveals all kinds of foods that require processing, such as bread, jam, or yogurt.

To understand what people really mean when they say "whole" foods, it's more instructive to look at the marketing images used on food labels: idyllic farm scenes of red barns, smiling cows, and endless crops as far as the eye can see. In practice, "whole" foods really means what humans used to eat prior to the dawn of the Industrial Age: agricultural foods.

So the advice to "Eat more whole foods" really means "Eat more agricultural foods."

Whole grains? Grains are the ultimate farmer food. Whole milk? Dairy is the ultimate herder food. Eating whole foods means eating a herder-farmer diet.

2a. "Eat Organic"

Many people use the word "organic" as a synonym for "healthy"—even though that's not necessarily true. Organic sugar is still sugar. Organic cookies are still cookies. This foolishness has even spread to cigarettes: American Spirit advertises a variety rolled with organic tobacco and no chemical additives. While it's less unhealthy to inhale fewer chemical additives rather than more, it's not as if smoking organic cigarettes is healthy in any conceivable sense of the term.

"Organic" actually means "not industrial."

The organic movement attempts to distance itself from industrial ingredients and farming methods (chemical fertilizers, pesticides, antibiotics), though industrial manufacturing is often used to create and distribute organic goods. Similar to the push for whole foods, the injunction to eat organic is another way of rebelling against the industrial food system and embracing a traditional agricultural diet.

Back in Medieval times, when most of humanity lived as peasant farmers, all food used to be organic. This wasn't exactly a wonderful era of human existence marked by vibrant health and long life spans. (Of course, it makes as much sense to criticize a herder-farmer diet based on Medieval longevity, much of which had nothing to do with diet, as it does to criticize a hunter-gatherer diet based on Paleolithic longevity, much of which had nothing to do with diet.)

To the extent that eating more whole foods or organic foods means eating fewer industrial foods, most people can expect health improvements from adopting an agricultural diet.

2b. "Eat Low Calorie/Low Fat"

This last bit of advice warns us away from eating high-calorie, fatty foods. Before getting into fat, let's start with calories and the widespread belief that weight management is simply an easily controlled function of "calories in" (diet) and "calories out" (exercise).

One major problem with "calories in, calories out" is that the body is actually pretty good at matching energy intake to expenditure. Anyone who has done a hard workout has experienced the subsequent increase in appetite. If losing weight were as easy as cutting back on a tiny, tiny fraction of calories each day (*Three potato chips! One jelly bean!*), it would be impossible for anyone to maintain a normal weight. Lean people don't stay lean by measuring their caloric intake to the nearest jelly bean. Given how many calories are at our disposal, it's a wonder that we aren't even more overweight than we already are—or that obese people don't perpetually grow heavier throughout their lives but instead usually plateau at some point.

Another problem is that our sense of satiation is far more complicated than consuming a certain number of calories, and varies by macronutrient, the presence of micronutrient deficiencies, and even psychological effects such as serving size. Even the body's own unconscious mechanisms are attuned to more than just calories, so too should our conscious choices.

On the "calories out" side of the equation, most people focus exclusively on exercise, completely ignoring the body's largest source of energy expenditure: heat. This happens to be something that few people, aside from a few Buddhist monks, have any conscious control over.

It is difficult, if not impossible, to completely control our caloric balance through sheer discipline. Counting calories is a short-term tactic, not a long-term strategy. Attempting to count calories on an ongoing basis is a Sisyphean task, expressly designed for psychological torment and failure.

We Americans would have saved ourselves a lot of trouble if we had never discovered the (overly) simple fact that a gram of fat contains more calories than a gram of protein or carbohydrate, which seems to suggest that, all things equal, any overweight animal should eat more carbohydrate and less fat to lose weight. Yet carb-heavy grains are exactly what farmers feed to livestock to fatten them up as quickly and as cheaply as possible. Let me repeat that, just for good

measure: grains—the base of the USDA food pyramid for humans—
are what American farmers use to fatten up their livestock.

It's important to put the last half century of low-fat diet advice
in historical perspective. Atkins is often portrayed as a modern her-
etic rebelling against the low-fat consensus, but there's nothing new
about low-carb diets. When obesity first started appearing in Britain
soon after the Industrial Revolution, the first popular diet quickly
followed. Published in 1863, the Banting Diet was a low-carb diet,
restricting sweet and starchy foods.

If anything is a historical fad, it is low-fat diets. It was only in
1977 that the United States Senate Select Committee on Nutrition
and Human Needs, chaired by Senator George McGovern, released
Dietary Goals for the United States. The report put in place nutritional guidelines for all Americans, encouraging higher carbohydrate
intake and lower fat intake—the broad anti-fat consensus that still
exists today.

None of this is to say that carbohydrate is the be-all and end-all of
our dieting woes, but greater historical perspective calls into question
the wisdom of the current anti-fat orthodoxy. Again, any approach
that effectively reduces heavily processed industrial foods—fat, protein, or carbohydrate—can be expected to work, at least partially.

Much of the fat hysteria may boil down to a far simpler cause.
It's a shame that dietary "fat" is referred to by the same word used
to designate someone as being overweight. Encouraging modern
women to eat more fat is about as easy as selling them a makeup
called Ugly. Better terms for dietary fat would have been "lipids,"
"triglycerides," or "sexy"—as in, "Each spoonful of lard contains
13 grams of sexy."

Fat has become the boogeyman, not just of weight loss, but of
heart disease too. Most people have been trained to fear cholesterol,
saturated fat, and red meat.

Cholesterol has been villainized for decades, but the body
needs cholesterol. Cholesterol is an essential precursor to our sex
hormones—testosterone, estrogen, progesterone—and if the body

doesn't have enough, it makes more. We are given warning after warning about high cholesterol foods like eggs—but researchers can't actually find a significant, consistent connection between egg intake and cardiovascular disease. In fact, low cholesterol (intake and serum) is linked to higher mortality from cancer, mental illness, and suicide. Even statins, the popular class of cholesterol-lowering drugs, appear to gain their effectiveness by mechanisms unrelated to actually lowering cholesterol levels.

Saturated fat has been unfairly ostracized from our diet as well. Much as the body needs cholesterol, the body needs saturated fat. Roughly 40% of fats in human breast milk are saturated—as are a similar proportion of all fats in the body at all ages. The body uses saturated fat in cell walls and in the coating of the neurons in our brains. (Our ancestors who used stone tools to crush the skull cavity of an animal carcass got to eat a healthy dose of saturated fat: brains.) Saturated fat is good at these things precisely because it's saturated; the chemical structure doesn't easily react with free radicals and other molecules. Saturated fats are also great for cooking, since they are chemically stable even at high heat—unlike polyunsaturated fats (PUFAs), which oxidize easily and become rancid quickly.

In 2010 the *American Journal of Clinical Nutrition* published a meta-analysis on the link between saturated fat and heart disease. A meta-analysis pools data from multiple studies, and this one aggregated the results from twenty-one other studies covering 347,747 patients. The conclusion was unequivocal: "[T]here is no significant evidence for concluding that dietary saturated fat is associated with an increased risk of CHD [coronary heart disease] or CVD [cardiovascular disease]." It's a jaw-dropping conclusion considering what public health authorities have been telling us for decades.

When it comes to saturated fat and cardiovascular disease, public health authorities are failing to base their recommendations on scientific evidence. A recent Dutch study examined reports from three leading U.S. and European advisory committees and compared the reports to the underlying scientific articles they cited. The reviews of the scientific literature were woefully incomplete, and they systematically highlighted findings that fit the current consensus (the effects of saturated fat on LDL), while ignoring ones that didn't (the effects of saturated fat on HDL). The paper concluded, "Results and conclusions about saturated fat intake in relation to cardiovascular disease, from leading advisory committees, do not reflect the available scientific literature."

This does not instill faith in our public health authorities.

Among the increasing number of doctors who know about the tenuous connection between saturated fat and heart disease, many are afraid to change their dietary recommendations because they might lose credibility with their patients—or even get sued.

The so-called French Paradox isn't a paradox. The French have low rates of heart disease not despite eating so much saturated fat, but rather because of it, or at the very least independently of their high saturated fat intake. The widespread advice to replace saturated fat with polyunsaturated fats (PUFAs), which are commonly found in vegetable oils, is more troubling in light of the "Israeli Paradox." Israelis consume lots of PUFAs and little saturated fat—and they have notably high rates of heart disease. Perhaps these aren't "paradoxes" but evidence that the conventional wisdom is backward.

Red meat is another food we've been trained to view as unhealthy. Every few years a new study scares people about eating red meat. Since this happens on a regular basis, it's worth looking at one example. In 2012 *Archives of Internal Medicine* published just such a paper, which analyzed data collected during two large observational studies running over the past few decades: the Nurses' Health Study and the Health Professionals Follow-up Study. It concluded that one additional serving of unprocessed red meat each day increased the risk of overall mortality by 13%, rising to 20% for processed red meat.

The first problem with observational studies is well known: they can only reveal correlations, not prove causation. There were lots of differences between the people who ate the most red meat and those who didn't: the big meat-eaters also smoked more, exercised less, and took fewer vitamins. Even though the researchers adjusted for these effects, there were likely other confounding variables they missed. Additionally, the diet data are based on the participants filling out a Food Frequency Questionnaire *once every four years*. There are well-known food questionnaire biases, including people tending to underreport foods regarded as unhealthy—except for people with diagnosed conditions, who actually tend to overreport them. On average, the women in the lowest quintile of red meat consumption reported eating an average of 1,202 calories a day—so if the study was to be believed, many of the nurses were either extremely petite or starving to death.

At the same time, there are plausible ways in which eating red meat might be unhealthy. Insufficient cooking might not kill all viruses, parasites, or bacteria. Enough industrial processing can make anything unhealthy, and red meat is no exception. It's best to eat meat that has few industrial ingredients (flavorings, preservatives, and fillers), and that ideally comes from a healthy animal that was fed a natural diet. It's also probably not a good idea to cook meat at extremely high heat, as charred meat has many toxins. But there's good reason to be skeptical that red meat—the flesh of adult mammals—is inherently unhealthy. Until there's compelling evidence that carnivorous wolves, coyotes, and lions are dying prematurely from excess red meat consumption, I'll be enjoying my grass-fed steak medium-rare, thank you very much.

Not only has our calorie-driven fat phobia caused us to fear cholesterol, saturated fat, and red meat, but it has led to a general suspicion of eating animal products. This can be seen, in part, in the growth of vegetarianism, and the growing chorus of authorities who recommend a plant-based diet. Many health-conscious people now have a default predisposition that consuming whole plants is healthy while eating whole animals is not.

If either plants or animals should be regarded as "guilty until proven innocent," it's more appropriate to be suspicious of any given plant. The Plant Kingdom contains far more chemical diversity than the Animal Kingdom. Plants are the source of the vast majority of medicines, poisons, and psychoactive drugs. In contrast, mammals are built from pretty much the same stuff we are: muscle, sinew, bone, fat. There are no mammals with venomous flesh (even snake venom is edible), but there are countless toxic plants, each with its own style of biochemical warfare.

The chemical differences between plants and animals stem from different survival strategies. It's hard to walk up to a living animal and take a bite—they use hooves, horns, hides, and herds to evade predators. In contrast, plants can't run away from predators, so they evolved (organic) pesticides and poisons to stave off hungry insects and herbivores. Killing an animal is hard; digesting one is easy. Killing a plant is easy; digesting one is hard.

That said, the grocery store isn't filled with wild plants (or living animals). Domesticated plants have been bred to be more digestible (less fiber) and less toxic (fewer bitter-tasting compounds). Even so, it's far more problematic for an omnivore to eat a diet concentrated in a small number of plant species, which is what many people do, than it is to eat a diet concentrated in a small number of animal species.

One of the underlying sources of support for the anti-fat guidelines comes from the vegetarian lobby, which is motivated as much by ideology as it is by objective health science. Much of the fat in an industrial diet comes from animal sources, whereas the main alternative—carbohydrate—comes almost entirely from plant sources. Thus, railing against eating fat is a roundabout way of railing against eating animals. As a result, vegetarians have been particularly vocal supporters of the anti-fat orthodoxy.

Until 1990 McDonald's cooked its French fries in beef tallow (plus 7% cottonseed oil). Under pressure from the Center for Science in the Public Interest (CSPI), the fast-food chain switched to partially hydrogenated vegetable oils—as did most major fast-food and restaurant chains. CSPI was founded in 1971 by Dr. Michael Jacobson along

VEGETARIAN MYTHS

Myth #1: Humans did not evolve to eat meat.

Those who claim that meat hasn't been an important, long-standing part of the human diet seem to display willful ignorance of the considerable evidence to the contrary. Even frugivorous chimpanzees, our closest primate relatives, eat some meat. (Many primates eat insects too.) By 2.6 million years ago, our hominin ancestors were using stone tools to butcher animal carcasses. Paleolithic campsites are often littered with bones, and early humans hunted numerous animal species to extinction. Stable isotope analyses of some Paleolithic hominin remains show evidence of substantial meat consumption, particularly in high latitude locales like Siberia. There are no known vegetarian indigenous populations. Meat contains essential nutrients, such as vitamin B12, which are impossible for human beings to obtain in sufficient quantity from plant sources.

Myth #2: A meat-heavy diet is a modern phenomenon.

It's common to hear that meat used to be a side dish for thousands of years, until voracious Americans started eating Big Macs as the main course at every meal. To the extent that meat used to be viewed as a luxury, it was largely because people were poor. Invariably, wealthy rulers throughout history have eaten more meat than have peasants, and in greater variety. Increasing global prosperity is leading to a higher level of meat consumption—but the amount of meat consumed isn't out of the ordinary when viewed from a broader historical perspective. Of contemporary hunter-gatherer societies studied, most have gotten more than 50% of their calories from animal products.

Myth #3: Vegetarians are healthier than meat-eaters.

Vegetarians often are healthier than meat-eaters, but not necessarily because they avoid meat or fish. Vegetarians are less likely to smoke tobacco and drink alcohol, and more likely to exercise regularly—suggesting an overall greater concern with their health. These differences make it more difficult to isolate the specific health effects of avoiding meat or fish. Of five major studies conducted on vegetarians, two showed lower overall mortality relative to the general population (–17%, –20%), two showed higher (+11%, +17%), and one showed the same (all adjusted for age, sex, and smoking status). Both of the studies that showed vegetarians to have lower overall mortality were conducted on the Seventh-day Adventists, a close-knit religious group. Yet Mormons, who are similar except for eating meat, are also healthier than the general population. So it's hard to say.

It's important to remember that when people make a dramatic switch to a plant-based diet, they often make many other changes to their diet and lifestyle, such as avoiding soda, vegetable oils, white flour, and refined sugar; exercising more; and getting more sleep—recommendations sure to deliver health improvements independent of whether or not the person consumes meat. Vegetarians also suffer from certain distinct health problems related to avoiding meat, such as vitamin B12 deficiency. They tend to have lower bone mineral density (a big problem for women as they age), whereas consumption of animal protein has been shown to reduce osteoporosis and hip fractures. There is also some evidence to suggest that women on strict vegetarian diets are more likely to lose their period (amenorrhea) or become temporarily infertile.

Myth #4: *The China Study* says so!

The China Study is a bestselling book by Dr. T. Colin Campbell, who advocates a plant-based diet based on the results of a large observational study conducted in China. For critical analyses showing how the book misrepresents the study, see the work of Denise Minger (RawFoodSOS.com) and Ned Kock (HealthCorrelator.blogspot.com), which indicates that wheat consumption is strongly associated with overall mortality, whereas consumption of animal protein appears beneficial. Wherever the science nets out, the final answer will undoubtedly be more nuanced than the glib dogma "Plants good, animals bad!"

with two scientists and former co-workers from Ralph Nader's Center for the Study of Responsive Law. Longtime vegetarian Jacobson has been described as puritanical, imposing his personal eating ideology on employees of CSPI. As it turns out, McDonald's new vegetable oils contained synthetic trans fats, which CSPI defended at the time as a safe alternative to saturated fat (as did some mainstream health authorities). Synthetic trans fats, of course, were later discovered to be an extremely unhealthy type of fat that directly contributed to heart disease. In contrast, beef tallow is high in saturated fat, which means that it's not easily denatured or oxidized by cooking at high temperatures—a virtue in this case.

In a nutshell, an organization founded and led by a zealous vegetarian pressured McDonald's to re-engineer the preparation of French fries to fit its nutritional dogma, which resulted in making fries less healthy. Over the next few decades, the food movement excoriated McDonald's for cooking with trans fats, and advocates of a plant-based diet made condescending documentary films heaping scorn on ordinary Americans who got fat eating French fries cooked in *vegetable* oil. Nice.

If vegetarians didn't want to eat animals, they had a much simpler solution: don't order French fries. But instead CSPI imposed vegetarian ideology on everyone else—particularly the many working-class people who regularly eat fast food—to the detriment of their health.

While there are many legitimate ethical and environmental questions to be raised about the industrial food system, factory farming, and eating meat, those questions are separate from determining what is actually healthy for a human being to eat. Listening to vegetarians talk about the benefits of a plant-based diet, it can be hard to separate health claims from ideological, ethical, or environmental claims. At various times it has been claimed that vegetarianism can end world hunger; end food cravings; reverse global warming; reverse heart disease; reduce violent crime; reduce cholesterol; improve the sex drive; reduce the sex drive; end sexism;

cure cancer, and usher in the Age of Aquarius. Apparently soybeans grow best in bullshit.

Stepping back from modern health debates and taking a longer historical perspective, our fear of animal fat and protein is a rejection of herder diets, such as those of the Mongolian nomads in Asia, the Masai in Africa, or the early Jews in the Middle East. These ancient antecedents to Atkins tended to be high in animal fat and protein due to the consumption of milk, meat, and even blood. While herders face their own health challenges (infectious disease and infant mortality are high), studies of contemporary herders show low rates of cardiovascular disease relative to Western populations.

Our national fat phobia is also a rejection of the traditional diet of the American dairy "farmer"—who is also a herder of cows. Even as food companies plaster their low-fat products with idyllic farm scenes, they reject the very foods most valued by traditional farmers. American herder-farmer diets have traditionally been high in fat and animal products, which were usually considered the most wholesome (and valuable) foods on the farm: raw milk, whole cream, real butter, cheese, eggs, and meat.

By rejecting nutrient-dense herder diets in favor of a few staple cereal grains, the conventional advice to "eat low fat" actually means "Eat like a poor, malnourished farmer."

Here's what's on the menu: whole rye bread (no butter), lentil soup, an heirloom variety of apple, and a fist-sized portion of skinless chicken breast—all of it organic. It's a meal fit for a serf, sold for a princely sum to slavish Whole Foods shoppers.

Most health authorities aren't consciously attempting to push the "Poor Farmer Diet." But farm-fresh organic food is what most of humanity ate before the Industrial Revolution came along. It's what we remember. The Poor Farmer Diet is what comes from a combination of fat phobia and the increasingly popular rule of thumb: "Don't eat anything your great-grandmother wouldn't recognize as food."

But what if we had a longer memory?

Ten thousand years—about four hundred generations—takes us back before the Industrial and Agricultural Revolutions, back to our time in the wild living as hunter-gatherers.

What did that grandmother recognize as food?

Quite a lot, actually.

Large mammals—such as antelope, gazelle, and elephant—were definitely on the menu by 2.6 million years ago. Of these, she would have eaten more than just the muscle meat, happily devouring organs such as the liver, heart, brains, marrow, and bones. Fresh seafood was a popular choice where available, and evidence of eating shellfish and other aquatic species appears 1.95 million years ago. Both primates and contemporary hunter-gatherers eat insects, eggs, and honey, so Paleolithic people most likely did too. Birds, reptiles, and amphibians would have been options, though small game was almost certainly less desirable than big game, seafood, or honey. Fruit was eaten, though it wasn't the primary dietary staple as it is among chimpanzees. Starchy roots and tubers were an important food source, and nuts were an option as well. (We were on the menu too: cannibalism appears to have been fairly widespread among pre-agricultural peoples.)

In short, hunter-gatherers were opportunistic omnivores—eating mammals, seafood, roots and tubers, a diversity of plants, fruit, honey, nuts, eggs, birds, insects, reptiles, and amphibians. With the advent of cooking a million years ago, an even broader array of species became edible.

Eating such diets, hunter-gatherers were as healthy as any other wild species that is well adapted to its habitat. From their height, bone structure, and teeth, Paleolithic hunter-gatherers were quite a bit healthier than the poor, squat, miserable farmers who followed. Contemporary hunter-gatherers have virtually no obesity and diabetes, and low rates of cardiovascular disease and cancer. They require only minimal modern medicines to regularly achieve life spans into their sixties and seventies. There have been only a handful of small, short clinical trials testing approximations of Paleolithic diets, and initial results have been positive—but there simply needs to be more, larger, longer, and better-controlled studies.

None of this is to say that Paleolithic diets are the last word in nutrition science. The quest for a healthy human diet doesn't end in the Paleolithic—but that's the right place to start.

8

FOOD:

PRINCIPLES FOR A HEALTHY DIET

Just as tribes of hunter-gatherers ate different diets, so too will "tribes" of modern people. Here are four general principles to help establish a clear and specific starting point for healthy eating in the short term, coupled with general guidelines to create, maintain, and strengthen a healthy lifestyle over the long term:

1. **What to eat:** *Mimic a hunter-gatherer (or herder) diet.*
2. **How to eat:** *Follow ancient culinary traditions.*
3. **What not to eat:** *Avoid industrial foods, sugars, and seeds.*
4. **Make it meaningful:** *Experiment, customize, enjoy.*

Personally, I follow guidelines found in *Perfect Health Diet* by Drs. Paul and Shou-Ching Jaminet, and I have integrated many of their points into this framework.

1. What to Eat:
Mimic a Hunter-Gather (or Herder) Diet

To eat a Paleolithic diet, one doesn't need to live in the wild and hunt with stone tools. Mokolo and Bebac didn't eat wild plants flown in from Africa; the produce in the Cleveland grocery store was close enough. Eating a Paleolithic diet is not about historical re-enactment; it is about mimicking the effect of such a diet on the metabolism with foods available at the supermarket.

There was no one diet eaten throughout the entire Paleolithic, nor is there a single diet eaten by contemporary hunter-gatherers. Hunter-gatherer diets can vary substantially depending on the geography, season, and culture. Even so, the commonalities among hunter-gatherer diets provide useful parameters for a healthy modern diet.

Stop Counting Calories

Mimicking a Paleolithic diet does not require counting calories. There is no evidence that hunter-gatherers knew the meaning of a calorie, much less measured or counted them—yet obesity is nonexistent among extant tribes. Among nonhuman wild species (none of which count calories), obesity has not been observed when they consume their natural diet. In contrast, obesity is now common among pets, laboratory animals, farm animals, and zoo animals fed a variety of industrial diets. Efforts at teaching them to lose weight by counting calories have yet to succeed.

If anything, hunter-gatherers pursued the highest calorie and most nutrient-dense foods relative to the effort required to obtain them—usually large game and honey. While it's tempting to conclude that hunter-gatherers could "afford" to eat high-calorie foods due to their active lifestyle, a 2012 study of the Hadza tribe in Tanzania revealed that their total energy expenditure was comparable to that of modern Americans (after adjusting for body size). Even though the Hadza spent more energy on physical activity, it was offset by expending less energy on their base level at rest. The authors suggest that the primary cause of obesity is not our lack of energy expenditure, but eating novel foods that disrupt our metabolism. Thus we should eat the types of foods eaten by humans during the bulk of our evolution.

Eat the Right Food Groups

Hunter-gatherers ate a wide variety of species. Mimicking this means eating a varied diet of meat, seafood, roots and tubers, leafy vegetables, fruit, nuts, and eggs.

But which food groups were most important?

A review of the diets of 229 foraging societies estimated that nearly three-quarters of them obtained more than 50% of their calories from animals (though many of the tribes were involved in horticulture, limited agriculture, or hunting with advanced technology, including guns in some cases). In another study of nine contemporary hunter-gatherer tribes, food groups were exactly weighed and measured. Seven of them obtained more than 50% of dietary calories from meat and insects.

Among plants, starchy roots and tubers were most important, accounting for roughly 15% of calories on average. Fruit accounted for more than 10% of calories for only three tribes. For eight of nine tribes, nuts and seeds were not a source of calories at all; only the !Kung Bushmen, indigenous to southern Africa, ate large amounts, subsisting on mongongo nuts (which are high in fat).

Thus animal foods are the single greatest source of calories, but plant foods, due to their low caloric density, constitute greater bulk in the diet. Animal foods tend to come from fatty animals and seafood; plant foods tend to come primarily from starchy roots and tubers.

Don't Be Afraid of Fat

Hunter-gatherers show quite a bit of dietary flexibility depending on their habitat, and unsurprisingly their diets span many different proportions of protein, fat, and carbohydrate. For example, the Inuit eat an extremely high-fat diet mostly composed of animals (fish, seal, caribou), since few plants grow in the snowy Arctic. In contrast, the Kitavans, a tribe of Pacific Islanders, eat a high-carbohydrate diet, largely obtained from starchy tubers (yam, cassava, sweet potato, taro)—in addition to fish, coconut, fruit, and the

CANNIBALISM: THE HUMAN DIET

I have been assured by a very knowing American of my Acquaintance in London, that a young healthy Child well nurs'd, is, at a Year old, a most delicious nourishing and wholesome Food, whether stewed, roasted, baked, or boyled; and I make no doubt, that it will equally serve in a Fricassee, or a Ragoust.

—Jonathan Swift, *A Modest Proposal* (1729)

Though it has long offended the moral sensibilities of most people, cannibalism was a fairly widespread practice among pre-agricultural people. Paleolithic remains of both Neanderthals and *Homo sapiens* have, in some instances, shown signs of having been butchered just like any other prey species. Cannibalism has been observed in chimpanzees, as well as in a variety of more distantly related species—and not just during times of extreme food stress. Eating the departed most likely came to an end with the rise of infectious disease during the Agricultural Age.

Even though a strict reading of a Paleolithic diet would include cannibalism, it is a practice that I have to discourage. Modern people have a much higher ratio of omega-6 to omega-3 fatty acids due to their grain-based diets; carry a wide variety of chronic infections; have destroyed their liver with excessive consumption of alcohol and fructose; and contain many environmental toxins. That said, if one were to incorporate cannibalism into "eating paleo," it would be healthiest to eat people who strictly adhered to the guidelines in this book.

occasional pig. Studies of both tribes show them to be substantially healthier than typical Westerners.

A focus on macronutrients alone, like calories, is no silver bullet for modern health problems. However, thinking about macronutrients can still be useful for two reasons: (1) most people already hold strong and possibly mistaken opinions on fat, protein, and carbs; and (2) others may want to optimize their diet for weight loss or performance.

There are fairly uncontroversial parameters for healthy levels of protein consumption, and more important, the body seems to have a pretty good sense of how much protein it needs. Conventional guidelines usually recommend 10–20% of calories in the form of protein. There are limits to how much protein the liver can process, but most people never reach that threshold (unless you're a seventeenth-century American settler trying to survive a harsh winter only on ultra-lean rabbit meat). Protein is the most satiating of the macronutrients, and protein-fueled bodybuilders know it takes a lot of effort to eat large amounts of skinless chicken breast or tuna fish. The appetite quickly tires of it.

The debate over macronutrients largely revolves around fat and carbohydrate. Hunter-gatherers clearly valued concentrated forms of both, seeing as they pursued fatty animals and sweet honey.

The bulk of evidence suggests that most Westerners would benefit from less carbohydrate and more fat. Many hunter-gatherer tribes had a total fat intake that was as high or higher than the standard American diet—suggesting that a higher fat intake would be well tolerated. After the Agricultural Revolution, the shift to a higher carbohydrate diet contributed to widespread tooth decay, indicating that the first part of the human digestive tract was poorly adapted to consuming so much carbohydrate; the introduction of industrial refined sugar only exacerbated the problem. Today excess sugar and carbohydrate are directly implicated in cardiovascular disease, insulin insensitivity, and type 2 diabetes, a disorder of blood sugar regulation. Sugar is also the preferred fuel of many cancerous tumors.

In fact, the only truly nonessential macronutrient is carbohydrate. People can subsist on a fat and protein diet (called a ketogenic diet), but they can't subsist on a fat and carbohydrate diet (which lacks essential amino acids) or a protein and carbohydrate diet (which lacks essential fats). This doesn't mean that zero carbohydrate is optimal, of course, but it does mean that carbohydrate isn't essential.

Shifting to a low-sugar, lower carbohydrate diet is particularly important for people looking to lose weight or repair their metabolism, and it seems prudent for everyone. Learn to trust your natural instinct to eat and enjoy fatty foods: moist meats, potatoes with butter or sour cream. Don't be afraid of foods that contain fat.

Eat Nose to Tail

Being an omnivore—eating everything—extended to eating nearly every part of an animal. Brains, bone marrow, liver, heart, kidneys, skin, and tongue were all on the menu. Not only did hunter-gatherers eat organs and fatty cuts, they preferred them to the lean protein of muscle meat. For example, the Inuit had very specific methods of dividing carcasses between adults, children, and dogs. The rich, marrow-filled bones were for people, not dogs—the exact opposite of today's practices. The method of division varied by species, and scholars are just beginning to rediscover the nutritional wisdom embedded in such traditional practices.

Much of the aversion to nose-to-tail eating is largely cultural, in the same way that sushi was considered repulsive before being embraced by Western palates. Bone marrow is a food closely tied to what it means to be human, one that made us who we are today. Bone marrow should hold a revered place in the modern human diet.

Organ meats are some of the most nutrient-rich parts of the animal, which is why liver pops up as a uniquely nutritious food in culture after culture. Not only are fatty deposits like bone marrow a great source of energy, but they also contain a great deal of fat-soluble vitamins. Eating an entire mammal provides everything required to build another mammal. During expeditions to Alaska in the early twentieth century, explorer Vilhjalmur Stefansson survived on a meat-only diet in good health—but more than just muscle meat, his diet included fatty cuts, raw cuts (which contain vitamin C), and some organs.

Many zoos engage in a similar nose-to-tail practice called "whole-prey feeding." They simply feed the predators (lions, snakes, birds of prey) an entire carcass of their natural prey (goats, mice, fish). Some zoos gut-load the prey with supplements, but, in general, whole-prey feeding frees zookeepers from worry about nutrient deficiencies because the predator gets all the nutrients it needs by eating its natural diet: the entire prey animal, just as it would do in the wild. Eating nose to tail is the ultimate nutritional supplement.

Eat a Variety of Plants

As for eating plants, the key issue is to provide a diversity of nutrients while minimizing toxic load. The solution is to eat a variety of plants; this diversifies nutrition and also reduces toxicity since every plant has different toxins and each toxin usually isn't dangerous in a small dose. The most healthful plants are green leafy vegetables and seaweeds, fruits and berries, and roots and tubers (in contrast to grains, legumes, nuts, and seeds). For most people, roots and tubers are a good source of "safe starches" or "safe sugars"—safe because of the low levels of problematic antinutrients. These include sweet potato, potato, yam, taro, carrots, parsnips, rutabaga, beets, onions, and squash. Another good source of nontoxic starch is white rice.

Experiment with Dairy

Except during infancy, hunter-gatherers did not drink milk. After the domestication of animals, multiple herder populations independently gained a genetic adaptation to digest lactose into adulthood. Their milk-based diet must have been profoundly beneficial because these people were robust, their populations grew quickly, and they usually dominated their unlucky neighbors. Today people with the lactase persistence gene (about 35% of global population) are descended from one of those herder populations (though people without the gene can still thrive on high dairy diets). Even so, most people in the world are still lactose intolerant—and given milk's recent history in the human diet, it clearly isn't necessary for good health.

Dairy consumption is a point of contention among professional academics, as well as lay dietitians. Some scholars believe that proteins and hormones in milk are implicated in gut inflammation, cancer, and acne. That said, lactose and casein (a milk protein) are also found in human breast milk, so they aren't completely foreign compounds to the human metabolism. Furthermore, many herder populations who consume large amounts of dairy don't appear to suffer from diet-related health conditions, though traditional processing methods probably played a role in that. Milk and dairy were full fat, unpasteurized, and often consumed in fermented form, which is not quite the same as the milk and dairy one finds in a modern grocery store. Aaruul, a Mongolian food made of fermented curdled milk, dehydrated and dried in the sun, has yet to find its way onto the shelves at Whole Foods.

Dairy is one of those areas where personal experimentation is required—exclude it entirely for a time, then add it back in and see how you feel. Many people seem to do just fine with full-fat or fermented dairy, including real butter (very popular), heavy cream, sour cream, cheese, and yogurt. It's best to avoid low-fat, ultra-pasteurized dairy entirely.

2. How to Eat:
Follow Ancient Culinary Traditions

Ancient culinary traditions often exist for a reason: they don't just make food tastier; they often make food healthier. For example, scientists frequently discover that traditionally prized foods (seaweed, liver) often turn out to be rich in one or more key micronutrients. In a sense, these culinary traditions were the original "supplements"—but they were more effective than many of today's supplements, which are either poorly absorbed or taken in excessive quantities. When dealing in proverbs and old wives' tales, it can be hard to separate superstition from science, so it's a good idea to look for traditions that are old (persistent), widespread (pervasive), and originated in multiple cultures (profitable).

Make Broths and Stocks

"A good broth can raise the dead" is a South American proverb. Bones are a great base for soups, and humans have been boiling bones for nearly as long as we've had fire and a container to hold water. Hot water leaches nutrients, collagen, and marrow out of bones, as well as nutrients from meat and skin. A similar injunction to "drink the spinach water" or pot likker gets to the same point with vegetables. The drippings from cooking are often quite nutritious and make a delicious addition to broths, stocks, sauces, and soups.

Eat Fermented Foods

Fermentation is a way to process food with bacteria. It is commonly used to brew beer, leaven bread, curdle cheese, pickle vegetables, culture yogurt, cure meats, and sour foods (like sourdough, sour cream, and sauerkraut). Found in cuisines all over the world, fermentation has been applied to just about every food group, including grains (alcohol, bread), legumes (soy sauce), vegetables (pickles, sauerkraut), fruit (wine, vinegar), honey (mead), dairy (cheese, yogurt), fish (fish sauce), and meat (salami, pepperoni).

Fermentation often makes foods healthier than they otherwise would be—or even edible at all. For example, fermented dairy products have less lactose (the sugar in milk), and thus are more easily digested by those who are lactose intolerant. Raw soybeans are inedible for humans, but fermented soy products (soy sauce, natto, tempeh) are common in Asian cuisines. Sourdough is made from fermented grains, which contain fewer problematic compounds, such as gluten, phytates, or lectins.

Some fermented foods contain active bacterial cultures, and eating them can help people maintain a healthy population of gut bacteria. Good options include sauerkraut or kimchi (fermented cabbage), pickles (fermented cucumber), and kombucha (fermented tea). For those who eat dairy, good options include full-fat Greek yogurt or aged cheeses. Unfortunately, industrial manufacturers often sterilize fermented foods, which means it's a good idea to buy them from a traditional source (farmers markets, health food stores) or ferment them yourself. The recent probiotics craze is a few millennia late to the game, but nonetheless it is a welcome corrective to the mistaken view that all bacteria are bad. Not only have humans cultivated external strains of bacteria for thousands of years; we have lived in synergy with internal bacteria in our body for as long as complex life has existed.

Fermentation is right up there with cooking as one of the most powerful methods to transform food. In a very real sense, the underlying process of fermentation—synergy with bacteria—is older than cooking; complex life forms have been co-evolving with microorganisms going all the way back to the first cellular organism teaming up with mitochondria, which used to be independent life forms. Humans have co-evolved with the bacteria in our gut since long before we were human, and fermentation simply externalizes that synergistic relationship.

Cook with Traditional Recipes

Traditional recipes and food pairings aren't simply arbitrary combinations chosen on the basis of flavor. People who happened to find these recipes delicious ended up more successful (reproductively) than those who did not. Mesoamericans combined lime and corn to release niacin, preventing pellagra. Wasabi—real wasabi, not dyed horseradish—is an antimicrobial agent, and thus is a good accompaniment to raw fish. Pairing olive oil, or another fat, with tomatoes helps make available a nutrient called lycopene. Don't ignore tradition.

Cook with Low Heat

Slow cooking is one of the oldest methods of cooking. A mix between steaming and baking, it relies on indirect, low heat for a long period of time. Hunter-gatherers often used simple earthen ovens: dig a fire pit, light a fire, let it go out, bury the embers along with the food, and dig it up hours later, ready to eat. The traditional form of cooking among Pacific Islanders (think Hawaiian pig roasts), it also finds a modern manifestation in the New England clambake, barbecue pit, and slow cooker. Heat is a catalyst for chemical reactions, and cooking at extremely high temperatures causes the food to react with oxygen more easily (oxidize), particularly sugars and polyunsaturated fats. The blackened part of heavily cooked meat or plants is carcinogenic. Buy a slow cooker.

Cook with Traditional Fats and Oils

Traditional animal fats include tallow (beef fat), lard (pork fat), butter, and ghee (clarified butter). Healthy plant oils include coconut oil and olive oil. Generally, tropical plants provide the healthiest oils. Choose cooking fats and oils that are low in polyunsaturated fats (PUFAs). Avoid industrial vegetable oils, such as canola oil or soybean oil.

Eat Raw Foods

While there are substantial benefits to cooking, there are also benefits to eating food in its raw state—plants and animals both. For example, cooking vegetables reduces their fiber content, and cooking meat destroys vitamin C. Just about every ancient ethnic cuisine includes a dish made from raw animal products: *sushi* and *sashimi* (fish, Japanese), *ceviche* (fish, Central and South American), *kibbe* (lamb, Middle Eastern), *crudo* (fish, Italian), *kitfo* (beef, Ethiopian), *yukhoe* (beef, Korean), *chee kufta* (beef, Turkish), and *poke* (fish, Hawaiian). Raw animal foods are usually accompanied by one or more antimicrobial agents (wasabi, acidic juice, vinegar, spices), and they are best consumed from a trusted source prepared in traditional ways.

Eat Your Colors
The different colors in plants indicate different chemical compounds, and each provides a different set of antioxidants and nutrients. Eating a variety of colors is a good way to eat a variety of micronutrients.

Sprout, Soak, or Ferment Grains, Legumes, Nuts, and Seeds
For those who keep grains in their diet, sprouting, soaking, and fermentation are three traditional ways to make them less toxic. For a wonderful exploration of fermentation, read the fourth part of *Cooked* by Michael Pollan.

Don't Throw Out the Yolk
According to the Talmud, "An egg is superior to the same quantity of any other kind of food." People who order egg-white-only omelets are missing out on the most nutritious part of the egg: the yolk. Dr. Chris Masterjohn points out that of all the nutrients in an egg, the yolk contains 100% of the fat-soluble vitamins (A, E, D, and K), essential fatty acids DHA and AA, and carotenoids. The yolk contains over 80% of nine nutrients (calcium, iron, phosphorus, zinc, thiamine, folate, B6, B12, and pantothenic acid), whereas the white contains over 80% of just three nutrients (magnesium, sodium, and niacin). Six other nutrients are split more evenly between the two. Of course, the yolk also contains 99% of the fat, which is why people avoid it. Despite the widespread fear of cholesterol, eating eggs has not been shown to cause cardiovascular disease. Egg yolks from pastured hens are a deep orange, unlike the pale yellow of conventional yolks, and are richer in nutrients. They taste better too.

Eat Liver
When Inuit hunters kill a seal they immediately cut it open and eat the raw liver first. Liver is one of the most famously healthy foods in the world: according to a Chinese proverb, "Eat liver, fortify your own liver"; chopped liver is prominent in Jewish cuisine; cod-liver oil is a traditional dietary supplement in Nordic countries; many American

families used to eat liver on Sundays; and pregnant women are often still advised to eat it.

Yet after millennia of good press, liver has recently fallen out of style. Some fear that the liver is like the lint trap on a dryer—clogged up with all sorts of nastiness. But the liver doesn't literally function like a filter; it's more like a well-functioning washer and dryer, which continually clean things up and flush dirtiness out of the system.

It's true that feedlot animals often have fatty liver disease (from excessive consumption of grains) and their livers shouldn't be eaten, so buy liver from a young animal (calf's liver) or, better yet, from an animal that was fed its natural diet. Many people make the mistake of overcooking liver, which actually gives it a stronger taste. Duck liver pâté, though associated with the upper crust, is surprisingly affordable, and it is an easy way to get liver into the diet without having to cook it.

Eat Oily Cold Water Fish

According to a Dutch saying, "A land with lots of herring can get along with few doctors." Small cold water fish such as mackerel, sardines, herring, and anchovies are amazing for just about everything except your breath. They are a rich source of omega-3 fatty acids, as well as vitamin D, calcium, and vitamin B12. Whether cooked, cured, or canned, whole fish are an underappreciated way to eat nose to tail, getting the skin, bones, and many of the organs.

Eat Seaweed

Seaweed refers to many large species of algae. The Japanese diet has long included many varieties of seaweed, such as nori (the seaweed sheets wrapping sushi), wakame (used in seaweed salad), and kombu (a brown kelp often used in soups). The sea is full of minerals, so perhaps it's no surprise that seaweed is an excellent source of minerals required by the body. Seaweed typically contains iodine, vitamin B12 (rare among nonanimal foods), and large amounts of protein—making sea vegetables particularly popular among vegans.

Eat Real Butter

According to an old Irish saying, "What butter and whiskey can't cure, can't be cured." In the mid-twentieth century butter came under fire for its high saturated fat content, and margarine—made from partially hydrogenated vegetable oils—was marketed as a healthier alternative. Decades later, real butter looks to be the healthier option, yet it still retains a stigma. Real butter is a great addition to vegetables, particularly for picky children. For extra flavor and nutrition, try butter made from the milk of grass-fed cows. Grass-fed butter is a rich source of vitamin A, a healthy fat called CLA (conjugated linoleic acid), and vitamin K2. Many grocery stores now carry Kerrygold, an authentic Irish grass-fed butter.

Drink Tea

According to an ancient Chinese proverb, "Better to be deprived of food for three days, than tea for one." The Chinese have been drinking tea for at least three thousand years, initially as a form of medicine and eventually for enjoyment. Tea spread to Japan and India, then from India to Great Britain and much of the Anglophone world. Not only was boiled water safer to drink, but the many varieties of tea contain a vast number of flavanols and other bioactive compounds that may help reduce the risk of cardiovascular disease, diabetes, and dementia. Green tea is also a good low-caffeine option for people who need a boost but don't want to disrupt their sleep cycle.

Salt to Taste

A folktale common in Europe and India features a king who asks his three daughters how much they love him; the youngest is exiled for her answer—"As much as meat loves salt"—though she is eventually recognized as correct. Not only is salt the most ancient food preservative, but salt is one of the basic human tastes—and it exists for a reason: salt contains minerals that are essential to human life. Naturally occurring salt (and salty foods) usually originate from the sea, and thus are a rich source of minerals: sodium, chloride, iodine, and

EATING EARTH

It may be that the world's oldest medicine is the earth itself.
—Dr. Timothy Johns, "Well-Grounded Diet" (1991)

G eophagy is the practice of eating clay. This seemingly odd behavior appears not only across human cultures, but also among a wide variety of species, including chimpanzees, birds, reptiles, and rodents. Among humans it has often been labeled a compulsive eating disorder called pica, particularly when cravings lead people to eat ice, chalk, cornstarch, or even toilet paper. In the nineteenth century, slave owners even affixed iron masks over the heads of slaves who ate dirt, believing that eating dirt was an attempt to commit suicide.

As it turns out, eating clay has health-related functions. Clay is "adsorptive," a property akin to microscopic static cling. (Adsorption is not to be confused with absorption, where a fluid permeates a solid.) This property causes clays to bond with certain toxins and minerals, and then are flushed out of the system. Geophagy happens to be most prevalent among pregnant women (particularly in their first trimester), children, and people of recent equatorial descent—all of whom are particularly sensitive to toxins or tend to be exposed to high levels of pathogens.

Today most people depend on clays without realizing it. Clay was one of the original active ingredients in Kaopectate, used to soothe an upset stomach. Most water filters are made with charcoal, and poison control recommends keeping activated charcoal in the house as an effective antidote to many poisons. One reason it's difficult to poison rats, even though they can't vomit, is that they nibble on protective clays. Similarly, Medieval European royalty, paranoid about being poisoned, would consume clay tablets with every meal.

Source: *Craving Earth* by Dr. Sera Young

many more depending on the source. Despite all the hysteria over the sodium added to industrial food, there is only meager evidence that low-salt diets significantly reduce blood pressure, heart attacks, or strokes. If you generally avoid industrial foods, then your own sense of taste should be a reliable guide to salt intake.

3. What Not to Eat:
Avoid Industrial Foods, Sugars, and Seeds

When you're lost in the wild, eating a handful of unknown berries or a mysterious mushroom can kill you, but there's nothing you can eat or drink that will dramatically or permanently improve your health. Poisons are real; the Fountain of Youth isn't.

The same principle applies in the grocery store: what *not* to eat can be more important than what to eat. The single most important way for many people to quickly improve their health is to subtract unhealthy foods, not to add healthy foods. Eating broccoli does not "cancel out" devouring three slices of pizza.

Top on this list are industrial foods (sugar, vegetable oils) as well as the seed-based crops they're made out of (cereal grains, legumes). Think of these as slow-acting poisons when consumed in large quantities.

Avoid Industrial Foods
In general, avoid things that are made in a factory, contain lots of ingredients you can't pronounce, and don't spoil. Avoiding sugar, vegetable oils, and cereal grains will also preclude most industrial foods.

Avoid Sugars
Sugar comes in multiple forms (glucose, fructose, sucrose, lactose), but none of them is healthy in large, concentrated quantities. Yet, because the body metabolizes sugars in different ways, different sugars bring different benefits and risks.

Glucose is the sugar found in starchy foods such as potatoes and rice, and it is used by the body in a wide variety of natural processes like fueling the brain. Too much glucose in the bloodstream is toxic, and the body releases the hormone insulin to store excess glucose in muscles, liver, and fat tissue. When people snack throughout the day ("to keep their blood sugar up"), they are attempting to maintain a consistent level of glucose in the bloodstream—although what they're often doing is slowly poisoning themselves.

Fructose is the sugar often found in fruit, as well as sweeteners like high fructose corn syrup. Unlike with glucose, the body does not use fructose directly, but shunts it from the bloodstream to the liver, where it is converted into glycogen (a stored form of energy). The liver has only a limited capacity to store glycogen, about the equivalent of a couple pieces of fruit—less than one can of soda. The rest must be converted into fat through a slower, less efficient, and more damaging process. Excessive consumption of fructose contributes to the development of fatty liver disease, kidney stones, and gout. Fructose also reacts with proteins in the body to form "advanced glycation end products" (AGEs), which, appropriately enough, cause a variety of symptoms of aging.

The best way to avoid large amounts of fructose is simply to avoid industrial foods, such as soda or pastries. Fruit is best eaten whole (not as juice), in small quantities, and in the morning when the liver's stores are more likely to be depleted. Those trying to lose weight may want to cut fruit out of their diet altogether.

Lactose is the sugar commonly found in milk, made up of glucose and galactose, another type of sugar. The body uses an enzyme called lactase to break down lactose into glucose and galactose. People who are lactose intolerant don't produce lactase, face digestive problems when drinking milk, and so usually don't drink it. Additionally, milk (particularly low-fat milk) initiates a strong insulin response from the body—much stronger than an equivalent amount of glucose from, say, a potato. Given that one of insulin's roles is to store surplus energy as fat, this is reason enough for lactose tolerant people to avoid it.

Sucrose is table sugar; it is a combination of glucose and fructose. Adding a large amount of table sugar to a meal or baked goods is a double hit on the metabolism.

Overall, it's a good idea to avoid any food with added sugar, no matter what kind. Even when eating whole foods, large quantities of sugar should be avoided. Some foods that aren't considered "sweet" can still have lots of sugar in them, such as milk. Of all the sugars, glucose is the one that, in moderate quantities, is most useful as an energy source, and starchy foods have a place in a healthy diet. Just choose roots, tubers, or rice over wheat, corn, or beans.

Avoid Vegetable Oils

Vegetable oils are liquid fats derived from plants. Many vegetable oils—including soybean oil, corn oil, peanut oil, rapeseed/canola oil, safflower oil, and sunflower seed oil—are extracted from grains and legumes. Though olive oil is thousands of years old, most vegetable oils are relatively recent industrial foods. Becoming common before World War I, they were favored for their low cost and supposed heart-healthiness relative to traditional animal fats. They are now widely used in all kinds of foods, including salad dressing, baked goods, and a vast number of industrial foods that require fat.

Not only do vegetable oils contain the plant toxins discussed below, but they are also notably high in omega-6 fatty acids. Omega-6 fatty acids, along with omega-3 fatty acids, are polyunsaturated fats (PUFAs). PUFAs are essential to the human diet since the body cannot derive them from other compounds—but they are toxic in large amounts. The typical industrial diet contains far more omega-6s than the body needs, and as a result the ratio of omega-6s to omega-3s is dramatically skewed toward omega-6s. Since omega-6s have a pro-inflammatory effect throughout the body, they exacerbate existing inflammation.

In a variety of laboratory experiments on mice, diets excessively high in PUFAs led to obesity, fatty liver disease, and metabolic syndrome. In humans, excessive omega-6 consumption has been associated with higher rates of obesity, mental illness, violence, allergies, asthma, and cancer. Simply avoiding vegetable oils goes a long way to reducing PUFA intake to nontoxic levels. Since excess omega-6 fat consumption prevents the body from properly utilizing omega-3 fats, avoiding omega-6 fats helps to restore a proper balance between omega-6s and omega-3s.

Avoid Cereal Grains

Cereal grains are the seeds of grasses. The top four—wheat, corn, rice, and barley—account for nearly 70% of global agricultural crops by weight. Along with sorghum, oats, rye, and millet, these grains account for 56% of all calories eaten by humans.

The seeds of cereal grains contain toxic proteins. Many of these toxic proteins are *intended* to make it difficult for a grazing mammal to digest the seed. From a seed's perspective, it doesn't "want" to get digested—it wants to make a new plant. The goal is to exit a mammal's digestive tract still intact, dispersed and covered in the manure that will fertilize the seed's growth. The toxic proteins are more heavily concentrated in the outer shell (also known as the "bran"), but are found throughout the entire kernel. Grains that contain the heavily toxic bran are described as "whole grains," and are often mistakenly viewed as entirely healthy.

In wheat, for example, gluten makes up the majority of wheat protein. Even though gluten is associated with the small percentage of people with celiac disease (about 0.4 to 0.8% in the United States), it causes gut inflammation in over 80% of people. The gut is the digestive tract, which plays a central role not only in digestion, but in metabolism and immune function as well. Persistent gut inflammation can damage the intestinal lining, and large molecules and bacteria can ooze into the bloodstream—which initiates a reaction from the immune system. Autoimmune disorders occur when the body chronically attacks itself, and a wide variety—lupus, type 1 diabetes, and multiple sclerosis—are associated with a leaky, inflamed gut and wheat consumption.

Though gluten gets all the attention these days, it is far from the only toxic protein in wheat or other cereal grains. Wheat also contains opioid peptides and wheat germ agglutinin. Opioid peptides are opiates (in the same family as opium, morphine, and heroin) and make eating wheat enjoyable, addictive, and difficult to stop. Wheat germ agglutinin also damages the gut and has a tendency to bind with other molecules. The immune system identifies these clumpy molecules as invaders and attacks them—often damaging the gut and other body parts in the process.

Consumption of wheat has been associated with a vast number of chronic health conditions, including cardiovascular disease, autoimmune disorders, and cancer. Corn contains many toxic proteins similar to those found in wheat and other cereal grains. Of all the cereal grains, white rice is the least toxic, largely consisting of pure carbohydrate. Therefore, depending on one's level of carbohydrate intake, white rice is a good low-toxicity option.

Avoid Legumes

Legumes are grain-like seeds. The most important legume in the industrial diet is the soybean, the fifth largest agricultural crop in the world. Other common legumes include peanuts, lentils, peas, alfalfa, and any variety of beans.

Legumes fill an ecological niche similar to that of grains and have evolved similar defenses against hungry insects and herbivores. In Australia and New Zealand, for example, female sheep that eat too many of certain pasture legumes that contain compounds that bind with estrogen receptors have difficulty with conception, miscarriages, and infertility.

For humans, many legumes are extremely toxic in their raw state;

the deadly poison ricin is made from castor beans. Legumes require significant processing before they are even edible, such as soaking, boiling, sprouting, or fermenting. In Asia, for example, soybeans are traditionally soaked and fermented beforehand (to make tofu, miso, and tempeh).

Legumes contain many toxins. Lectins are a class of proteins also found in cereal grains. Some lectins bind with nutrients and make them unavailable to the body. Since they prevent nutrients from being absorbed by the body, they are often called *anti*nutrients. Another antinutrient is phytic acid, which binds with zinc and other micronutrients in the gut. (Soaking can help break down phytic acid, and the bacteria used for fermentation help reduce the amount of antinutrients.) Lectins and phytic acid also inflame the gut and can cause diarrhea and bloating.

It has been known since ancient times that eating beans causes gastrointestinal distress and bad gas, a hard to ignore indication that digestion isn't going smoothly. Historically, many farmers have grown legumes not to eat, but as a cover crop to plow under due to the plants' ability to fix nitrogen from the air and act as a fertilizer.

Nuts and seeds—such as almonds, acorns, cashews, and sunflower seeds—fill an ecological niche similar to that of cereal grains and legumes, and thus often contain toxins in their wild state. Wild almonds contain cyanide, and eating just a few can be deadly. The almonds found in the grocery store are of a domesticated variety, with the gene responsible for producing cyanide deactivated. The seeds of many common fruits also contain a form of cyanide, including apple seeds, peach pits, and cherry stones. Many seeds come in strong casings or shells, which is nature's way of saying: "Stay out." Of the "big eight" food allergies, half involve a seed or seed-like part of a plant: peanuts, soy, wheat, and tree nuts.

Avoid Other Potentially Problematic Foods

Those with persistent digestive problems may want to follow an "elimination diet" by removing a wider range of foods from their diet,

WHAT TO DRINK

Thirst is the body's signal to drink—but what, how much, and how often? Take an approach similar to that for food: (1) start with the Paleolithic drink of choice (water) and let thirst dictate when and how much; (2) add traditional Agricultural beverages (wine, beer, tea, coffee, milk) but drink them in moderation; (3) avoid Industrial drinks (soft drinks, energy drinks, skim milk).

Water: It is the healthiest option in most situations, but there is no evidence that forcibly drinking eight glasses of water a day is beneficial.

Tea and coffee: Enjoy tea as desired. Coffee is fine too—studies consistently show positive effects—but don't let excessive caffeine intake interfere with sleep. (Biohacker Dave Asprey pioneered a seemingly odd but surprisingly delicious addition to coffee: grass-fed butter.)

Alcohol: Drinking alcohol is a bad idea for peoples recently exposed to alcohol, such as Native Americans or Pacific Islanders. For everyone else, it is sufficient to avoid excessive alcohol intake. While studies often show light alcohol consumption (a glass of red wine) can have slight health benefits, it's hard to imagine an academic risking his career by saying otherwise. For those who choose to drink, do it out of personal enjoyment, a cultural tradition, or socializing, not for any purported health benefits. Avoid sugary mixers. Gluten-free options include wine, hard cider, hard alcohol, gluten-free beer, or sake (rice wine). Author (and mixologist) Robb Wolf invented the "NorCal Margarita"—tequila, lime juice, and soda water—which is popular among those who follow a paleo diet modified to include alcohol ("alco-paleo").

Milk: More than half the world's population is lactose intolerant;

(continued)

WHAT TO DRINK (*continued*)

drinking store-bought milk isn't even an option. Even for those who can, modern milk is a far cry from the milk of their agricultural ancestors. Traditionally, milk has been consumed raw (unpasteurized) and whole (with full fat), and unhomogenized (unblended fat molecules). While there is controversy in the United States over drinking raw milk due to lack of pasteurization and the risk of disease, advocates swear by it, pointing out that the modern re-engineering of milk was necessitated by an industrial food system, not an agricultural one. Raw milk consumption is common in Europe (where it's known as "farm milk"), especially in France where it and products made from it are considered an essential part of the cuisine. Experiment with milk, particularly the more it approaches a full-fat, raw, and unhomogenized state. Also, avoid anything that pretends to be milk, but isn't, such as soy, almond, or rice "milk."

Juice: Many fruit juices have lots of added sugar, and even natural juices are extremely sweet. Cutting back on juice is a good way to reduce sugar intake (though passing up freshly squeezed anything would just be silly).

Industrial beverages: Avoid soft drinks (regular and diet), energy drinks, sports drinks, low-fat milk, sweet tea, and other industrial beverages.

particularly plants. Common culprits include nightshades (tomatoes, eggplant, peppers, potatoes), eggs (particularly the whites), charred foods (the black stuff is toxic), and sugar-cured meats.

4. Make It Meaningful:
Experiment, Customize, Enjoy

Everyone is a little different. Each of us has a unique genome inherited from our ancestors. Each of us had our own formative time in the womb and in childhood. Each of us has our own gut bacteria. Each one of us has our own allergies, injuries, infections, deficiencies, and conditions. Each of us has different sources of motivation and meaning. Each of us has our own goals—whether to lose weight, build muscle, or get pregnant. All of us face different constraints: our jobs, our budgets, locally available foods.

That is to say, each of us is a unique organism living in a unique habitat. Therefore each of us will end up with a unique diet too.

Start "Orthodox"

I recommend that beginners start with a month of "orthodox" paleo completely free of industrial foods as well as agricultural newcomers. So that means avoiding sugars (added or otherwise), vegetable oils (canola oil, soybean oil, corn oil), grains (wheat, corn, oats, barley), legumes (soy, peanuts, beans), and dairy (milk, cheese). Eat seafood (salmon, sardines, shellfish), meat (beef, lamb, poultry, pork), vegetables (spinach, cabbage, broccoli), roots and tubers (carrots, sweet potatoes), eggs, a little fruit (particularly berries), and a few nuts (walnuts, almonds). Eat fermented foods (sauerkraut, kimchi); cook with real animal fats and tropical oils (coconut oil, butter, beef tallow, olive oil); and try some organ meats (liver, marrow, heart). Some people may find that they do fine by including full-fat dairy (heavy cream, sour cream). Limit indulgences (alcohol, dark chocolate).

Some people with high levels of inflammation, allergies, or digestive problems may want to eliminate all nuts, seeds, nightshades (peppers, potatoes, eggplant, tomato), and eggs. This will give the body time to heal—and after establishing a new healthy baseline, it will become easier to feel how the body responds when reintroducing specific foods. At this point, a wider variety of foods may be well tolerated.

For those getting started, the single best online resource is Marks DailyApple.com. Published by Mark Sisson, author of *The Primal Blueprint*, it has excellent introductory material on just about any health topic. For those with a need or desire to take a deeper dive into diet, I highly recommend *Perfect Health Diet* by Drs. Paul and Shou-Ching Jaminet (PerfectHealthDiet.com). They seem to have an encyclopedic knowledge of nutrition science, and their work contains extensive citations to the underlying science—without being boring or losing sight of the big picture. Like other open-source communities, biohackers like to share odd solutions to unique issues. The best resource is PaleoHacks.com, founded by tech entrepreneur and best-selling author Patrick Vlaskovits.

Experiment and Customize

Experiment by trying new foods and cooking methods. Reintroduce foods one at a time to try to isolate how your body responds to them. There's no reason to permanently eliminate foods that don't cause problems for you; at the same time, you may need to eliminate foods that others tolerate if they cause you problems. Or start with a moderate carbohydrate diet, try an ultra-low-carb diet for a few weeks, then try a higher carb diet. Track your performance over a few weeks.

Eventually you can customize your diet to you and your goals. Aboriginal peoples may want to strictly avoid industrial foods, cereal grains, and alcohol. Athletes and women trying to get pregnant may want to increase carbohydrate intake. Those trying to lose weight may want to lower carbohydrate intake. People with gut or autoimmune problems may want to focus on eliminating more foods from their diet, usually plants, or adding fermented foods with live cultures.

Enjoy Life

Living well starts with "living," and it's healthy to bend the rules sometimes. Personally, I try not to let the way I eat grow into a rigid ideology that distances me from other people or the good things in life. If I'm not going to eat like a vegan, I sure as hell don't want to act like one.

If I am a guest at dinner, I politely eat what is served. If a friend goes through significant effort to make a dish, I certainly try it. I don't try to "convert" people (aside from speaking, blogging, and writing books on the topic). I don't obsess over the occasional indulgence. In a business situation where it would be distracting, I don't eat in a way that elicits looks. And if I have the opportunity to experience something truly unique—the best pizza place in Brooklyn, the signature dish of an ethnic cuisine—then I eat it and don't feel guilty about it. My outlook is nourished as well as my body, and excessive guilt would be counterproductive.

At the same time, I don't use these exceptions as excuses to go back to my old ways. Based on how easily you revert to an unhealthy diet or respond to specific foods, you will have to set your own guidelines.

Make It Meaningful

Even if science eventually answers the tough questions—"What is a healthy diet?" "Why am I so constipated?"—are people going to drink their prune juice?

Probably not.

That's because leading a healthy lifestyle is a two-pronged problem: (1) *knowing* what's healthy, and (2) *doing* what's healthy.

Science has focused on the first—figuring out what's healthy—while neglecting the second: motivating people to make healthy decisions. The prescriptions of our diet culture, based on reductionist science, just aren't meaningful to most people. The B vitamins never got anyone out of bed in the morning. There's something else missing from our diets, and it's not a macronutrient or a vitamin. It's something deeper: meaning. Meaning is the secret ingredient that turns a diet into a lifestyle. So find ways to care about the way you eat.

Make food part of your identity as an individual. Hunt, gather, grow, or prepare it yourself. Hunt a wild animal, kill it, thank it, gut it, and get your hands bloody—then share the meat with others. Get your hands dirty: plant a vegetable garden, grow herbs on a windowsill, or gather wild berries. Raise some chickens or learn to butcher an animal. Fish.

Cook food that is distinctive to your lineage. Learn some family history. Dig up your great-grandmother's cookbook or look up traditional recipes from your ethnic heritage. Learn how to cook one dish better than anyone else in the family. Find out how your ancestors died, and see if you can uncover any hereditary conditions. Get your genome sequenced. Do some ancestor worship. Fasting is a part of most religious traditions, so look up traditional forms of fasting in yours. Observe those holidays.

Another good way to create meaning is by using food to foster personal relationships. Make chicken broth for someone who is ill. Invite friends over for dinner and cook together. For mothers, having a healthy pregnancy is a good motivation to eat well, as is breast-feeding. Teach children where food comes from. Go meet a farmer or visit a farmers market. Participate in a "pig share"—buying an entire pig from a farmer and splitting it among a group. Better yet, organize a pig share.

It's also just fun to try new foods. Admire the color of egg yolk from a pastured chicken. Try grass-fed beef. Buy butter from grass-fed cows—take a bite of it, on its own, without any guilt. Love fat again. Ferment something: beer, wine, yogurt, sauerkraut, kimchi. Try bone marrow, liver, an insect, and raw milk. Try seaweed. Make your own jerky. Break open a coconut.

Whether for identity, family, relationships, or fun, finding a way to make eating meaningful is a time-tested way to make eating healthy. And you might just find that rather than restricting your diet, you broaden it.

FASTING

In wealthy nations the eradication of hunger has been replaced not by satiation but by incessant cravings. The longest period most people go without eating is eight hours during sleep. Some can't even make it through the night, raiding the fridge for a midnight snack.

Breakfast literally means "breaking the fast," and presumably it is the most important meal of the day. But breakfast, lunch, and dinner have all declined in importance relative to snacking—a diet soda here, a slice of pie there. Some nutritionists even encourage "grazing" in order to "keep blood sugar up." The natural conclusion of this line of thinking is found in hospitals. There it goes unquestioned that ill patients with a reduced appetite should be put on a glucose drip, delivering sugar directly to their bloodstream.

But is all this food on demand a good idea? How often should we eat? Obesity has become so common, it's worth asking: does *hunger* play a role in a healthy diet?

Wild animals eat at different intervals depending on their diet, life cycle, health, and ecological context. Herbivores eat almost constantly (it takes a lot of grass to power a cow), whereas carnivores eat more sporadically (a cow can power a wolf pack). Many species hibernate for the winter months and don't eat at all. An unchecked deer population means that many deer barely scrape by, subsisting on the edge of starvation—and starvation is extremely common throughout the Animal Kingdom. A wide variety of species, including humans, lose their appetites when wounded or diseased. Clearly, there are plenty of instances in nature in which not eating is a normal part of an animal's life cycle, which suggests that organisms have long-standing adaptations in the face of a diminished food supply.

What makes for healthy eating frequency depends on the species.

Mokolo and Bebac, the western lowland gorillas at the Cleveland Metroparks Zoo, suffered from eating too *in*frequently. When they were fed gorilla biscuits, they could eat all of them fairly quickly, early in the day. Under this regimen, they regurgitated their food and re-ingested it—but the regurgitation behavior didn't begin until just after they ran out of gorilla biscuits. When Mokolo and Bebac were switched to a plant-based diet, it took them much longer to eat all their food—and the regurgitation behavior stopped entirely.

In contrast, carnivores in captivity often suffer from eating too frequently. In 1993 the Topeka Zoo had five overweight lions. They were fed on a regular schedule (once a day, six days a week), but the zoo decided to switch to a "gorge and fast" feeding schedule (once a day, three days a week) modeled after wild lions, which typically eat every two to three days. The food was kept the same—a ground mixture containing horsemeat—and each lion received the same amount of food over the course of a week as it had before; they now received larger portions on feeding days. The lions were allowed to eat until they had their fill and walked away from their food. Only then were leftovers removed from the enclosure. The four weekly fasting days were chosen at random, which meant that the lions sometimes experienced four days in a row of fasting.

Previously, the lions had always finished their meals, but now four of the five routinely left portions of their meal uneaten. The result was a decrease in weekly overall caloric intake—and significant weight loss. Four of the five lions lost from 9 to 16% of their total body weight (the fifth lion injured her leg and had been under veterinary care leading up to the measuring period). However, the benefits weren't simply due to eating fewer calories; based on fecal samples, the lions digested their food more thoroughly and efficiently under the gorge and fast model.

Both captive gorillas and lions suffered from the same issue: we forced them to accommodate our regimented workdays. They were being fed on a human schedule, not a schedule based on how their species naturally eats in the wild.

So what's a natural eating frequency for humans?

Humans are omnivores. That means we probably fall in between a pure carnivore eating frequency (gorge and fast, regularly going a day or more without eating) and a pure herbivore eating frequency (consistent eating throughout the day).

But with our constant snacking these days, we're eating more like herbivores—it's referred to as "grazing" for a reason. Compared with how most people eat today, the correct direction is clear: *we should eat less frequently and less predictably than we currently eat.*

There's not a lot of evidence from Paleolithic remains on eating frequency, and fruit-eating chimps aren't much help either. Most of what we know comes from anthropological accounts of contemporary hunter-gatherers. It's common to see fewer than three prepared meals a day. Communal meals focus on sharing animal foods, since the kills are often large and would spoil if left uneaten. It's also common to see sex differences in eating patterns, with women eating more frequently throughout the day than men. When food is plentiful it's uncommon for hunter-gatherers to go a full day without eating, and thanks to communal food sharing, unlucky hunters don't have to (though when a day without food does occur, it's usually not treated as a big deal). When food is scarce, such as in temperate or arctic climates during winter, hunter-gatherers may go days without eating and then gorge on a buffalo or caribou.

The !Kung Bushmen in southern Africa are one example. In the morning, "breakfast" consists of leftovers, if there are any—and frequently there aren't. The women head out to dig for roots or gather berries or nuts. The men either go hunting or prepare to do so (repairing weapons, gathering grubs used for arrow poison). Women will sometimes eat what they gather throughout the day—berries are gathered and eaten on the spot; otherwise birds get them. Spoils of the hunt are communally shared, whereas what a woman gathers belongs to her and her family. Dinner is thus partially communal (any hunted meat) and partially individual (anything gathered). There are other social obligations regarding eating, and food availability varies by the season.

The limiting factor to eating at will isn't usually scarcity of food, per se, but the time it takes to hunt, gather, or process the most desirable types of food. Among the Aché tribe in Paraguay, men pass up lots of edible plants and small game while hunting for large game. The only food that they'll stop to gather is honey; the rest just doesn't measure up to the caloric and nutrient value of large game.

Overall the anthropological literature seems to boil down to a few basic principles. There is nothing quite as exact or frequent as "three square meals a day." The most important meal of the day does not precede the day's activities (breakfast), but follows their completion (lunch/dinner). Eating is often opportunistic—driven by spoilage (meat), seasons (harvest, migrations), and competition with other species (ripe berries). Hunter-gatherers experience low-level hunger on a fairly regular basis; they eat when they're hungry, when food is ready to eat, and when social norms allow for it.

DURING THE Agricultural Age, a cultural tradition of purposeful abstention from food and drink emerged around the world: fasting.

Fasts commonly last from daytime (twelve hours) to a day (twenty-four hours), but the most famous ones have lasted weeks. Mohandas Gandhi used long fasts (hunger strikes) as a nonviolent form of protest and as personal purification. His fasts lasted anywhere from three days to three weeks. Many religious and spiritual traditions stipulate fasting as an explicit part of their rules. Mormons, for example, fast on one Sunday each month and give the money they would have spent on food to the needy. Traditions vary as to what constitutes fasting, including abstaining from meat, all meat and seafood, all solid foods,

FASTING AROUND THE WORLD

Judaism: Traditionally Jews observe six fast days a year: two
major fasts (dusk to dusk) and four minor fasts (dawn to
dusk). Yom Kippur is considered the holiest day of the year.
No food or drink can be eaten for roughly twenty-five hours,
from just before sunset on the first day to just after sunset
on the next. No sex or bathing either.

Islam: Fasting during the month of Ramadan is one of the five
pillars of Islam. During Ramadan, Muslims fast from dawn
(*fajr*) to dusk (*maghrib*), consuming neither food nor drink.
These daytime fasts are broken with nightly feasts.

Catholicism: Catholics abstain from meat and only eat one
full meal on Ash Wednesday, Good Friday, Fridays in
Lent, and, until the mid-twentieth century, Fridays year
round. Lent itself, the forty-day period leading up to Easter,
commemorates the forty days Jesus spent fasting in the
desert; Catholics still give up something for Lent, often a
food.

Eastern Orthodox: Fasting is a strong element of the Eastern
Orthodox tradition, which stipulates four extended fasting
seasons, as well as fasting on Wednesdays and Fridays—
adding up to 174 days of fasting on the 2013 calendar. The
complicated rules require abstention from meat (100% of
fasting days); dairy and eggs (96% of fasting days); fish,
except shellfish (82%); and oil and alcohol (72%)—as well
as complete abstention from sex. Strictly observed, these
fast days amount to a form of celibate veganism (plus
shellfish) for one out of every four days of the year.

Hinduism: Fasting is important in Hinduism, but practices
vary considerably. In addition to full-day fasts during
festivals, it is common to fast from dawn to dusk on a
particular day of the week (Tuesday, Thursday), each of
which is devoted to a different deity. Fasting typically

(continued)

FASTING AROUND THE WORLD *(continued)*

entails no food or drink of any kind, though sometimes liquids are consumed.

Buddhism: Some Buddhist monks do not eat anything from the noonday meal until dawn the next day, resulting in sixteen to eighteen hours of abstention from solid food and most liquids. Lay Buddhists are instructed to do the same once a week. Fasting is practiced during certain holidays, and some Buddhists undergo supervised fasting for multiple weeks at a time.

Taoism: Early Taoist texts prescribe periods of fasting described as air or spirit swallowing *(fuqi),* which requires breathing exercises. An initial period of abstaining from solid foods is followed by an extended period of complete fasting. Early Taoist ascetic traditions influenced Confucianism, as well as Japanese practices.

Religions of the American Indian Nations: Fasting is a common feature of Amerindian spirituality, from the Inuit to the Pueblo. The vision quest, an important rite of passage, typically entails solitary fasting for many days in the wilderness.

Common exemptions from fasting include prepubescent children, pregnant women, nursing mothers, the severely ill, the elderly, and in the case of Islam, menstruating women.

everything but water, or everything altogether. Secular fasts, such as cleanses and juice fasts, follow similar guidelines.

Religious and spiritual traditions typically explain fasting as a time of sacrifice, atonement, or meditation—an opportunity to purify the body and reach a higher state of spiritual consciousness by rising above the needs of the flesh. All that may be true, but new scientific findings suggest there are substantial health benefits to fasting as well.

Fasting helps the body fight infection.

One indication of this effect comes from the behavior of sick animals, including humans, who often lose their appetite until an illness has passed. Farm animals, pets, zoo animals, and wild animals often just stop eating altogether when facing an acute infection or a serious injury. The widespread nature of this phenomenon suggests it's an adaptive response. Loss of appetite isn't a bug, it's a feature.

Like attacking the supply lines of an invading army, dietary restriction weakens pathogens while the immune system mounts a counteroffensive. Tiny pathogens don't have large nutrient reserves and rely on the host for nutrition—therefore manipulating *our* nutrition is a way to manipulate *their* nutrition.

A low- or zero-protein diet can have a number of beneficial effects in the war against infection. Many pathogens are dependent on specific amino acids for their metabolism, such as tryptophan, and depriving the pathogens of these amino acids stops them in their tracks. In fact, many modern-day antibiotics are effective because they bind to the receptors that bacteria use for protein synthesis, short-circuiting their metabolism.

The absence of dietary protein has another beneficial effect: it initiates a cellular protein-recycling process called *autophagy*, which literally means "self-eating." When cells receive signals that protein is scarce, cellular organelles called lysosomes begin to recycle junk and debris that ordinarily accumulate in the cell. In addition to gobbling up debris, they also gobble up intracellular pathogens like viruses and bacteria. Autophagy also recycles mitochondria, the power plants of the cell—even targeting "the biggest polluters" that are emitting molecules that cause oxidative damage.

Iron is another nutrient that bacteria and other pathogens need to acquire from their host. During fevers, iron levels in the blood drop, suggesting that this is part of the body's coordinated and adaptive response to infection. In a study of Kenyan children, those with iron deficiency were less likely to be suffering from acute infections. Studies on rabbits and hamsters have also shown that iron restriction impedes the growth of pathogens.

The human body needs iron too, and persistent iron deficiency has negative health consequences, particularly for children and pregnant women. Periods of low iron levels (anemia) may be a trade-off: a brief attack in an attempt to dislodge pathogens. Geophagy, the practice of eating clays, has often been viewed as the cause of iron-deficiency anemia—but it may actually be better understood as a short-term attempt to starve stomach pathogens that are siphoning off iron on a long-term basis.

There are benefits to limiting carbohydrate too. Glucose is the preferred fuel of many pathogens, as well as cancer cells, and so restricting intake of glucose is a good way to slow their growth. Limiting carbohydrate inhibits the growth of another problematic infection: *Streptococcus mutans,* one of the bacterial strains leading to tooth decay and gum disease. Viktor Frankl, Holocaust survivor and author of *Man's Search for Meaning,* recounts a surprising effect of forced starvation on prisoners: "I would like to mention a few similar surprises on how much we could endure: we were unable to clean our teeth, and yet, in spite of that and a severe vitamin deficiency, we had healthier gums than ever before." The nutritional status of host and microbe are intimately linked.

The effectiveness of fasting as a weapon against infection may partially explain why religious fasting, as distinct from appetite loss during illness, rose to prominence during the Agricultural Age. Fasting may have been an effective way to attack chronic infections, which had multiplied since the Agricultural Revolution. This is not to say that all methods of religious fasting were equally effective, or even effective at all. Nor is it to say that fighting infection was the only reason people fasted. But in a sense, religious fasting actually *was* a form of bodily purification—purification from pathogens. (An enterprising academic may want to test the hypothesis, purely speculative and quite possibly wrong, that an entire population fasting or washing at the same time, coordinated by religious calendars, functioned as a society-wide assault on pathogens that had a greater impact than the sum of its parts—in the same way that vaccinations are more effective when enough of the population participates.)

The health benefits of fasting go beyond fighting infection; fasting is also one of the most promising areas of cancer research.

Chemotherapy is the most common anticancer treatment, but the drugs don't just kill malignant cancer cells; they kill any cells that reproduce rapidly, including healthy ones like hair and bone marrow cells. Chemo drugs are only partially effective at destroying enough tumor cells to make patients well, but they are fully effective at causing toxicity in enough healthy cells to make people sick. Some chemo patients find the side effects so unpleasant that they elect to let advanced tumors run their course.

Fasting alters the playing field by activating ancient starvation defenses in the cell. Fasting is a *signal* to the body that resources are scarce. Healthy, nonmalignant cells take the hint and stop dividing as often, focusing instead on cellular repair mechanisms that conserve resources. So even as chemo damages healthy cells, they are hard at work repairing chromosomal damage. But malignant cells don't stop dividing; they're "cancerous" because they refuse to do anything but grow and grow. Not only does fasting sensitize malignant cells to chemo drugs; it also defends healthy cells against chemo toxicity.

In an intriguing 2008 study, two groups of mice, one fasting and the other fed, underwent chemotherapy. The fasting mice were allowed to consume only water for forty-eight to sixty hours before treatment, while the fed mice were allowed to eat at will. The results were striking: the fed mice experienced the typical unpleasant side effects of chemo, whereas the fasting mice "showed no visible signs of stress or pain." Forty-three percent of the fed mice died (ten of twenty-three), whereas only 6% of the fasting mice died (one of seventeen). In a separate trial in the same study, fasting was also shown not to interfere with killing the tumor cells. Additional work has shown that fasting kills tumor cells on its own. In combination with chemotherapy, it improves the effectiveness of both.

Uncontrolled case studies in ten human cancer patients also showed encouraging results. Patients consumed only water (or water plus vitamins) and fasted for 48–140 hours prior to treatment and for 5–56 hours afterward. All patients reported fewer and less severe side effects, and "[n]ausea, vomiting, diarrhea, abdominal cramps, and mucositis were virtually absent . . ." Not all patients survived, but everyone who underwent chemo both ways—fasting and fed—chose to stick with fasting as a way of dealing with the side effects of chemo.

In an era when potential blockbuster drugs get caught up in lengthy and expensive trials, fasting is free, entails no high-tech equipment, requires zero government approvals, and offers hope for many people who have nothing to lose.

Fasting is also beneficial for metabolic health, protecting against heart disease, diabetes, and obesity.

Regular fasting looks like one reason that Mormons have notably lower rates of coronary artery disease (CAD) than other Americans and Utahns. In an uncontrolled observational study of 4,629 patients, Dr. Benjamin Horne of the University of Utah found that those who fasted once a month had an even lower incidence of CAD than Mormons in general (even when taking into account known risk factors). Additionally, in that study and a subsequent one, regular fasting was associated with a lower incidence of diabetes. This should be unsurprising: whatever foods contribute to insulin resistance and diabetes, fasting necessarily cuts them out, improving insulin sensitivity.

A *ketogenic diet*—a very low carb or zero-carb diet—has been found to be an effective treatment for a number of neurological conditions, including seizures and Alzheimer's. High blood sugar is toxic—so when we eat carbohydrate, our body disposes of it as quickly as it can. However, once the carbs have been burned for energy, stored in the liver and muscles as glycogen, or turned to fat and stored in fat cells, most of the body switches back to burning fat for energy. Then, since the brain and blood cells need some glucose in order to function, the liver turns glycogen back into glucose and releases it back into the bloodstream. Ketones are a by-product of both fat burning and glycogen burning, and an elevated level of ketones in our blood is called *ketosis*. Ketosis can result from fasting, or from eating a diet very low in carbohydrate. If the body stays in ketosis long enough, the brain will start using ketones too, decreasing its requirement for glucose. Since ketones are products of dietary fat, eating fat doesn't interrupt ketosis—and fats (e.g., coconut oil, MCT oil) are particularly efficient at generating ketones and maintaining ketosis.

Given this inside look at human metabolism, it's fair to say that all successful diets are high-fat diets. How so? When dieters try to lose weight, they almost always mean lose *body fat*. The only way to lose body fat—short of liposuction—is for the body to burn fat stores as fuel, instead of food. Even to the extent that low-fat diets are successful, it's because the metabolism turns to body fat. All successful diets are high-fat diets.

So is breakfast really the most important meal of the day?

Breakfast is important to many people for the same reason that fasting is hard: they're addicted to sugar. Consider all the sources of sugar in a typical breakfast, one that probably seems healthy to most people: a bowl of Kellogg's Corn Flakes, skim milk, a little table sugar sprinkled on top, and a glass of orange juice. The cereal contains glucose but is sweetened with a little high fructose corn syrup, the skim milk contains lactose, the table sugar (sucrose) breaks down into glucose and fructose, and the orange juice contains fructose. Then there's toast, waffles, syrup, muffins, Pop-Tarts, or French toast. The typical American breakfast is a sugar bomb.

Nighttime is the longest period many people go without eating sugar, and that means they wake up starting to slip into sugar withdrawal. (Some people don't make it through the night.) Skipping breakfast leads to intense cravings, inability to concentrate, shaky hands, and light-headedness. It's no wonder that people show better performance after eating breakfast; going through withdrawal isn't exactly good for productivity. Smokers like a cigarette in the morning, too. Breakfast is a fix.

Like missing breakfast, most people find their first fast to be somewhat difficult and mildly unpleasant. However, once people have switched to a fat-based metabolism, their body has no problem producing the energy it needs from its fat stores. Hunger pangs quickly subside—if they come at all—and the mind is clear. Many people like to start their fast after an early dinner, go to sleep, skip breakfast, and then eat a late lunch or early dinner.

Intermittent fasting—fairly regular, short fasts lasting sixteen to twenty-four hours—amounts to skipping one or two meals on either side of sleep; it doesn't require a lot of special attention and can be safely performed on a regular basis. Fasts longer than twenty-four hours might draw notoriety, but they aren't common as cultural traditions. Beginners and those undergoing longer fasts should read up on the topic and discuss any existing medical conditions with their doctor.

Just as food intake patterns vary between the sexes, fasting is likely to have different effects on men and women. Fasting is a signal that resources are scarce, and that signal almost certainly inhibits female fertility faster than male fertility since women bear more of the direct costs of pregnancy. The female body knows that it's a really bad idea to get pregnant when food is extremely scarce, and the issue is sufficiently important that the body takes no chances. Women who chronically diet, restrict their caloric intake, and vegan/vegetarian women are known to suffer amenorrhea (lose their period)—or just don't get pregnant. Women who start adding back animal foods, fats, and carbs often regain their period and their fertility. Women should keep a closer eye on the effects of intermittent fasting on their health. It can be great for weight loss, dealing with chronic infections, and healing the metabolism—but getting pregnant is a whole lot easier during a feast than a famine.

Fasting for young children may be problematic for a similar reason—fasting signals scarcity. Chronic nutrient deficiencies at a very young age certainly send the body down a different developmental path, though it is unclear to what extent acute deficiencies do the same. Skipping a meal is no big deal, but extended fasting does

FASTING FOR THE FIRST TIME

Fasting type: Most of the known benefits of fasting accrue from avoiding protein and carbohydrate. One option is to eat nothing, but still drink water, unsweetened tea, or black coffee. A second option, easier for many people, is to eat only pure fats, such as coconut oil or heavy cream. Or follow the fasting rules specified in your religion.

Length: Sixteen-hour fasts appear to be long enough to trigger autophagy, and fasts up to twenty-four hours can be safely completed on a regular basis. It's not clear that longer fasts deliver additional benefits.

Before: Find a time to fast that doesn't require working, driving, or dealing with stressful situations. Bingeing before a fast, particularly on sugary foods, will make the eventual withdrawal that much harder. Just eat a well-balanced meal with lots of healthy fats.

During: The more sugar in one's typical diet, the more difficult fasting will be. Expect strong hunger pangs at regular mealtimes, light-headedness, shaky hands, or an inability to focus. Effective distractions are drinking water, herbal tea, or having a spoonful of coconut oil (for those eating fats). Typically the hunger "breaks" a couple of hours after the first missed meal. If hunger doesn't subside during the entire fast, that may indicate that you have a nutrient deficiency. In those cases it's wise to identify and rectify the nutrient deficiency before fasting again.

After: The longer the fast, the more gradual the transition back to eating. Do not gorge on the first meal, particularly with processed or sugary food. Eat slowly and savor the food. Breaking a fast with someone else is a good reason to slowly enjoy a meal together.

Cautionary notes: Children, pregnant women (or those trying to get pregnant), the elderly, those with eating disorders, or the severely ill should not fast.

not seem wise. There's a reason that North Koreans are a few inches shorter than South Koreans, despite coming from the same genetic stock.

The signals sent by fasting and food intake are also tied to circadian rhythm, which isn't just based on light and dark. Animal studies suggest that when food is available, light/dark is the main driver of circadian rhythm, but when food is scarce, avoiding starvation is more important than whether it's night or day. Bats are nocturnal during hot months when insects are out at night, but they become diurnal during colder months when insects are out only during the day. That insight has led to fasting as a method to mitigate the effects of jet lag and adjust to new time zones more quickly.

Over the past few years I incorporated eighteen- to twenty-four-hour fasts into my life, but I decided I wanted to try for something longer. Appropriately enough, the opportunity presented itself during Lent. During the week between Passover and Easter, my father was visiting a Trappist monastery, the Abbey of Gethsemani located about an hour south of Louisville, Kentucky. I decided to use the opportunity to conduct a three-day fast, starting on midday on Tuesday and ending at midday on Good Friday. It wasn't forty days in the desert, but it was long enough to make it interesting. I would eat no food at all—no solid, liquid, juice, tea, coffee, caffeine, cayenne pepper, maple syrup, medications, supplements—nothing. Only water.

Gethsemani may be best known for being the home of the monk Thomas Merton, an author, poet, and activist—described as "part Augustine, part Emerson, and part Gandhi." Founded in 1848 by monks from France, it is the oldest monastery in use in the United States and the "mother house" of American Trappist monasteries.

The Trappists are a Roman Catholic monastic order that follows the *Rule of St. Benedict,* a set of guidelines for ascetic living written by Saint Benedict of Nursia around A.D. 530. Monastic life is a simple existence of peace, work, and prayer. Contrary to popular belief, the

FASTING TO BEAT JET LAG

A 2002 study by the U.S. military suggested the effective-ness of the Argonne Anti–Jet Lag Diet. This program stipulated four alternating days of feasting and fasting leading up to a trip, with the fourth day (fasting) taking place on the day of travel. Of 186 soldiers deployed to Korea, 9% of soldiers on the diet got jet lag, whereas 49% of those not on the diet got jet lag. On the more difficult return trip from Korea, 26% of soldiers on the diet got jet lag, whereas 83% of those not on the diet got jet lag.

Dr. Clifford Saper, a neuroscience researcher at Harvard Medical School, has suggested an easier way: figure out when breakfast will be served in your eventual destination and then work backward and fast for more than sixteen hours in advance of that time. That means no food, alcohol, caffeine, or sleeping pills—just water or decaf herbal tea. Then eat breakfast at the time it is being eaten at your eventual destination, even if that happens to be on the flight itself.

There are lots of other good reasons to fast when flying. Airport food is usually unhealthy and always expensive. Air travel also exposes people to lots of germs—and since fasting strengthens the body's response to infections, you are less likely to get sick if you fast.

monks do not actually take a vow of silence, but talking is strongly discouraged—some monks even use a simple sign language for necessary but routine communication. The monks typically make a living by producing simple crafts or artisanal foods, such as fudge, cheese, jam, or the world-famous Trappist beers. According to an old saying, "To a Trappist, work is a form of prayer."

To a non-Trappist, prayer is a form of work. The Trappists adhere to the Liturgy of the Hours ("the hours"), which means formal prayer, readings, songs, and Psalms in the church seven times a day: Vigils (3:15 A.M.), Lauds (5:45 A.M.), Terce (7:30 A.M.), Sext (12:15 P.M.), None (2:15 P.M.), Vespers (5:30 P.M.), and Compline (7:30 P.M.). This was in addition to celebrating the Eucharist (6:15 A.M.), reciting the Rosary (7:00 P.M.), and private prayers. I planned to use the time to be as silent as possible, spending my time thinking, reading, writing, meditating, and praying—exploring both the physical and the spiritual aspects of fasting and the ascetic tradition.

After arriving in Louisville I met my father and a friend of his at the airport then drove south. After a quick lunch at a local diner, we arrived at the Abbey. A sign greeted us where the parking lot ended and the path to the Abbey began: "Silence beyond this point." The entire Abbey was plastered with reminders to curb our chatty instincts: "Silence is spoken here" and "The porch and gardens are places of silence."

We found our rooms and unpacked. Before I knew it, it was time for None, the fifth of the hours. Thus began a series of days of making something from nothing.

The first day of my fast was familiar territory, and I used the time to explore a foreign one: the ascetic tradition. Christian monasticism, including the *Rule of St. Benedict,* sprang out of hermits living in the Egyptian desert around the third century A.D., called the Desert Fathers and Desert Mothers. They eschewed material possessions, isolated themselves from the outside world, and lived a minimalist existence. Common ascetic practices included long fasts, silence, prayer, and meditation—sharing many similarities with the Eastern ascetic tradition, such as in Buddhism. In essence, they were early biohackers, exploring the frontier of human physical experience.

If there was one thing they discovered, it was this: there is more to be gained by subtraction than by addition. The ascetics also knew the benefit of making life harder.

My own fast was easier and less unpleasant than I thought it would be. As the fast went on, my hunger decreased: It was strongest on the first day but quickly subsided after the first two missed meals. I had a few stomach grumblings, but my thoughts generally weren't fixated on food. I attended all the meals except breakfast, reading a book and watching everyone else eat. That probably sounds like torture, but it wasn't—I had a clear purpose for fasting, which allowed me to persevere much more easily.

I didn't have any headaches, light-headedness, shaky hands, or grouchiness. Despite not being able to cut out caffeine in advance, I didn't have any caffeine withdrawal symptoms. In these respects, my experience diverged from that of an average person with a sugar-heavy or caffeine-heavy diet. Through the first day and into the second, I felt awake, alert, and active. I had no desire to move much on the second and third days, and I definitely didn't feel like hunting any wild animals in order to feed myself. In fact, even going on some long walks was tiring, and I lagged behind a few others who weren't fasting.

By the end of the second day, my alertness downshifted into a more meditative state. I wasn't drowsy per se, but my mind lost the desire to work on complex tasks. I wanted to zone out a bit more: stare at the leaves moving in the breeze, look at the colors of pebbles on the path, and enjoy the sun shining on my face. It felt like a mild high. This was fine in a relaxed setting, but it would not have been ideal if there had been things to get done.

In terms of health, I noticed a number of changes.

My skin felt amazing. My sinuses cleared up. Sinuses are my first indication of inflammation—two beers and they get slightly stuffy. But I couldn't remember my nasal passages and breathing ever being so clear.

I felt a little cold at times, though not severely so—just enough that I decided to throw on a sweatshirt a few times. My body was clearly conserving energy by turning down the heat. I developed slightly bad breath. I also noticed lower libido (that also could have been due to the absence of young women). I forgot to weigh myself before and after, but by the fit of my jeans I could tell that I lost a couple pounds.

At 3:07 A.M. on the final morning (night?), my alarm went off. I was used to going to bed at this time, not waking up.

I put on pants and a shirt, slipped on a pair of sandals, and shuffled out the door. I tried to close it gently, but the sound traveled loudly in the uncarpeted hallway.

I walked out onto the balcony at the back of the church. Ten or so pews lined either side of the balcony, sprinkled with other tired-eyed retreatants. I took a seat in the front and looked down to the floor of the church. Since it was Good Friday, the church was almost entirely dark.

I waited—tired, silent, fasted.

To an outsider, the hours is perhaps the most arresting aspect of the monks' life: chant-like recitations of the Psalms, singing, and formal ritual. I was entranced by the monks' entrance and exit at each of the hours. Out of the darkness a small, white-robed figure would emerge from one of the wings near the altar and quietly walk up the aisle toward our balcony, then turn and find his place in the pew. Each individual took his own unpredictable path, arriving at his place at a slightly different time from the others—but all the monks moved at the same speed, slowly and deliberately, and resolved to the same formation.

The bells began to toll. One or two more hurried in right under the wire.

It was 3:15 A.M., and the monks began to chant. It was Vigils, the first of the hours. Twenty minutes later, after the recitation of Psalms, singing, ritual, and prayer, it was done. And I, already in a dream-like state, shuffled back to my room and went to sleep.

When I broke my fast later that morning, I didn't eat out of hunger or habit, but by my own conscious choice. It was the most deliberate meal I had ever eaten. Breakfast isn't the most important meal of the day; breaking a fast is.

And what is a fast without a feast?

All cultures celebrate feast days—when we put down our labors, slaughter the fattest calf, gorge and indulge, drink and dance, mate and make love—banishing hunger for a time. And I'm pretty sure that's healthy too.

10

MOVEMENT

When I first moved to New York City I was one of those people who paid for a gym membership but hardly ever used it. I had selected the gym based on what I thought was the most important motivating factor for working out: physical proximity to my bed. It was two blocks away and was open twenty-four hours. Despite the convenience, I consistently found excuses not to work out. Part of my lack of motivation stemmed from the gym habitat itself. It provided everything I needed to exercise—except a reason to move.

Until very recently in history, humans—both hunter-gatherers and herder-farmers—needed to move quite a bit in order to survive.

Consider the Paraguayan Aché tribe, as witnessed by anthropologist Dr. Kim Hill. The men hunt nearly every day that it's not raining. This entails about six miles in slow tracking and a mile in fast pursuit through the dense jungle—before returning with the prey. Hunter-gatherer women cover less ground than the men, but they engage in lots of walking while carrying heavy loads. Women carry children (no strollers), fetch water, dig up roots and tubers, pick fruit, trap small game, and help with butchering animals—and carry back their haul, children and all. That may sound exhausting, but hunting and gathering is their job—which leaves plenty of time for leisure. It was farmers who really had toil day in and day out; subsistence agriculture requires even higher levels of physical activity than foraging. Anyone who has grown up on a farm knows that the chores begin before sunrise and end after sunset.

But the Industrial Revolution replaced human power with machine power, which meant fewer physically demanding jobs. That trend has accelerated with the Information Revolution as more and more people find themselves sitting at a desk and typing away at a computer. Now not only is it possible to survive without moving, but modern success increasingly depends on sitting for decades of education and employment.

The problem is that humans have lost the motivation to move. What, then, is the solution? It isn't some new exercise protocol that people aren't going to follow, or some new machine that is just going to collect dust.

The solution is to rediscover a motivation to move.

Consider the two definitions of the root word "motive":

mo·tive / ˈmōtiv/
1. (*noun*) A reason for doing something
2. (*adjective*) Producing physical or mechanical motion

The first definition of "motive," as a noun, is frequently used in the courtroom. One of the core principles of the legal system acknowledges that having a motive—"a reason for doing something"—makes it more likely that someone has, in fact, done something. The second definition of "motive," used as an adjective, means "producing physical or mechanical motion"—as in the motive power of an engine. It is the same root in "loco*motive*" and "auto*motive*."

Motivation literally means *a reason for physical motion.*

No motivation, no movement. So how can we become motivated to move?

The best ways to motivate human beings are the oldest ways, tapping into timeless needs and emotions: hunger, thirst, fear of death, sex, beauty, identity, status, respect, honor, shame, love, compassion, community, fun. All of these tie back, directly or indirectly, to those most fundamental and evolutionary of motivations: survival and re-production. The secret is learning how to tap these ancient motivations, and harnessing them to achieve modern goals.

Sports are the most obvious example. The actual movements required by football, baseball, and basketball are often completely arbitrary and would be useless in any other context—but that just underscores their power to motivate. Sports have long been associated with ancient tribal warfare—as preparation, imitation, and prevention—and they harness those deeply rooted human motivations. Not much has changed: one side wears blue face paint, the other side wears red, they try to kill each other, and the winners get a lot of booty (both kinds).

Modern society is set up to encourage sports during youth, but access to sports participation drops off dramatically after college. Many people lose their primary athletic activity and resign themselves to watching their favorite team on television or playing fantasy sports online. For personal fitness they resort to gyms or jogging—if they exercise at all.

In contrast with sports, the fitness world is marked by a widespread failure to motivate. As in the diet world, calories are king—but most people don't care about calories on a deep level. All the gym equipment in the world is pointless if people aren't motivated to use it.

Every year around New Year's, millions of Americans make a resolution to get in shape. They sign up for a gym membership, work out for a few weeks, then fall off the wagon and go back to their sedentary habits. Regular gym goers know that the exercise machines will be crowded for the first three weeks in January—after which the gym will empty out again. Not only does this happen every single year, but the business model of many gyms actually depends on people quitting. They advertise heavily in late December and early January and rake in revenue from people who sign up but don't show up.

The gym I joined looked like just another impersonal big box gym. Two rows of treadmills and ellipticals lined one wall, along with a couple of StairMasters, a few rowing machines, and one lonely stationary bike that looked more like an art installation than a functional piece of exercise equipment. The opposite wall was covered by a giant mirror with a waist-high rack of free weights in front of it. The middle of the gym contained several weightlifting machines and a few stations with a barbell for Olympic lifting. A padded nook was good for stretching, sit-ups, and using medicine balls; and even better for watching women in yoga pants stretching, doing sit-ups, and using medicine balls.

The gym provided only one form of external motivation: mirrors. Mirrors were everywhere. I couldn't help but see my own reflection (and steal glances at others'). Mirrors reinforced the motivation to "look good naked." Since men and women have different ideas about what that means, they self-segregated: bros hit the weights, wanting to bulk up; chicks stuck to aerobics, wanting to slim down. While I wanted to have a healthy body that looked good, that motivation alone wasn't sufficient to get me to the gym on a regular basis.

Other than mirrors, I was responsible for motivating myself. As a competitive person, I was limited to measuring a few abstract numbers (weight lifted, calories burned) and comparing them to my prior workouts. There was no team to join; I exercised alone. There were no challenges to overcome, no sense of community or accomplishment from having achieved something meaningful. There were no skills to hone, no enemies to defeat, no trophies to win. There was no spirituality, no beauty, no deeper meaning. There was no danger or play.

Working out was boring and unstimulating. Individual exercises were monotonous, and my workouts hardly changed from visit to visit. I felt self-conscious trying new exercises and didn't want to do something stupid in front of strangers. My intensity level was predictably moderate: I set the treadmill to a constant speed when running. When lifting I took plenty of time to rest between sets. The machines forced a robotic regularity on my physical motions. The exercises themselves were abstractions, unmoored from any functional objective in the real world, completed in pursuit of the vague, general goal of "conditioning." This conditioning turned out to be a rather narrow one, since I always trained in perfect conditions: surfaces were flat, temperatures unchanging, water always close at hand. Nothing novel or unexpected ever occurred.

The gym seemed to be organized on the principle of minimizing anything that might constitute contact with another human being. I never learned the names of more than a couple of people; most were simply strangers to be avoided. That was easy to do, since most people were enveloped in their iPod. There was little speaking aside from the bare minimum of self-interested gym etiquette: "You done using that?" Any sound that might suggest physical exertion—a grunt, a shout, heavy breathing—was frowned upon. Sweating was an unfortunate by-product of exercise and was merely tolerated. The gym seemed designed to make it appear as if people *weren't actually working out*.

When I started eating paleo, I rededicated myself to getting to the gym. I tried to change things up with greater variety, intensity, and fun. I even introduced a survival motivation into my workout. I sprinted on a treadmill while imagining that I was being chased by a hungry lion. I had to psych myself up beforehand, hitting my head with my hands, envisioning that I actually might die. It worked, but onlookers were alarmed. A staff member asked me if I knew what I was doing; he had never seen anyone sprint on a treadmill before.

I tried to find creative ways to use the equipment—otherwise known as "misusing" the equipment. I did pull-ups on a stand-alone pull-up station and then climbed on top of it. It started to wobble and almost tipped over. When I started running up and down the stairs, I was told it might interfere with people walking up and down the stairs. When a buddy and I designed a "circuit" in the gym and raced to complete it, we were told that we were being disruptive and had to stop. The gym rules were as restrictive as the exercise machines; both prescribed a narrow set of acceptable movements and speeds.

It's hard to fight your habitat, and eventually I left.

In January of 2007, three months into my paleo experiment, I joined CrossFit—a new fitness movement that billed itself as the antithesis of big box gyms.

CrossFit was founded in 2000 by Greg Glassman, a former gymnast who had been hired to run a training program for the Santa Cruz Police Department. When I came across it in late 2006, CrossFit was still a tiny fringe movement, relegated to a scrappy website, a few obscure Internet forums, and a dozen or so affiliates on the West Coast. Today CrossFit is a global fitness juggernaut with thousands of affiliates worldwide, a long-term partnership with Reebok, and competitions that are broadcast on cable.

I joined CrossFit NYC—the Black Box, the first CrossFit affiliate in New York City and one of the first twenty worldwide. The first day I showed up I wasn't sure I had come to the right place. It was just an empty room on the fourth floor of a nondescript building. There was no treadmill, no elliptical, no bench press, no mirrors, and no pop music—in fact, there was no sign that it was a gym at all. It had a white tile floor and was lit by fluorescent lights, one of which was flickering. I saw some PVC pipes, a dry erase board with weird formulas scrawled on it, and a couple of jacked guys standing around a bucket of chalk.

CrossFit started with a fundamentally different philosophy of fitness from most exercise programs—it actually *had* a philosophy of fitness. Rather than idealizing the endurance athlete (marathoners, triathletes) or the hyper-specialist (most professional athletes), CrossFit venerated the ultimate generalist (Navy SEALs, special ops). Generalists needed to be prepared for anything—so they had to train for everything.

But how do you train for everything?

The answer, according to CrossFit, is a combination of three things: (1) high intensity interval training, (2) constant variation, and (3) functional movements. By the outfit's own admission, these concepts had been borrowed from a wide variety of existing disciplines in order to deliver well-rounded athleticism.

High intensity interval training means short but intense workouts alternating with brief moments of rest. It promises strength and power (anaerobic gains) without sacrificing endurance (aerobic conditioning). An eight-minute workout, done at top speed, leaves people lying on the ground gasping for breath.

Constant variation among exercises prevents overspecialization and plateaus in progress. Each day CrossFit HQ posts a Workout of the Day, or "WOD," which prescribes a different set of exercises, weights, repetitions, and rules. Exercises are drawn from a variety of disciplines, including Olympic lifting and gymnastics. Each person is instructed to scale the weight and intensity to his or her personal fitness level.

Functional movement means approximating movements used in real-world situations. Rather than relying on machines that dictate the same narrow range of motion, workouts favor exercises that require greater coordination and full-body motion.

CrossFit didn't just change the exercise protocol; they also completely redesigned the motivational habitat. Each day was a new prescribed workout, and workouts didn't repeat for weeks. All workouts were performed in a group. Everything was timed and scored. It was competitive and intense, but also cooperative with a lot of camaraderie. There was no fancy equipment, no mirrors, and no cushy amenities. It felt like something out of *Fight Club*.

As the years went on, CrossFit exploded in popularity. There was no advertising—it was all organic, driven by word of mouth and the Internet.

As CrossFit grew, so did its critics.

Some said CrossFit was *too* intense. Adrenaline-driven workouts caused some people to overdo it, giving priority to intensity, not form, and leading to injury. There were a few reported cases of a serious condition called rhabdomyolysis, when damaged skeletal muscle tissue causes vomiting, muscle spasms, and potential kidney failure. But rather than discouraging hyper-intensity, CrossFit glorified it. Two cartoon clowns acted as mascots: Uncle Rhabdo, shown hooked up to an IV and crapping out his intestines, and Pukey the Clown, drawn vomiting.

Others said CrossFit was *too* varied. If there was no planned progression to the programming, then athletes training for an event wouldn't achieve optimal performance. Variety might be healthy and natural, but total randomness was less effective at accomplishing specific athletic goals.

Still others claimed that CrossFit's most common exercises weren't *actually* functional. What real-world situation requires throwing a medicine ball at the ceiling? Or doing handstand push-ups? Arguably, CrossFit still emphasized conditioning, just as did other methods, except it used a broader set of arbitrary exercises.

These criticisms had merit, but nearly all the critics were missing the bigger picture. CrossFit wasn't a revolution in exercise *physiology* so much as a revolution in exercise *psychology*.

CrossFit was a revolution in motivation.

For most people, the biggest obstacle to exercising on a regular basis isn't the minutiae of exercise protocol—it's having the motivation to exercise at all. Something about CrossFit clicked for certain types of people. Yes, they got their ass kicked, but they came back for more.

CrossFit was so successful at creating a tight-knit community of believers that outsiders started to describe it as a cult. In the most sedentary era of human history—with unprecedented rates of adult and childhood obesity, health-care costs going through the roof, and countless failed public health efforts—these people were *too* committed to health and fitness. Every gym in America should be banging down the door trying to understand how CrossFit motivated people to exercise.

CrossFit's design showed a sophisticated understanding of human psychology—particularly masculine psychology.

Workouts are competitive. Everyone competes against the clock. Since everyone keeps track of his previous times, people compete against themselves. And since others are in the class, people compete against each other. At CrossFit competitions, each box fields a team to compete against other boxes.

Workouts are team oriented. All workouts are performed in groups. For typical workouts, people aren't on actual teams, but there is a sense of team-like camaraderie that comes from doing the same workout together. The harder it is, the stronger the bond—the Band of Brothers effect. The fittest people finish early, and then hang around to cheer on those who have yet to finish, further motivating them. After a workout everyone can commiserate over how hard it was.

Workouts are hard. Even though all workouts scale to one's own fitness level, they're still intended to be challenging for everyone. Not only do demanding workouts deliver better physical results for most people, but they also create a reputation for elite fitness. That reputation, in turn, attracts not only top athletes and competitive people, but also average athletes who want to associate with elite fitness. To maintain this status hierarchy, CrossFit workouts must always be a challenge for the best athletes, but scale down to the worst. This status hierarchy, like an unending escalator, propels people of all fitness levels upward.

Workouts foster real human relationships. It's hard to be anonymous when everyone has to write his name up on a whiteboard, and some exercises require a partner. A lack of anonymity means that everyone has a reputation to maintain during workouts. At CrossFit NYC I actually learned the names of the people I worked out with, got to know the instructors, and we even socialized with each other outside the gym. Not only is it more fun to work out with friends, but it's more difficult to leave.

CrossFit built a common culture. I could travel across the country—across the world, really—drop in at a random box, and immediately feel welcome. People know the same workouts, read the same blogs, and many even eat paleo. People share values.

The hardest workouts are named, and thus, meaningful. Names have always had the power to imbue something with meaning, and workouts are no different. At a conventional gym, a typical workout might be ten pull-ups, thirty sit-ups, and fifty push-ups—arbitrary numbers of abstract movements that don't *mean* anything. But at CrossFit, when the workout says "Fran," everyone knows it means something more than just a bunch of pull-ups and thrusters. It's *Fran*. It is an important benchmark, and a good time on Fran earns status and respect.

The named workouts come in two varieties: girls and fallen heroes, both tapping into two decidedly male sources of motivation. How could a workout be that hard if it was named after a girl? Of course, only someone who had never completed "Fran," "Helen," or "Cindy" would think that.

The Hero WODs are named after CrossFitting soldiers or first responders who died in the line of duty. The first Hero WOD was named "Murph" after Michael Murphy, a Navy lieutenant who was killed in Afghanistan. The message was simple and undeniably powerful: if Mike Murphy gave all, then anyone could put it on the line for a single workout. "Murph" is usually scheduled for Memorial Day.

Workouts strive to be functional. Functional movements are imbued with meaning by the immediate context and goals. They give training a concrete purpose beyond the abstract goal of conditioning and looking good naked. The original emphasis on functional fitness was intended for the real-world demands of military, firefighters, and the police—people who needed to be strong and fast to save a life or serve others. Ordinary people would have peace of mind from being at least somewhat physically prepared should they unexpectedly be faced with an emergency physical challenge.

In fact, CrossFitters seem to be preparing for a time when they might be called upon to be a hero: escaping a burning building or saving someone from drowning. Many CrossFitters unironically sport t-shirts with slogans like HEROES DO EXIST. That might sound silly to some, since civilization insulates us from the risks of life, but it didn't sound silly to New Yorkers only a handful of years after 9/11. CrossFit tapped into a deep desire to regain control over their lives even in small ways—one of the most effective ways to cope with

MURPH

In memory of Navy lieutenant Michael Murphy, twenty-nine, of Patchogue, New York, who was killed in Afghanistan on June 28, 2005.

This workout was one of Mike's favorites, and he'd named it "Body Armor." From here on it will be referred to as "Murph" in honor of the focused warrior and great American who wanted nothing more in life than to serve this great country and the beautiful people who make it what it is.

For time:
- 1-mile run
- 100 pull-ups
- 200 push-ups
- 300 squats
- 1-mile run

Partition the pull-ups, push-ups, and squats as needed. Start and finish with a mile run. If you've got a twenty-pound vest or body armor, wear it.

Source: CrossFit.com

traumatic events. And more than just coping with the past, working out at CrossFit felt like preparing for the future—the off chance situation where being physically fit might be the difference between life and death, between being a hero or a burden.

And there I was, walking down the streets of New York City on a beautiful sunny day, getting all worked up thinking about heroism, honor, shame, life, and death—all in relation to my gym. CrossFit had found a way to re-create the most basic motivations felt by our hunter-gatherer and herder-farmer ancestors.

Yet if these methods really did tap into something deep, then they shouldn't be unique to CrossFit—and in fact, they aren't.

According to legend, in 490 B.C. the Greek warrior Pheidippides ran from the Battle of Marathon to Athens to alert the Athenians of their victory over the Persians, giving a name to the race we call the marathon. The race, as we know it, is largely a product of modern times. It was added to the first modern Olympics in 1896, and the distance was only fixed in the early twentieth century. By 2011 over half a million people ran a 26.2 mile race.

Why?

Well, 26.2 miles isn't just 26.2 miles—it's *a marathon*. It isn't just a number, it has *a name*. And the name commemorates *a military hero who died* while doing something *functional*, not just burning calories. The marathon is a Hero WOD. CrossFitters, who notoriously dislike endurance running, have to live with the knowledge that the marathon will always be the most famous Hero WOD in the world (though they can take solace from the fact that Pheidippides supposedly died right after delivering his news to the people of Athens).

Running 26.2 miles can be meaningful for many reasons—because it's *a marathon*, because of *what it commemorates*, because it's the *Boston* Marathon, because it's someone's *first* marathon, because it's raising money *for a good cause*, because two friends trained for it *together*, because it's *hard*, and because completing a marathon brings *status and respect*. All of these sources of meaning are why so many people are motivated to run a marathon—and more impressively, train for one. It's also why no one rolls out of bed to go run 17.4 miles or 19.6 miles. The difference between just so many miles and a marathon is meaning.

Both the early-twentieth-century promoters of the Olympics and the early-twenty-first-century creators of CrossFit did the same thing: they turned physical activities into a sport. It's the same psychology of sport that's found in football, baseball, basketball, or any other sport the world over—all of which do a good job of motivating people.

Sport motivates so effectively that athletes regularly sacrifice their health to achieve success. NFL players wreck their bodies with injuries, and every sport has characteristic injuries resulting from overuse. That's because the competitive impulse isn't designed for health per se; it's designed for victory. And it's difficult to harness the motivational power of war-like competition without some people overshooting. That's just the nature of the beast. In fact, the best way to know whether people find a physical endeavor meaningful is if some people push the boundaries of what's possible, far beyond what is strictly healthy. So it should come as no surprise that the most competitive CrossFitters take it too far; that is a sign of CrossFit's success.

If sport imitates war, that might explain the growing popularity of military-style obstacle courses, adventure endurance races, and all-terrain mud runs. According to *Outside* magazine, in the United States in 2011 "roughly a million people signed up for events in the four most popular series: Spartan Race, Tough Mudder, Warrior Dash, and Muddy Buddy." Tough Mudder is a 10–12 mile obstacle course interspersed with dozens of different challenges, such as climbing walls, crawling through tunnels, and crossing a rope bridge over water— part military boot camp and part *American Gladiators*. Based on a race in the United Kingdom called the Tough Guy, Tough Mudder was founded by Will Dean and Guy Livingstone as a more fun, varied, and team-oriented alternative to marathons and triathlons. I participated in the first Tough Mudder in Pennsylvania in early 2010. Whereas at the end of a marathon people have nothing to talk about but their time, at the end of the Tough Mudder there was a lot more to laugh about. The event attracts teams of friends and co-workers who are bored with marathons, bored with triathlons, bored with gyms— bored with modern approaches to fitness.

If the motivational power of sport is derived from the *psychology* of violence between *groups* of men, then martial arts are the *skill* of violence between *individual* men.

Rule bound forms of fighting (wrestling, boxing, karate) are as old as time. Though critics view them as testosterone-fueled acts of unrestrained barbarism, practitioners tend to be incredibly disciplined athletes who learn to self-impose constraints on their own power—which ironically makes them more powerful still. Learning how to control oneself (i.e., control one's testosterone) has always been the most important lesson of the wise old sensei, often achieved through meditation, humility, and practice. For that reason alone, martial arts can be an incredibly productive activity for young boys, particularly high-testosterone ones who might otherwise struggle to control their power. But it usually takes a strong older male to keep them in line, command their respect, and impart that wisdom.

External rules are just as critical to martial arts as internal ones; otherwise men just end up crippling each other by gouging out an eye. (A "low blow" is intentionally attacking another man's crotch; the first gentleman's agreement not to do so was the birth of sportsmanship, the result of mutual vulnerability.) Since any martial art requires both fighters to abide by at least some rules, over time these rules become ritualized and diverge from the fighting techniques that would be most effective in real-world, unconstrained, "no-holds-barred" brawls. The long history of martial arts alternates between periods when a single art becomes increasingly ritualized (to the point where it can become largely ineffective in an actual fight, or at least contains fatal weaknesses), and periods when practitioners synthesize multiple disciplines and reground them in functional fighting techniques.

The last twenty years has witnessed an astonishing synthesis of disciplines under a single banner: mixed martial arts (MMA). MMA largely sprang out of the Gracie family, a Brazilian clan who founded Brazilian Jiu-Jitsu (itself a synthesis of disciplines), and who moved to the United States in 1993 and helped start the Ultimate Fighting Championship (UFC). Two decades later, MMA bouts on pay-per-view regularly outstrip boxing.

The rise of MMA has been so utterly fascinating to watch *not* because of the brutality—or not *only* because of the brutality—but because MMA was the greatest synthesis of bare-handed fighting techniques at any point in the history of the world. The UFC was criticized for its "anything goes" approach (no low blows, of course), but the absolute minimum of rules and ritual was a feature that allowed the most effective martial arts and fighting techniques to emerge. The early UFC bouts, which can be watched online, actually pit sumo wrestling against boxing; kickboxing against karate; judo against Brazilian Jiu-Jitsu.

And no one knew who was going to win!

Karate didn't fare too well in the UFC. Millions of American men—who, as boys, had flocked to see *The Karate Kid*, dressed up as Daniel-san for Halloween and begged their parents for karate lessons—were disabused of their boyhood fantasies in a few short minutes of bloody reality. As it turned out, karate was light on "martial" and heavy on "art."

The rise of MMA was a rejection of abstract ritual and a return to functional, purposeful movement in the realm of fighting. This is the exact same trend that is causing a backlash against big box gyms, where exercise machines enforce abstract, ritualized movements as stringently as Mr. Miyagi forced Daniel-san to "wax on, wax off." Messy reality teaches its own lessons.

Without question, sports, military obstacle courses, and martial arts don't appeal to everyone, and these aren't the only ways to motivate human beings. Ritualized and real violence tends to appeal to more masculine, high testosterone personalities (male or female). These types of activities also tend to be fairly high intensity and involve a lot of force—ideal ways to put on muscle bulk. (Don't worry, ladies—most women don't have the hormones to put on as much muscle as men. However, you may be at risk of developing a really nice butt.)

Others may gravitate toward low to moderate intensity exercises that require greater endurance (echoes of gathering?). These types of activities are ideal for appreciating qualities other than fierce competition—socializing, enjoying nature, meditating—and as a result, end up attracting more feminine, lower testosterone personalities (male or female).

The motivational habitat of a typical yoga class couldn't be more different from that of a CrossFit workout or UFC bout. Many people find yoga to be deeply meaningful and thus have no difficulty integrating it into their long-term lifestyle. Yoga draws on a New Age spirituality rooted in Eastern philosophy and offers a holistic worldview inclined toward vegetarianism, environmentalism, and peace. Hatha yoga sprang out of Tantra, which was associated with early Indian sex cults. Yoga is undeniably more sensual than other athletic endeavors, as any healthy heterosexual male in the back row of a yoga class can attest.

While yoga is very physically demanding (much more than it sometimes looks), the motivational habitat in a yoga studio is, in some ways, entirely opposite that of a sport. It is quiet, not loud. There are no teams (or rather, people profess that there is one big team, whether or not there actually is). It's almost inconceivable that there might be a scoreboard placing people into a status hierarchy, and a yoga studio that did so would quickly demotivate its egalitarian members. Competition just doesn't feel right: an article on the New York Regional and National Yoga Asana Championship revealed that despite the impressive flexibility on display, the practitioners felt awkward positioning yoga as a competitive sport.

Yet similar to sports teams, CrossFit boxes, or MMA gyms, in yoga there is community, a common culture, and shared values. Like martial arts or fasting, yoga is conducive to meditation, self-discipline, and introspection. It is a temporary withdrawal from the intense realities of the outside world before re-engaging with them, rejuvenated and refreshed.

Therein lies the promise and potential danger of yoga: under its deceptively soft exterior lies a deep, sensual strength that calms and rebalances; but because it does not ground itself in functional physical challenges in the real world, its practitioners have a tendency to get twisted up into knots. For yoga to return to the realm of functional fitness, rather than simply perpetuate abstract movements that one yogi passed down to another, it would have to be regrounded in some real-world activity. Given yoga's history, the natural choice would be sex. Based on a number of high-profile sex scandals between male yogis and their female students, that process appears to be well under way.

Dancing is another ancient form of human movement. Tribal dances often took place at important moments, such as coming-of-age rituals or the changing of the seasons. Today dancing may attract a female clientele, but historically tribal dancing has not been the exclusive province of women. Male dances were often intense and lasted for hours (even days), demonstrating a man's health and vigor. Contemporary examples include the Hawaiian hula or the Maori Haka, one of which is performed by the New Zealand All Blacks before their rugby matches. For both men and women, good dancing broadcasts sex appeal. Dance is another effective way to tap into an ancient form of movement—even if it is performed in more recent ethnic styles and geared toward modern goals.

Whether it's a sport or yoga, the most important thing for people to do is move—any way, any how—and to integrate physical activity into their life on an ongoing basis. To do that, "optimal exercise protocol" is less important than finding physical activities and goals that are meaningful, above and beyond any health benefits.

BEYOND MOTIVATION, where is fitness headed? What is the future of the gym?

A hint lies in a seemingly unlikely place: the playground.

There has always been a certain wildness to children at play. Kids don't run at a steady pace on a treadmill; they sprint, pivot, and dodge during a game of tag. They are born with an instinct to run, wrestle, roughhouse, climb, crawl, and jump. Kids have to be taught how to play sports; they don't have to be taught how to play.

Humans are not the only species in which the juveniles play. Lion cubs pounce and wrestle, and baby antelope run away from each other and kick. Playtime isn't a frivolous pursuit at all but actually has an important biological function. It's an adaptive behavior to prepare juveniles for the challenges of adulthood. Play is a way to practice essential survival skills.

Different species face different survival challenges and, unsurprisingly, there are different types of play. *Predatory* play (such as pouncing, nipping, or pawing) is found among predator species like felines, canines, and otters. *Locomotor* play (such as running, leaping, or kicking) is observed in prey species like horses, zebras, and goats. *Object* play (such as grasping, holding, or throwing) is seen in humans, as well as chimpanzees. *Social* play (make-believe, mock aggression, or playing at being adults) is also seen in human beings, who have complex social lives and depend heavily on learning local culture.

Play is skill development, and skill development requires neurological wiring—not simply raw aerobic capacity or muscle strength. That takes time, practice, and focus.

Hunting an antelope isn't easy. Though cheetah cubs will grow up to become the fastest animals on land, they still need to practice for years before they become successful hunters. Biologist Dr. Tim Caro documented how cheetah cubs practice on actual prey. Initially, the mother cheetah will bring back dead hares and gazelles, and the cheetah cubs will pounce on them. Over time, the mother will bring back wounded animals, which the cubs will chase and attempt to kill. When the prey (almost inevitably) gets away, the mother will go catch it and bring it back again. This may continue a few times before the mother finally kills the prey. Occasionally the prey escapes entirely, which underscores the importance of practice—the benefits of play are worth the risk of losing dinner.

Zoos have learned the hard way that skill development is essential to successfully reintroducing animals into the wild. The wild population of golden lion tamarins, a beautiful monkey native to Brazil, had declined to just a few hundred individuals. In the 1980s, conservation efforts at the National Zoo in Washington, D.C., led to a re-introduction program: captive-born tamarins would be raised at the zoo, trained for the wild, and then flown to Brazil and released.

At the National Zoo the tamarins were split into two groups. A free-ranging group was given access to zoo grounds. With that came exposure to natural surfaces, aerial predators, and weather conditions. A captive group remained in their enclosure and had fixed feeding times, fixed travel routes, and access to a limited number of obstacles—most of which were made out of sterile, rigid PVC pipe.

Upon re-introduction in the Brazilian rain forest, the sky rained monkeys. The monkeys would slip, lose their grip, and fall out of the trees—golden bundles of fur streaking down through the green canopy like fiery comets hitting the jungle floor.

The free-ranging group showed better balance than did the captive group, but both groups showed a variety of behavioral deficiencies compared with wild tamarins: they fell more, moved less often, didn't climb as high, spent more time on the few artificial surfaces provided by the scientists, and spent less time foraging for food.

Over the following year, both groups of re-introduced tamarins made rapid gains. Sadly, the tamarins that adapted their behavior least were also the most likely to die. The population that adapted best? The young.

Children's job is to play. Many schools now prevent young boys from roughhousing, but to a certain extent, boys *need* rough-and-tumble play as part of proper physiological development. Girls too! (Nor is playing dress-up or make-believe a frivolous "girly" activity; it is learning how to deftly navigate the social world.) Yet our society seems to have become ever more risk-averse, full of helicopter parents who try to shield their children from all risks—which is impossible—rather than purposefully exposing them to reasonable risks.

Unfortunately, it's easier to build an innovative new playground for monkeys in a zoo than for kids at a park or a school. Says Jon Coe, a pioneering habitat designer of zoo enclosures, "Zoo design is such an open field, we can try all kinds of things. Free-form playground for chimpanzees? Easy. We can build it in a day. But start to plan a playground for kids, and there'd be twenty-five regulations why you can't do it."

The conventional gym habitat for adults is hardly any better, with almost a complete absence of any kind of movement-based skill development. Balance? Accuracy? Coordination? Nowhere to be found. Furthermore, conditioning-based exercises are monotonous. In contrast, skill development requires an active and engaged mind.

The gym of the future will create (1) a richer motivational habitat and (2) habitat features that facilitate skill development.

Imagine a playground for adults with a variety of sources of motivation: competition, cooperation, status, looks, community, fun. It has ever-changing conditions and challenges: uneven surfaces, wobbly balance beams, accuracy targets, different temperatures, and functional goals—all of which require constant adaptation.

It won't be a gym, so much as a *jungle gym*.

One of the pioneers of wild fitness is a charismatic and athletic Frenchman named Erwan Le Corre—a modern day Tarzan with a Gallic accent. Le Corre is founder of a fitness method called MovNat, short for "natural movement." Rather than paying exclusive attention to conditioning, MovNat focuses on the skill of movement. Le Corre identifies three domains of fundamental, universal human movements: *manipulative* (lifting, carrying, throwing, catching); *locomotive* (walking, running, balancing, jumping, crawling, climbing, swimming); and *combative* (striking, grappling).

Le Corre sees his mission as similar to that of a zoo reintroducing a species into the wild—except Le Corre wants to rehabilitate the "human animal" from the "zoo" of civilization.

When Le Corre announced his first MovNat fitness retreat back in 2009, I immediately signed up. The weeklong retreat was located in Mexico, about four hours south of Cancún, beyond the typical tourist resorts.

The week before I arrived, Le Corre, his team, and a gang of locals hacked our campsite out of the jungle with machetes. On the edge of a crystal-clear lake, a clearing had been covered with palm fronds and served as a practice area for various skills. It was also a sparring area for grappling, striking, and self-defense. Our exercise "machines" were logs, branches lashed together, and stones.

This really was a jungle gym.

On our first day of "rehabilitation" a few things became immediately apparent. Even though getting dirty was inevitable, I tried to avoid it. I was so accustomed to working out in spotless gym attire that I was psychologically unprepared to get muddy. There were a lot of distractions: the main clearing wasn't flat; roots and rocks came out of nowhere; scratches started appearing on my arms and legs as I got bitten by bugs.

When it came to the actual movements, I learned that I was weaker in nature than I was in the gym. Trying to walk across a few logs in succession revealed a poor sense of balance. I couldn't jump two feet and land on a target. Deadlifting a log was harder than deadlifting a gym weight, since logs don't come evenly balanced with a perfect grip. I had to reconcile my situational goals (move this log) to the environmental context (poor grip, unsure footing), and struggled to adapt.

The jungle gym changed my perspective in another subtle but important way. In the gym I tried to expend as much energy as possible—in fact, that seemed like the whole point of working out. But out in the jungle gym, with a long day ahead of us, Le Corre taught us to expend as *little* energy as possible while completing a challenge.

That meant learning how to move efficiently.

In a gym I might do pull-ups with the conditioning-based goal of total exhaustion. But given a functional goal of getting into a tree, Le Corre taught us to generate momentum and swing on top of the branch with a minimum of effort. The emphasis on efficiency elevated the importance of form and skill.

One day we traveled to a nearby set of Mayan ruins, our practice area for the day. It was almost entirely deserted—just mown grass surrounding ancient stone edifices. We learned martial arts and practiced barefoot running in the shadow of pyramids.

After a few days I started to notice changes. I became more resilient to annoyances like dirt and scratches. It became second nature to scan the terrain for good footing. Each day the conditions were a little different—the rain changed everything—but the more the conditions changed, the easier it became to adapt to each new change.

Part of our progress stemmed from changes to our entire lifestyle. We fell asleep not long after nightfall, completely exhausted, and woke to the sun—often getting nine hours of sleep. We didn't sabotage our training with heavy drinking or a poor diet. We ate paleo meals: ceviche, grilled chicken (and not just skinless chicken breast), salad, fruit, coconut, avocado. We recovered faster and retained more of what we learned. We got plenty of sun. We had time to relax and didn't have any chronic stress.

The whole of the habitat was greater than the sum of its parts.

On the last day, Le Corre had prepared a final challenge: an obstacle course. His team had cut a long loop through the jungle. It wasn't something we had seen before, much less trained on. The rules were simple: follow the leader. Try to keep up with Le Corre as he wended his way through the jungle, crawling under branches, balancing across logs, sprinting, climbing up obstacles, jumping off them, swimming out into the lake, and doing it all over again—differently.

We didn't know the length of the course—"It lasts as long as it lasts," said Le Corre—but we still had to keep up with him. This forced us to be fast but efficient.

An hour and a half later, utterly exhausted, I found myself waist-deep in the lake, grappling with Le Corre. I could barely raise my arms.

"Okay, you're done," he said. "Nice job."

Dirty, bloody, wet, bitten, bruised, and sore—I had never felt so alive.

11

BIPEDALISM:
STAND, WALK, RUN

If there is a single form of movement that defines humanity, it is traveling upright on two feet. Bipedalism is over four million years old and long predates stone tools, fire, and large brains.

The demands of standing, walking, and running have literally shaped the entire human body from head to toe. The human head is stabilized by the nuchal ligament, a ligament in the back of the neck found in species that run long distances (horses, wolves) or have oversized heads (elephants). Since we use our toes for balance and not grasping, they are shorter than those of other primates. Though humans are quite slow sprinters, we are excellent endurance runners—the only primate with that capability—and we can run as far as animals that specialize in endurance running, such as horses and wolves. Under certain conditions we can even run further.

Humans are built to stand, walk, and run.

We are not built to sit, however—even though sitting has become humanity's preferred form of non-movement. The rise of sedentarism resulted from the same historical forces as the demise of movement. The machines of the Industrial Revolution replaced human labor and led to more sedentary professions; the Information Age is quickly turning every job into a desk job. Having been comfortably ensconced on the sofa for over a generation now, humans have lost the motivation to stand and walk—and have forgotten how to run.

There isn't too much controversy over *how* to stand or walk—the challenge is motivating people to stand and walk more, and integrating these activities into our daily lives on an ongoing basis.

Running is more of the reverse problem: millions of people *are* motivated to run—more Americans run than participate in any other athletic activity—but runners are plagued by chronic running injuries and confusion over proper form and equipment. We have been caught up in decades of running fads, having forgotten how humans ran for over a million years: barefoot, or in minimalist footwear such as sandals or moccasins. The growth of barefoot running has refocused attention on proper running form and foot health.

Standing and Walking

Hunter-gatherers cover long distances on foot each day. A review of multiple tribes found that hunter-gatherer women traveled about 6 miles per day, on average, whereas men covered 9 miles. In contrast, the average American travels about 1.5 miles on foot each day.

Not only do we cover less ground, but we rest differently. When hunter-gatherers aren't on the move, it's common to see them squat. Young children instinctively know how to squat. It's the natural way for humans to defecate, many indigenous cultures use it as a position during childbirth, and squatting is still prevalent in Asian countries.

In contrast, the average American spends most of the day sitting—in the car, at work, on the La-Z-Boy, at the dinner table, and on the toilet. It should come as no surprise that sitting causes poor posture: a hunched back, tight hamstrings, and a shortened Achilles tendon. When we finally stand up, we move like broken marionettes. And people wonder why their back hurts.

A common view is that the occasional vigorous exercise is a sufficient antidote to a sedentary lifestyle, the notion that a couple hours of cardio a week somehow counteracts days of sitting. But a number of studies suggest that sitting is unhealthful in its own right, independent of the occasional visit to the gym.

In 1953 Scottish epidemiologist Dr. Jerry Morris conducted a clever study on the relationship between a sedentary profession and heart disease. He analyzed the health outcomes of roughly 50,000 male employees of the London transportation system (bus, trolley, tram, underground). He compared the drivers, who sat all day long, to the conductors, who were on their feet collecting fares. The drivers and conductors came from a similar social class and led similar lives—Morris's attempt at a controlled comparison—but what primarily differed was the physical activity required by their job.

Morris found that "the conductors had less coronary heart-disease than the drivers, and the disease seemed to be appearing in them at a later age. What disease the conductors had was less severe: they had a smaller early case fatality as well as a lower incidence, and therefore they had a substantially lower early mortality-rate." Morris found similar results when comparing over 100,000 men who worked for the postal service. Civil servants with desk jobs had worse outcomes than the postmen who delivered the mail on foot or on bike.

More recently, scholars have begun to study this new field of "in-activity physiology"—the impact of sedentary lifestyles on human metabolism and health. The metabolism changes when people sit down for long stretches of time. Muscles stop firing, and the body's natural calorie burning rate drops by about two-thirds. A protein called lipoprotein lipase (LPL), responsible for regulating triglycerides and cholesterol, drops substantially. Low levels of LPL are associated with metabolic syndrome (obesity, heart disease, etc.) and correlate more closely to the amount of time spent sitting than whether an otherwise sedentary person does a short workout.

Even small breaks from sitting can make a big difference. An Australian study showed that after every twenty minutes of sitting, two minutes of light walking significantly reduced blood glucose and insulin levels. Long, uninterrupted stretches of sitting appear to be worse than the equivalent time interspersed with short breaks.

The challenge, then, is to sit less—and when we do sit, to take small breaks.

Dr. James Levine, a leading researcher at the Mayo Clinic, is on a crusade to get people to move more, even in small ways. That means re-engineering the two habitats where adults spend most of their time sitting: at work (usually at a desk) and at home (usually watching TV).

While watching TV, Dr. Levine suggests people make a point to get up during commercials. Video games and books also contain natural breaks (completing a level, finishing a chapter) that can serve as reminders to stand up for a minute or two. On a computer, it's easy to set up a recurring reminder to stand up every twenty minutes. Wearing a pedometer makes it easy to track your daily walking distance; one initiative set the goal of taking 10,000 steps a day, which comes out to about five miles. More radically, Dr. Levine suggests replacing the couch with a walking treadmill—an interesting convergence with gyms installing TVs in front of treadmills—perhaps even synchronized to turn off the TV when the treadmill is not in use. Something tells me this idea will be most popular with people who don't actually watch very much TV.

Personally, I'm skeptical that many people will change how they spend their leisure time (though I'd be happy to be proved wrong). Pedometers have been around for a while, as have gym treadmills with TVs attached. The key problem is motivation. "Being healthy" or "burning calories" just isn't a strong source of motivation, particularly in the privacy of home (where few others can witness what an awesomely healthy person you are) and when the exercises (standing, walking) may not change one's physique in a dramatic way. Also, many people like to rest and relax during their leisure time, even if they work a desk job. Even hunter-gatherers like to take it easy after a day spent foraging.

Whether people were foraging or farming, the most active part of the day has always been devoted to earning a living—that is to say, earning a living has always been a reliable source of motivation. Workplaces are often public spaces, where slackers are frowned upon. Thus the workplace seems like the most promising place to motivate more standing and walking.

The simplest way to combat the effects of a sedentary job? Turn it into an upright job and work standing up. Some professions still require people to stand up, including bartending, waiting tables, nursing, security, or delivering mail. People in these professions acclimate fairly quickly to being on their feet all day. But for people with desk jobs—who need a desk—that means using a standing desk.

UPSTANDING AUTHORS

Victor Hugo (1802–1885), French author of *Les Misérables.* "Close to the window, Hugo, who always wrote standing, established his standing desk, and in this room he appeared, as ever and everywhere when writing, in the early hours of the morning."

Nathaniel Hawthorne (1804–1864), American author of *The Scarlet Letter.* "[His] stand-up writing desk . . . faced bookshelves rather than the south-facing window, which offered a beautiful and therefore distracting view."

Henry Wadsworth Longfellow (1807–1882), American poet. Longfellow was the first American to translate Dante's *Divine Comedy,* which he did while standing: "It was his habit during the boiling of his coffee-kettle, to work, at a standing-desk, upon a translation of Dante. So soon as the kettle hissed, he folded his portfolio, not to resume that work until the following morning. In this wise, by devoting ten minutes a day, during many years, the lovely work grew, like a coral reef, to its completion."

Charles Dickens (1812–1870), English author of *A Christmas Carol.* Dickens's study was described as "books all round, up to the ceiling and down to the ground; a standing-desk at which he writes; and all manner of comfortable easy chairs."

Friedrich Nietzsche (1844–1900), German philosopher. Nietzsche writes, "The sedentary life is the very sin against the Holy Spirit. Only thoughts reached by walking have value."

Virginia Woolf (1882–1941), English author of *A Room of One's Own*. "She had a desk standing about 3 feet six inches high with a sloping top; it was so high that she had to stand to do her work." According to her nephew and biographer, Woolf wrote at a standing desk in order to compete with her sister Vanessa, a painter who stood at an easel.

Ernest Hemingway (1899–1961), American author of *For Whom the Bell Tolls*. Hemingway writes of "the typewriter which is in my bedroom on top of a book case so can write standing up. Writing and travel broaden your ass if not your mind and I like to write standing up."

Vladimir Nabokov (1899–1977), Russian author of *Lolita*. Nabokov writes, "I generally start the day at a lovely old-fashioned lectern I have in my study. Later on, when I feel gravity nibbling at my calves, I settle down in a comfortable armchair alongside an ordinary writing desk; and finally, when gravity begins climbing up my spine, I lie down on a couch in a corner of my small study. It is a pleasant solar routine."

August Wilson (1945–2005), Pulitzer Prize–winning American playwright. "For years, an Everlast punching bag was suspended from the ceiling about two steps behind. When Wilson was in full flow and dialogue was popping, he'd stop, pivot, throw a barrage of punches, then turn back to work."

Other upstanding citizens include statesmen Thomas Jefferson, Benjamin Franklin, Otto von Bismarck, Benjamin Disraeli, and Winston Churchill; jurist Oliver Wendell Holmes Jr.; composers Johannes Brahms and Richard Wagner; and authors Anthony Trollope, Lewis Carroll, E. B. White, and Philip Roth.

Standing desks are also known as executive desks, drafting desks, or architect's desks. As can be seen from their names, active and assertive people—executives, CEOs—have been drawn to standing desks, as have certain creative professions, such as architects and painters. In fact, standing desks have a long and distinguished history among writers, one of the oldest sedentary professions. Writing requires little physical activity but lots of mental activity, and many great writers and thinkers throughout history have discovered that standing, pacing, and walking spur creativity. According to bestselling author Nassim Taleb, "To become a philosopher, start by walking very slowly."

Standing all day may sound like torture to many people. In fact, standing for more than four hours actually *was* considered torture when guidelines were drawn up for prisoners at Guantánamo Bay. In 2002 Secretary of State Donald Rumsfeld—who uses a standing desk—signed off on the guidelines in a now-infamous memo, on which he scribbled in the margin: "However, I stand for 8–10 hours a day. Why is standing limited to 4 hours?"

Standing at work doesn't have to be torture, but it does take time to adjust. On the first day many people can tolerate only a few hours. Initially it's tiring, and some find it harder to focus. However, after a week or so, standing starts to feel natural, and the mind actually feels more engaged. Not only is it easier to stay awake while standing, but standing all day makes it easier to sleep at night. Dr. Seth Roberts, an emeritus professor at Berkeley and an early experimenter with standing desks, found that standing for more than eight hours a day substantially improved his sleep. (Subsquently, he found that standing on one leg until exhaustion, then switching legs, requires far less time and achieves a similar improvement in sleep quality.) Switching to a standing desk helped Zoe Piel, my research assistant, to mitigate the symptoms of Raynaud's syndrome, a circulatory condition that caused her hands (and feet, ears, and nose) to be cold to the point of numbness, even when the rest of her body was warm. When she reverted to a sitting desk, her Raynaud's got worse.

UNCLASSIFIED

GENERAL COUNSEL OF THE DEPARTMENT OF DEFENSE
1600 DEFENSE PENTAGON
WASHINGTON, D. C. 20301-1600

2002 DEC -2 AM 11: 03

ACTION MEMO

GENERAL COUNSEL

OFFICE OF THE
SECRETARY OF DEFENSE

November 27, 2002 (1:00 PM)

DEPSEC_____

FOR: SECRETARY OF DEFENSE

FROM: William J. Haynes II, General Counsel

SUBJECT: Counter-Resistance Techniques

- The Commander of USSOUTHCOM has forwarded a request by the Commander of Joint Task Force 170 (now JTF GTMO) for approval of counter-resistance techniques to aid in the interrogation of detainees at Guantanamo Bay (Tab A).

- The request contains three categories of counter-resistance techniques, with the first category the least aggressive and the third category the most aggressive (Tab B).

- I have discussed this with the Deputy, Doug Feith and General Myers. I believe that all join in my recommendation that, as a matter of policy, you authorize the Commander of USSOUTHCOM to employ, in his discretion, only Categories I and II and the fourth technique listed in Category III ("Use of mild, non-injurious physical contact such as grabbing, poking in the chest with the finger, and light pushing").

- While all Category III techniques may be legally available, we believe that, as a matter of policy, a blanket approval of Category III techniques is not warranted at this time. Our Armed Forces are trained to a standard of interrogation that reflects a tradition of restraint.

RECOMMENDATION: That SECDEF approve the USSOUTHCOM Commander's use of those counter-resistance techniques listed in Categories I and II and the fourth technique listed in Category III during the interrogation of detainees at Guantanamo Bay.

SECDEF DECISION

Approved ____ Disapproved _____ Other _____

Attachments
As stated

However, I stand for 8-10 hours a day. Why is standing limited to 4 hours?

cc: CJCS, USD(P)

D.R.   DEC 0 2 2002

Declassified Under Authority of Executive Order 12958
By Executive Secretary, Office of the Secretary of Defense
William P. Marriott, CAPT, USN
June 18, 2004

UNCLASSIFIED

X04030-02

When standing for long periods, avoid wearing shoes with elevated heels—men's shoes have elevated heels too—since they put the feet and spine in an unnatural position. Wear flat shoes, socks, or just go barefoot. It's best to avoid locked knees or not moving for long periods. From time to time, flex the knees a little or shift your weight. I find it comfortable to stand on one leg for a little while, placing my other foot on my ankle or calf; then I switch. Some prefer to stand on a soft mat instead of a hard floor, as Ernest Hemingway did. According to a 1954 interview by George Plimpton in *The Paris Review,* Hemingway "stands in a pair of his oversized loafers on the worn skin of a lesser kudu"—a species of African antelope—"moving only to shift weight from one foot to another." Kudu-hide mats work too (though they're probably more comfortable if you hunted the kudu yourself).

It's also okay to sit if your body is tired; being in any position for too long is probably not a good idea. Supreme Court Justice Oliver Wendell Holmes knew it was time to stop writing when he grew tired of standing: "If I sit down, I write a long opinion and don't come to the point as quickly as I could. If I stand up I write as long as my knees hold out. When they don't, I know it's time to stop." Everyone is different, and experimentation is essential.

It's not necessary to buy an expensive standing desk. The great German composer Johannes Brahms worked "at a simple standing desk which would not have fetched more than two shillings at an auction as the utmost of its intrinsic worth." Hemingway placed his typewriter on top of a bookcase, and novelist Thomas Wolfe was tall enough to use the top of his refrigerator as a writing platform. You can simply place a platform—a footstool, small table, milk crate—on top of a standard desk. It doesn't take much to support the weight of a laptop. Countertops become ideal working locations. Desktop computers may require a sturdier and more permanent setup. Some people may want to devise their own—as did Thomas Jefferson. The State Department displays one of Jefferson's drafting desks, said to be of his own design. The desk stood in Jefferson's Philadelphia apartment from 1775 to 1776, so he may have used it while drafting the Declaration of Independence.

In addition to standing desks, there are other variations on the desk that encourage movement. Treadmill desks—or "walkstations"—are a great opportunity to walk, though they tend to be a little expensive and difficult to set up. A. J. Jacobs, editor at large at *Esquire,* walked over 1,100 miles at his treadmill desk while writing his book *Drop Dead Healthy* (he didn't actually drop dead). A young software engineer (and cyclist) named Daniel Young founded a company called Kickstand Furniture, which makes "cycling desks." The desk accommodates a bicycle and is set up so that a person can cycle while working. When not cycling, one can simply use the desk as a typical standing desk. Others have found that sitting on a flexible exercise ball is a way to maintain good posture and engage more muscles than simply slouching in a chair.

Phone calls are also great opportunities to stand. As any actor or singer can attest, posture has a profound effect on the depth and strength of one's voice. One study found that simply using confident, strong posture caused hormonal changes that increased "feelings of power and tolerance for risk." Personally, I feel more active, assertive, and confident on the phone when I'm standing (often pacing) than when I'm sitting in a chair hunched over in the fetal position. I almost never take phone calls sitting down anymore, particularly when they concern business.

Another way to decrease time spent sitting is to conduct standing meetings, particularly for routine updates. Meetings are notorious for eating up time. Instead of everyone settling into a comfy chair and sitting through a meeting that drags on and on, standing up gives everyone an incentive to get to the point. It's both healthier and more productive.

Similar to the standing meeting is the walking meeting. When a meeting doesn't require written materials, the team can take a walk to discuss the topic. Though this may sound like a break— and it certainly wouldn't work for all types of meetings—the idea is to spur creativity and *increase* productivity. In fact, another well-known way to spur creativity also takes place standing up—taking a shower—and one can only imagine the creative output of group showers with the entire team. It's a seminal idea whose time has come.

Standing and walking are exactly the sort of low-level movement missing from most people's workday. Forget about calories and focus on accomplishment: don't take life sitting down.

Then, when the day is done, you've earned your rest.

Running

"Why does my foot hurt?" That simple question began Christopher McDougall's bestselling book *Born to Run*. For a species that supposedly evolved to run, we sure get injured a lot: a third or more of runners sustain some sort of injury each year. For decades the running industry has pitched products claiming to protect runners from injury, such as motion-control shoes, extra cushioning, better arch support, and orthotics. Yet amazingly there is no serious scientific evidence that these features actually prevent running injuries. This would be less consequential if injury rates among runners were low, but they're not. In its current form, modern running is a high risk contact sport.

The modern running shoe has relatively recent origins. In 1972 Nike released its first shoe to the public. It had a new "waffle sole" design, originally made by Oregon track coach Bill Bowerman when he poured liquid urethane into his wife's waffle iron. Nike and other athletic shoe companies have now created "more shoe"—more cushioning, more arch support, more lift—for just about every athletic endeavor. Prior to the last half century, runners generally wore racing flats, thin shoes without much structure or arch support. Around the world, runners wore leather sandals or moccasins—or just went barefoot.

Harvard professor Dan Lieberman—the same professor who showed me Skhul V—has published a series of studies that, it's fair to say, have upended the conventional wisdom in the running world. Modern running shoes have an elevated, heavily cushioned heel, which causes most runners to land on their heel, called "heel striking." Whereas most shod runners heel strike, barefoot runners tend to land on their forefoot (or midfoot). This seemingly small difference in form has profound implications for the impact on the body.

Running with a forefoot strike generates a lower peak force than a heel strike, and the impact takes place more gradually. This holds even for forefoot strikers who don't run barefoot. In a study of runners on the Harvard track team, forefoot strikers got injured at less than half the rate of heel strikers.

Barefoot runners avoid heel striking for a simple reason: it hurts. The pain of heel striking is a message from the body: *"Stop running that way!"* If one had to jump from a bench or chair to the ground, no one would land on his heels with locked knees—it would be incredibly painful. Reflexively the brain just won't allow it. Yet when people put on heavily cushioned running shoes, they deaden the signal coming from their feet. As a result they begin to heel strike—the heel pain is masked by the cushion, but the shock still travels up their legs—to the long-term detriment of their knees, shins, ankles, and feet.

The human foot does a superlative job of supporting the body, absorbing impact from the ground, and re-releasing it—when the foot is used as designed.

Athletes at the highest levels of performance have competed barefoot—and won. Abebe Bikila, gold medal winner of the marathon in the 1960 Olympics, ran the entire race barefoot through the streets of Rome; he had trained barefoot in his native Ethiopia. Zola Budd, a South African runner who also trained and raced barefoot, twice broke the women's world record for 5,000 meters. More recently, Tegla Loroupe drew international attention when she won major races running barefoot. In 1994 she was the first African woman to win the New York City Marathon (though she ran it in shoes).

Runners who are curious about barefoot running should start gradually. Most people have very weak muscles, bones, and tendons in their feet—precisely because shoes prevent their feet from getting enough exercise. Running too much, too soon is the most frequent way people injure themselves while transitioning to barefoot or minimally shod running.

Barefoot running is often described as a fad—one that will fizzle

---

TOP TEN TIPS TO BAREFOOT RUNNING

1. **Start slow!** The most common mistake is doing too much, too soon. Feet need time to strengthen. Drastically reduce your running distance. Start with a few hundred yards, then take a day off. Over the course of a month, gradually increase to a couple of miles.
2. **Learn barefoot, not shod.** Don't try to "transition" with a minimalist shoe. You want to learn the skill of running gently, and the best way to do that is barefoot. The ground gives better feedback when you're totally barefoot; heel striking will hurt. Furthermore, the still sensitive skin on your feet will prevent you from going too far before your body is ready.
3. **Learn on a hard, smooth surface.** A common misperception is that one should avoid hard surfaces. However, hard surfaces give clearer feedback on form, and form is a greater determinant of impact force than surface hardness. Barefoot running is most difficult on rough surfaces (gravel) or soft, uneven surfaces that allow bad form or hide obstacles (sand, grass).
4. **Use a forefoot strike, not a heel strike.** Modern high-heeled running shoes encourage a heel strike, and heel striking increases the impact with the ground and can lead to running injuries. Instead of landing on your heel, make contact with your forefoot first (or midfoot).

---

after a few years. But as Dr. Lieberman says, "If barefoot running is a fad, then it's a two-million-year-old fad. From the perspective of evolutionary biology, I can assure you that running in cushioned, high-heeled, motion control shoes is the real fad."

To most people the idea of going barefoot—standing, walking, or running—has always been hard to separate from the social signals it sends. In the Western world there has long been a stigma associated

5. **Don't run on tippy-toes.** Don't run with an exaggerated forefoot strike. Running all the way up on your toes is a good way to get a stress fracture. Allow the heel to come down and "kiss" the ground.

6. **Run with shorter, faster strides.** Among recreational runners, long strides encourage heel striking; short strides make it less likely. Many overstriding joggers run at a cadence of 150–170 steps per minute, and increasing your cadence by 5–10% is an effective guideline. Though it's not a magic number, some barefoot runners aim for 180 steps per minute.

7. **Zone in, not out.** Barefoot running requires attention, particularly to scan the ground for obstacles. Never run with earphones; barefoot running is mentally stimulating, so you won't need a distraction. Silent running is gentle running. Shod joggers are loud, smacking the ground with their feet.

8. **Don't run through the pain.** Pain is a signal that something is wrong. Adjust and see how it goes. If it still hurts, stop for the day. Tight calves and muscle soreness are normal at first; bone, joint, and soft-tissue pain are not.

9. **"Relax, relax, relax!"** —Barefoot Ken Bob Saxton, barefoot guru extraordinaire.

10. **Enjoy the freedom.**

with going barefoot: it signaled that one couldn't afford shoes and was lower class or even uncivilized. Slaves in the antebellum South were often barefoot, as were rural, backwoods people. Over time, shoes became less expensive and people became wealthier until virtually everyone could afford them; at that point going barefoot became a matter of choice—even defiance. In the 1960s, hippies increasingly went barefoot (or wore sandals), which created a new social stigma.

Even the recent rise of barefoot running was hard to separate from social signals: wearing a pair of Vibram FiveFingers—the odd looking "toe shoes"—makes quite the fashion statement.

Independent of these social considerations, there is quite a bit of evidence that going barefoot or wearing minimalist footwear is generally quite healthy. Habitually barefoot societies have lower rates of just about every major foot problem—flat feet, athlete's foot, plantar warts, plantar fasciitis, bunions, corns—many of which are practically nonexistent.

Shoes even change the very shape of our feet. A 2009 study in *Footwear Science* compared the feet of habitually barefoot Indians with shod Indians and Westerners and found striking differences. The barefoot group had wider feet, whereas the Westerners in particular had narrower feet. If form follows function, then malformations cause malfunctions. The barefoot group experienced more evenly distributed pressure on their feet than did the Westerners, who had more intense pressure focused on the heel, big toe, and metatarsals (the small bones leading to the toes).

It's well known that the shape of the foot responds to footwear, particularly during childhood—as shown by the extreme example of traditional Chinese foot binding. Even in the West, many women wear shoes that are too small for their feet, and a 1993 study found that an astonishing 80% of women had a foot deformity of some kind. All this calls into question the validity of much of the biomechanics research conducted on Westerners. As the authors of the *Footwear Science* paper asked, "[I]s the Western foot, used in most studies, not 'natural' any more, and is our current knowledge of foot biomechanics clouded by the effects of footwear—in other words, are we studying 'deformed,' but not biologically 'normal' feet?" In what must have been a moment of great cognitive dissonance, the paper won the Nike Award for Athletic Footwear Research in 2009.

Clearly, shoes are useful and going barefoot has some major drawbacks. The feet are more exposed to cuts, scrapes, burns, and frostbite. In equatorial countries, bare feet can expose someone to hookworm larvae living in mud or feces (though the larvae are so small they can even pass through canvas shoes). The solution is a minimal shoe or sandal that protects or covers the foot without constricting the foot or damaging it. For example, Barefoot Ted McDonald founded Luna Sandals, a company that produces comfortable and versatile sandals built with a traditional, minimalist design (LunaSandals.com). Many large shoe companies have jumped on the minimalist bandwagon—a welcome development.

Well-designed shoes let the foot do the work. A foot doesn't need arch support if it has a strong arch; the best way to have a strong arch is to use it. Patients with orthotics often become dependent on them rather than trying to strengthen their feet. No other part of the body is prescribed a permanent brace for a temporary injury. Neck braces are used for neck injuries, crutches are used for a broken leg—but neither is thought to be a permanent measure. All muscles, bones, and tendons grow stronger with use and atrophy without it; those in the foot are no exception.

Feet are our primary connection with the ground and thus are the foundation of most forms of human movement. The feet are filled with nerve endings and are absolutely core to the sense of balance. One study even showed that wearing thin socks caused worse balance than going barefoot. Consider how much more difficult it is to balance with forms of footwear that increasingly constrict or separate the foot from the ground: barefoot; socks; moccasins; running shoes; high heels; stilettos; ski boots; ice skates; stilts.

Shoes are a very useful tool, but a tool nonetheless. They are a tool in the same way that ice skates are a tool: both help humans deal with certain terrain more effectively. Wearing ice skates in all circumstances would be absurd. We should start thinking of shoes in the same way: using them when appropriate (rough terrain, cold weather), but not as the default option.

There is only one other species that we outfit with shoes: horses. In eerily similar fashion, even horse owners are re-evaluating the benefit of horseshoes.

BAREFOOT HORSES

Horses may be the only other animal besides humans to wear shoes, and we're the ones who put them there. Yet more and more horse owners are questioning the benefit of horseshoes. Over the last decade, the mounted unit of the Houston Police Department has transitioned to barefoot horses, having learned that they end up with fewer injuries and behavioral problems if their hooves are properly cared for.

Wild horses do just fine without horseshoes. A horse's hooves are well adapted to traveling long distances, over many types of terrain, in variable weather conditions. More than being well adapted to such exercise, it actually helps horses develop and maintain healthy hooves.

But when a horse is kept in a damp stall and doesn't get to move freely, the hoof is more likely to weaken, split, and rot. Many shoed horses have latent injuries or deformed hooves, which cause them to walk with a modified gait or react fiercely to unknown sources of pain. These problems can be made worse by a condition called laminitis, which causes systematic inflammation of the hoof. Laminitis has been linked to diet, particularly the excess sugars in grain-based feed, and bears similarities to type 2 diabetes.

Horses require a transition period as their hooves regain a natural shape and injuries heal, and sometimes a rubber boot is used. Barefoot horses require open pasture, free range of movement, a variety of surfaces, and the opportunity to graze.

Source: *Barefoot Running Step by Step* by Barefoot Ken Bob Saxton and Roy Wallack

Children, in particular, should be encouraged to go barefoot whenever possible. Their feet are growing and, like any other body part, they require use in order to develop properly. It is usually adults who force children to put on their shoes—often with the misguided intention of protecting their feet—whereas kids are often quite happy to run around without them. Unlike adults, tots aren't worried about whether going barefoot makes them look low status or weird. Many children's shoes are terribly engineered, often with half an inch or more of a hard rubber sole that does nothing but make it harder to balance and easier to fall. Those skinned knees aren't as inevitable as we were raised to believe.

The human foot contains twenty-six bones; together, the feet contain a quarter of all the bones in the body. Each foot has twenty moving joints and more than a hundred muscles, tendons, and ligaments. It is a work of anatomical brilliance, and we would be wise to heed the words of a brilliant anatomist:

> Though human ingenuity may make various inventions which, by the help of various machines answering the same end, it will never devise any inventions more beautiful, nor more simple, nor more to the purpose than Nature does; because in her inventions nothing is wanting, and nothing is superfluous, and she needs no counterpoise when she makes limbs proper for motion in the bodies of animals.

—Leonardo Da Vinci, *"Studies on Speech"* (c. 1508–10)

THERMOREGULATION

Of all the possible days of the year to roll out of bed and go for a dip in the ocean, New Year's Day is inarguably the worst. It was January 1, 2010, and my head was throbbing from too much cheap champagne and too little sleep. The ultimate hangover was about to go head-to-head with the ultimate hangover cure: the Atlantic Ocean in winter.

I was on the beach at Coney Island, the boardwalk and old amusement park where Brooklyn meets the Atlantic. Coney Island is the home of Nathan's Hot Dog Eating Contest, a rickety wooden roller coaster called the Cyclone, and a large population of Russian immigrants.

It's also home to the New Year's Day Coney Island Polar Bear Swim, during which more than a thousand otherwise sane people ring in the New Year by jumping into the icy cold ocean. More than five thousand others had come to watch the spectacle, gawking at the odd personalities that Coney Island always seems to attract. There was a three-hundred-pound hairy guy wearing only a Viking helmet and a red Speedo; a lady outfitted as a bikini-clad Wonder Woman and covered in colorful tattoos; a fully dressed Asian man caressing a large stuffed animal, which appeared to be half duck and half rabbit; and some idiot wearing a neon-green thong stretched up over his shoulders, Borat style, which simultaneously caught the eye and seared the retina.

At the appointed time I walked into a giant chute on the beach, along with all the other boisterous swimmers. After a dramatic countdown . . . well, I just stood there. I was at the back of the herd, but I could hear the people in front screaming as they ran into the water. As I slowly inched toward the ocean, it felt like a roller coaster ascending to the top of the first drop. And then there it was: the dark Atlantic.

Unless you have a heart condition, the best way to enter a 40°F body of water is at a full sprint. That way your momentum carries you forward into the water even after you have begun to feel how cold it is. It's hard to breathe at first, but then the body kicks into gear, pumping adrenaline and blood through the body. To the uninitiated, a minute or two is more than enough. Upon emerging from the water, first-timers are struck by an odd sensation: the air that felt so cold just a few minutes ago now feels practically balmy. And no hangover.

The annual event is hosted by the Coney Island Polar Bear Swim Club, the oldest cold water swim club in the nation, founded in 1903. To outsiders, the New Year's Day plunge is a big deal; for members it's one swim out of many. The Polar Bears go for a dip in the Atlantic every Sunday from the beginning of November to the end of April, the coldest six months of the year. The most memorable swims are when the water temperature dips below freezing or a blizzard is in progress. In club memory, stretching back decades, no swim has ever been canceled due to the weather.

To become a Polar Bear I had to participate in twelve swims in a season—nearly every other Sunday for half a year. My girlfriend at the time couldn't understand why I would wake up early on a snowy day, ride the subway for an hour and a half to a less than pristine beach, and jump into the freezing cold ocean for a few minutes—only to come right back.

To me, the appeal was obvious: I wanted to earn the Polar Bear patch awarded to members. But it was also an adrenaline rush. After a swim, not only did I feel amazing for the rest of the day, but I also felt impervious to the cold for a few weeks after. The other Polar Bears claimed all kinds of other health benefits, such as improved immune function and better circulation. I enjoyed hanging out with the seventy-five or so regulars, many of whom had been Polar Bears for decades. A jovial bunch—the cold seemed to stimulate warmth in people.

Every few weeks we'd get a visit from foreigners traveling in the United States: Germans, Finns, Japanese, Australians. Everyone had a story about their cold water swim club back home. We received an invitation from a Chinese group to attend an international competition of cold water swimmers in Jinan, the "City of Springs" (all expenses paid for two swimmers). However, I didn't have to travel to China to experience a foreign tradition of extreme temperature exposure; all I had to do was walk down the boardwalk to the Russian baths.

When Russians and other Eastern Europeans immigrated to the United States, most of them Jewish, they brought along their traditional methods of bathing. Inside the baths, there is a sauna (dry heat), a steam room (wet heat), a hot tub, a cold plunge (with ice floating in it), and a Russian *banya* (dry heat with a big stone oven in the middle). People spend hours switching from hot to cold to hot again.

The baths make people ravenously hungry, especially the cold plunge. There is a large indoor eating area often filled with entire families, speaking Russian, enjoying beer, vodka, smoked herring, and borscht. Outside there is a backyard. No matter the ambient temperature, it feels comfortable after an hour in the baths: the hottest summer day isn't as hot as the banya; the coldest winter air doesn't suck heat out of you like the cold plunge does.

So while the Polar Bears shivered in the 40°F degree ocean, just down the beach the Russians were sweating in the 200°F degree banya—a temperature difference nearly spanning water's freezing point (32°F) and boiling point (212°F). And both groups swore by the practice.

Why?

THERMOREGULATION IS the process by which an organism regulates its internal temperature in relation to the temperature of the external environment. Temperature measures heat, heat is a form of energy, and regulating energy intake and expenditure is central to any organism's survival and reproduction. Thermoregulation is a big deal.

Humanity's deep ancestry is intimately tied to temperature: first as furry warm-blooded mammals (Animal Age); then as hairless and sweaty hunters on the hot savannah, eventually harnessing clothing and fire to migrate into colder climates (Paleolithic Age); next, as sweat bath enthusiasts who purposefully created temperature extremes (Agricultural Age); and finally, as modernists who sought to eliminate temperature variation altogether, both externally—with heating in winter and air-conditioning in summer—and internally, with fever-reducing medications like aspirin (Industrial Age).

Humans are warm-blooded mammals and maintain a core body temperature that doesn't fluctuate more than a couple of degrees. Though 98.6°F is often reported as the "correct" human body temperature, there's natural variation depending on the body part measured, the individual, time of day, or activity level. We have methods of creating heat (shivering) and of disposing of heat (sweating). Thermoregulation is predominantly controlled by the hypothalamus in the brain, and the mechanism is far more complex and sophisticated than any man-made thermostat.

The evolution of warm-bloodedness brought with it a truly remarkable ability: maintaining core body temperature within a narrow range even as the outside temperature fluctuates wildly. This opened up cold parts of the planet (high latitude) and niches (night) that were unpopulated by sun-dependent cold-blooded animals.

(To be precise, the terms "warm-blooded" and "cold-blooded" are somewhat misleading. A "warm-blooded" mammal in hibernation can have a lower body temperature than a "cold-blooded" reptile basking in the sun. Biologists prefer the terms *ectothermic* and *endothermic*. "Cold-blooded" ectotherms predominantly rely on external sources of heat, usually the sun. "Warm-blooded" endotherms produce heat by internal means, such as a high metabolic rate or shivering. Both types of animals have evolved a suite of thermoregulatory mechanisms to regulate body temperature based on their ecological niche.)

There are trade-offs between cold-bloodedness and warm-bloodedness. By relying on external heat sources, cold-blooded animals have dramatically lower food requirements than do warm-blooded animals, since producing heat requires so many calories. For example, crocodiles can go for long periods without eating, sometimes more than a year, making them a very resilient species during times of food stress. The downside for cold-blooded animals, like crocodiles, is that their metabolic rate and activity level are far more sensitive to changes in temperature: they are less active at night (when it's colder), have difficulty surviving in cold climates, and are less able to sustain movement over an extended period of time.

In contrast, mammals are quite active, generally have a high metabolic rate, can more easily live in cold climates using adaptations like fur, and are more easily nocturnal. Some warm-blooded animals even adopt a cold-blooded strategy during times of low food availability, such as hibernation in winter. A hibernating mammal's metabolic rate and body temperature drop, allowing it to subsist on far fewer calories.

Around the Paleolithic Age, our ancestors lost their fur and gained a prodigious ability to sweat. Both of these adaptations improved their ability to get rid of excess heat, which was critical for scavenging and hunting over long distances on the hot savannah. Later in the Paleolithic humans figured out how to harness technology to control temperature: fire and clothing. Fire was a metabolism-like technology that generated heat from fuel; clothing was a fur-like technology that acted as an insulator. Fire and clothing allowed humans to migrate away from the equator into colder climates. Once there, projectile weapons helped people to hunt for food in the middle of winter, when plants were largely unavailable.

By the Agricultural Age, humans already had the ability to survive in hot or cold climates; the next challenge was to thrive. It was during this era that a similar set of cultural practices emerged independently among diverse groups around the world: brief, purposeful exposure to extreme temperatures in the form of sweat baths, often alternating with exposure to cold in water or snow. Even though the ancients had significant temperature variation in their daily lives, they pushed it even further.

If the Paleolithic wave of temperature-control technology (fire, clothing) helped people to *reduce* the variation in external temperature over *long* periods (night, winter), the innovations of the Agricultural wave (sweat baths, cold exposure) enabled people to *increase* the variation in external temperature over *short* periods (minutes, hours).

The baths went by different names, but the bathing practices were similar. There was some sort of enclosed structure heated by a fire, though usually by an indirect mechanism such as hot rocks, in order to avoid smoke. (Bathing complexes were also built around naturally occurring hot springs.) Water or herbs were placed on the hot rocks to create steam or herbal vapors. It was common to apply mud (recall the adsorptive properties of clay), oils, or poultices to the skin—or even stimulate and heat the skin by whipping it with bunches of leaves, an animal tail, or a similar implement. These sessions were sometimes interrupted or ended with forays into the cold (snow, lake, cold plunge).

These sweat baths were sufficiently important to be incorporated into the religious beliefs of many cultures. Early Japanese *mushi-buro* were built in temples, and religious rituals were carried out in Native American sweat lodges. According to an old Finnish saying, "In the sauna one must conduct himself as one would in church." Bathing in ancient Greece and Rome was practically a civic religion. The major exception was Christian Western Europe, where bathing

SWEAT BATHS AROUND THE WORLD

Laconica (Greek): Hot air baths from ancient Greece, *laconica* were named for their alleged origin in Sparta in a region called Laconia. Excavations show that *laconica* were often attached to gymnasiums. Like the Spartans, renowned for their athleticism, modern athletes still use both heat and cold to recover after sporting events.

Balneae/Thermae (Roman): *Balneae* were small baths located all throughout Rome. Over time, emperors commissioned and subsidized larger and more extravagant baths called *thermae,* which could accommodate thousands of people. *Thermae* contained a *tepidarium* (warm bath), *caldarium* (hot bath), and *frigidarium* (cold bath)—as well as a *sudatorium* (wet heat) and a *laconicum* (dry heat).

Hammam (Islamic/Middle Eastern): The Islamic *hammam* ("spreader of warmth") were derived from Roman *thermae,* but built on a smaller scale. Though often referred to as Turkish baths, hammams were common throughout the Islamic world after Muhammad endorsed their use.

Temazcal (Aztec): Spanish explorers described Aztecs using a *temazcal* ("bathhouse," "house of heat"), a domed structure filled with hot rocks; similar structures have

was uncommon and the Catholic Church frowned on the nudity or seminudity involved in sweat baths. (In one of the first European descriptions of the Aztec *temazcal,* a sixteenth-century Spaniard wrote, "Many Indians, men and women, stark naked, took these baths and committed nasty and vile sins within.") But wherever it was practiced, sweat bathing was seen as a practice that promoted good health.

Piecing together past accounts and modern research, brief exposure to extreme temperatures brings some clear benefits and hints at a wider range of potential ones.

One obvious benefit to the ancients was hygiene, and sweat

been unearthed in Mayan ruins dating to 2,500 years ago. An eighteenth-century Jesuit missionary observed that "the temazcalli is still so common that there are no Indian villages where many baths of this type are not seen." Sweat lodges were also commonly used by the many Amerindian tribes, from the Inuit *kashim* to the Lakota *Inipi*.

Mushi-buro (Japanese): The *mushi-buro* ("steam bath") is found in Japanese bathhouses called *sentō*. Similar bathhouses exist in Korea, called *jjimjilbang*, as well as in China.

Banya (Russian): The Russian banya is distinguished by a large stone oven and is known for particularly high temperatures.

Sauna (Finnish): In Finland, a country of 5.4 million people, there are more than two million saunas. Finland is best known for the wood-paneled, dry-heat sauna that is now common around the world. Finns enjoy dashing from the sauna and jumping into a cold lake or rolling around in the snow, often naked.

Similar traditions include the African *sifutu*, Swedish *bastu*, Karo (Indonesian) *oukup*, Indian *swedana*, and Celtic *teach alluis*.

Source: *Sweat* by Mikkel Aaland

bathing addressed infectious disease in a way that normal bathing couldn't—with temperature. As both pasteurization and refrigeration show, temperature can be an effective weapon against bacteria and other pathogens. Like Goldilocks and her porridge, bacteria have a preferred temperature: not too hot, not too cold, but just right. The preferred range varies from strain to strain. Two common misconceptions are that water *must* be brought to a boil to kill bacteria and that *all* bacteria are killed once water is at a boil. In reality, most bacteria die at temperatures lower than 212°F, and a few can survive at even higher ones. Since the air in saunas typically ranges from 158°F to

212°F, the temperatures are hot enough to kill off most bacteria external to the body.

In an era rife with infectious disease, sweat baths were sterile sanctuaries. During the fifth century B.C., the Greek historian Herodotus wrote about the use of sweat baths by the Scythians, nomadic people living north of the Black Sea in modern-day Ukraine and Moldova. They would use the sweat bath as "purification" after burying a corpse (long-standing practices surrounding burials are a tip-off to methods that address infectious disease). On the other end of life, Finnish women actually used to give birth in a sauna. Not only did the sauna provide warmth, privacy, and a source of hot water, but it was the most sterile place available—long before infectious disease was well understood. Russian women used to give birth in saunas too. After childbirth, Mesoamerican women were to remain isolated in the *temazcal* for three or four days and return nightly for the next three weeks. (In many cultures, sweat baths were closely tied to all aspects of female reproductive health.)

Another benefit is reducing inflammation. In 1841 the American painter and author George Catlin described the "vapour bath" of the Mandan, a Native American tribe in North and South Dakota. They would build a small lodge tightly covered in animal skins, then carry hot rocks inside and throw water on the rocks to create steam. Afterward they would jump in the Missouri River. Catlin writes, "[The vapour bath] is resorted to both as an every-day luxury by those who have the time and energy or industry to indulge in it; and also used by the sick as a remedy for nearly all the diseases which are known amongst them . . . The greater part of their diseases are inflammatory rheumatisms, and other chronic diseases." This description of the therapeutic uses of sweat baths is fairly typical across cultures.

The application of heat and/or cold is still a common treatment for inflammation. One study of patients with rheumatoid arthritis, osteoarthritis, and fibromyalgia showed that using a sauna reduced pain temporarily but pain actually increased twelve hours later. Other studies—and common practice—suggest that adding an intense cooling-off may be a more effective treatment than the use of heat alone. That the combination of heat and cold is superior to either one alone should come as no surprise to trainers of professional athletes, who regularly undergo cycles of both.

Today it's common to read warnings that sick people should not use a sauna or steam room. While in some cases that's probably sound advice (ask your doctor—who probably won't actually know much about the issue, and will just say don't do it), it stands in stark contrast to the practices in many ancient cultures, where sweat bathing was considered a remedy to illness. It's intriguing that many ancient cultures encouraged heat exposure for sick people, who presumably had a fever (i.e., elevated body temperature)—whereas today it's common for people to take fever-reducing medications, which have been shown to actually slow recovery.

It doesn't take a study to know that exposure to extreme temperatures increases adaptation to them; like muscles, the body's thermoregulatory mechanisms become stronger with repeated stress. A study of winter swimmers found they were slower to shiver than non-adapted controls, and thus could survive a greater temperature difference between their body and the environment. The adaptations from repeated cold exposure might last longer than adaptations to exercise; one study found reductions in the initial shock of entering cold water persisted more than seven months after initial adaptation.

The people who stand to benefit the most from improved adaptation to the cold are the ones who most resist it, usually just because they "hate the cold." That's like someone complaining about being weak but refusing to lift weights. My friend Uji Bluet, a rail thin Korean woman, complained of being cold all the time, until I dragged her to the New Year's Day Polar Bear swim and an afternoon at the Russian baths. She reported not feeling cold for the entire month of January.

Heat and cold exposure is beneficial for another reason: it's enjoyable and relaxing. In a modern era when people are chronically stressed, this practice is of greater benefit than it used to be.

Personally, there is no single activity that reliably relaxes me and puts me in a good mood than a nice hot sweat and cold plunge. Whatever combination of hormones cause stress, this reverses them. My friend Richard Nikoley refers to cold exposure as his "reset button"—I couldn't agree more.

Going to the sauna, banya, or baths has always been a great opportunity to socialize—whether among the thousands in the extravagant Roman *thermae* or with a handful of friends squeezed into a tiny Finnish sauna. According to Dr. Harald Teir, president of the Finnish Sauna Society, "The idea is not to have the best sauna on the block, but to get the entire block in the sauna." The baths are one of the few remaining spaces that have resisted the incursion of TVs, computers, and cell phones; the wet and heat act as insulators against the Information Age. And unlike many other forms of socializing—holiday dinners, drinking alcohol, going to a sporting event—this one leaves you feeling more relaxed and healthier.

Studies of populations that regularly participate in sauna bathing reveal few risks. A 2001 paper reviewed mortality statistics from Finland: "Of all sudden deaths (6,175) in Finland within 1 year, only 102 (1.7%) occurred within 24 hours of the sauna bath. One third of these were accidental, due to consumption of alcohol or drowning; the majority of the non-accidental deaths were due to acute myocardial infarction [heart attack] in which alcohol intake was an important contributing factor." A separate review concluded that "both the absolute and relative risks are small." Among pregnant women (with no complications), no ill effects have been observed on either mother or baby. On average, Finnish children are introduced to the sauna at five months old (though just for a couple of minutes, once a week or so). The most common risk to young children is accidental burns from hot water or equipment. However, because children do not have the thermoregulatory capacity of adults, they often sit at a lower level and stay in for a shorter period of time. Old people lose the ability to thermoregulate as well, and so should also be more mindful.

These guidelines hold true for cold exposure, with the addition that fingers and toes should be closely monitored since they lose heat the fastest, and one should never swim alone in cold water. People with heart problems should avoid a sudden shock to the system—hot or cold—and should enter gradually. Overall the risks associated with appropriate hot or cold exposure do not appear any greater than with other forms of physical exercise.

DURING THE Industrial Age, humans developed ever more effective and affordable methods of controlling external temperature: gas furnaces, inexpensive fuel, indoor plumbing (no trips to the outhouse), and air-conditioning. The average American lives a completely temperature-controlled existence. Whether in the home, car, or office, the thermostat is always set to a narrow, comfortable range. Today, in an odd reversal, it's not uncommon to feel chilly during a Texas summer due to air-conditioning on full blast, and a touch warm during a Minnesota winter, as a result of the coldest person controlling the thermostat.

We have only a poor understanding of how these changes may be influencing human health—perhaps even contributing to the rise of obesity. Modern health authorities admonish people to burn more calories, but they completely neglect the body's largest source of caloric expenditure: heat.

In *The 4-Hour Body*, author Tim Ferriss features a story about Ray Cronise, a former NASA researcher who began investigating the effects of cold exposure on weight loss. Cronise was puzzled that Olympic swimmer Michael Phelps could eat 12,000 calories a day yet, seemingly impossibly, burned it off through exercise. The answer, Cronise realized, is that Phelps spent hours in the pool, and his body had to burn thousands of calories just to stay warm. Furthermore, water conducts heat better than air—about twenty-three times better (40°F air is cold, but 40°F water is *cold*. 100°F air is hot, but 100°F water is *hot*). Swimming is a particularly draining activity—not simply because of the movement required, but because of the heat loss.

Human movement requires remarkably few calories. Treadmills

that report "calories burned" contain a fatal deception: they include the calories burned by the body even by lying on the sofa. Subtract the basal metabolic rate and the number of calories burned on the treadmill is depressingly low. In fact, running an entire marathon burns only about 2,600 calories, the equivalent of a day's worth of food. Even worse, body fat is a remarkably good way to store energy: a pound of body fat contains roughly 4,000 calories. That means losing a mere ten pounds is the caloric equivalent of running 13.5 marathons.

Far more calories are used to heat the body than to move it.

Polar explorers and mountain climbers lose a lot of weight during their expeditions and sometimes resort to eating sticks of butter. The ever-indulgent Romans used this phenomenon to their advantage: going to the baths, which included the *frigidarium,* was a way to whet the appetite. Not only does the body increase (or decrease) appetite in response to heat expenditure, but it also raises (or lowers) body temperature in response to caloric intake: starvation victims have lower than normal body temperatures. In the face of a severe caloric deficit, the body attempts to conserve energy.

Since the body is adaptive, trying to use cold exposure as a weight loss strategy may end up being as successful as running on the treadmill (not very). On the other hand, there are metabolic benefits to exercise above and beyond burning calories—and so too with cold exposure.

The body creates heat in a process called *thermogenesis.* One method is shivering, when muscle fibers quickly contract in order to generate heat. When shivering isn't sufficient, the body turns to specialized fat cells called brown adipose tissue (BAT). BAT gain their color from containing many mitochondria (used to produce heat), in contrast with the more common and familiar white adipose tissue. In some ways, it may be useful to think of BAT as a muscle—one that grows stronger with use and atrophies without it. The great thing about BAT is that it turns directly to body fat as a source of fuel. Short of liposuction, thermogenesis is probably the fastest way to reduce body fat.

HOW TO BE COOL

Swim. Most swimming pools are quite a bit cooler than the body; lakes and oceans definitely are. Incorporate swimming into your regular exercise regimen.

Do a polar bear plunge. Many cities have cold water swim clubs; look one up and join it. Cold water plunges are more fun with other people.

Visit the baths. Russian, Turkish, or Korean, proper baths have cold plunges. Some gyms have cold plunges too—if they don't, a cold shower will do.

Take cold showers. If it's too intense to start cold, then start warm and gradually turn it colder. It helps you wake up, too.

Build a cold plunge. Fill a bathtub or large plastic tub with cool water. Add ice. Enjoy.

Turn down the thermostat. Let the air be a touch cold rather than a touch hot. Others can choose to wear extra clothing if desired. This also improves alertness and saves money.

Exercise outdoors. Whatever the activity, do it outside. With gloves and a hat you can wear only a t-shirt, even in winter.

There are lots of little ways to encourage thermogenesis, even by doing something as simple as swimming in a cool pool. After an initial adaptation period during which the cold is uncomfortable, many come to enjoy it quite a bit.

During the Industrial Age we also increasingly began to fiddle with our internal temperature—in particular, by reducing the frequency, duration, and intensity of fevers. The rise of medications with fever-reducing effects (antipyretics)—such as aspirin, acetaminophen, and ibuprofen—meant that modern people have experienced shorter and less intense fevers. And with the rise of antibiotics and the decline of infectious disease, people have experienced fewer acute fevers. While the decline of infectious disease was unquestionably beneficial, few people stopped to question whether there might be drawbacks to the decline of fevers.

Fevers have an adaptive function: a fever is a natural immune response to infection, not just an unpleasant side effect of being ill. Fever isn't a bug, it's a feature.

Fevers are metabolically expensive, yet they are still quite common throughout the Animal Kingdom. Even "cold-blooded" animals, which rely on external heat sources, figure out a way to raise their body temperature when infected. In one experiment, fever specialist Dr. Matthew Kluger infected thirteen iguanas with bacteria. All but one sought out the warmth of a heat lamp, raising their body temperatures by a few degrees—essentially, giving themselves a fever. Eleven of the twelve lived, and the other one did not. When he injected more iguanas with bacteria and gave them a fever suppressant, the ones that still developed a fever survived, while the rest did not. Other animal experiments have shown an inverse relationship between fever and mortality. Similarly, people with aquariums have long used the trick of heating up their tanks to speed up the life cycles of pathogens, thereby pushing their pets to recovery.

The salutary effect of a fever is not a recent discovery. The ancient Greek physician Parmenides is alleged to have said, "Give me a chance to create a fever and I will cure any disease." More recently, Austrian physician Dr. Julius Wagner-Jauregg won the Nobel Prize in Medicine in 1927 "for his discovery of the therapeutic value of malaria inoculation in the treatment of dementia paralytica." That is to say, Wagner-Jauregg cured syphilis patients by infecting them with malaria. The malarial infection caused a lengthy, high temperature fever—clearing the syphilitic infection in the process—after which quinine was used to treat the malaria. This entire approach to fighting infection was abandoned after the discovery of penicillin.

More recent studies have shown minor drawbacks to fever-reducing medications: children take about a day longer to recover from chicken pox when given acetaminophen, and the common cold lasts about a day longer too. That may seem like a reasonable trade-off for greater comfort, but the indiscriminate use of fever-suppressing drugs, routine in hospitals, may actually be quite a bit more serious.

A compelling but more speculative line of reasoning suggests that the decline of fever has contributed to the rise of cancer. What's uncontroversial is that chronic infections cause many types of cancer. A paper in the prestigious medical journal *The Lancet* estimated that globally one in six cases of cancer are caused by infection, the most prevalent being gastric cancer (*H. pylori*), liver cancer (hepatitis B and C), and cervical or uterine cancer (HPV). It's highly likely that additional chronic infections will be implicated as cancer-causing agents.

Chronic infections become chronic in the first place due to an insufficient initial immune response. Once malignant tumors begin to grow, they release compounds that further suppress an immune response. Clearing the latent infection, therefore, is of the utmost priority.

What's also uncontroversial is that eliciting an immunological response—via injection of a vaccine, accidental infection, or purposeful infection—can result in tumor regression. The heightened sensitivity of the immune system targets not only whatever caused the initial response but other foreign invaders as well—be they bacteria, viruses, or malignant cancer cells. This general approach of stimulating the immune system forms the basis of a field called immunotherapy.

Though using immunotherapy to fight cancer stretches back into antiquity, it is most closely associated with the early-twentieth-century work of Dr. William Coley, a New York City oncologist. He observed spontaneous remission of tumors after accidental infections, and eventually he developed a generalized vaccine called Coley's Toxins. Made from killed bacteria, it stimulated a strong fever and immune response. Wagner-Jauregg took advantage of the same general process: using a malarial infection to trigger a strong fever, thereby harnessing the body's natural immune response to clear a syphilis infection. As Wagner-Jauregg put it, "We have listened to nature; we have attempted to imitate the method by which nature itself produces cures." (Da Vinci would have approved.) But with the rise of antibiotics, nature's cure—the fever—became something to be completely avoided.

Fevers are a mixed blessing. They damage good tissues in the body, and some runaway fevers end up killing people. Also, for as long as people have had fevers, they've used herbal medicines (including ones containing the active ingredient in aspirin) to relieve them. But it's also possible that ancients knew something we don't: that helping along a fever may actually be beneficial.

Overall, a certain amount of natural fluctuation in temperature—internal and external—is a good thing. Goldilocks was wrong: "too hot" and "too cold" are sometimes just right.

13

SUNRISE, SUNSET

Life would not exist without the sun. Ancient people saw the sun as a source of life, yet modern people are just as likely to view it as a source of death. What used to be wholesome sunshine has now become "sun exposure," a phrase that evokes vulnerability and disease.

Like plants, people need the sun to stay healthy. The skin uses sunlight to generate vitamin D, which the body uses to build bones and teeth, maintain a strong immune system, and to fight cancer. It is essential to a surprisingly wide variety of bodily systems. Our health depends not only on the presence of the sun, but also on its absence. Light and dark are signals that set our biological clock, influencing sleep quality, energy levels, alertness, and mood. The cyclical sun enforces its own rhythmic balance on life.

Yet we have lost all sense of balance toward the sun. We hide indoors during daytime and then replace the sunshine with artificial light at night. We confuse our biological clock and try to live by electronic ones. We rarely get much sunshine, but when we go on vacation we move closer to the equator and make up for lost time. White people live in Australia, black people live in Alberta. We slather on sunscreen yet go to tanning salons. We try to reduce the sun to just so much vitamin D, as if those golden rays could somehow be captured in capsules of fish oil.

If our attitudes toward the sun have become unhinged, perhaps it is because our lives first became unhinged from it.

To re-establish a balanced relationship with the sun, it helps to understand how our relationship with the sun has changed over time. Important transitions include vertebrates leaving the sea for dry land (Animal Age); the evolution of dark skin (Paleolithic Age); the evolution of light skin (Agricultural Age); and the movement indoors, the rise of clocks and electric lighting, and the rise of tanning and sunscreen (Industrial Age).

Day

Microscopic phytoplankton and zooplankton have generated vitamin D from the sun for well over 500 million years. When vertebrates left the seas some 350 million years ago, vitamin D took on new importance. Previously, bony fish could absorb usable calcium for their skeleton directly from the calcium-rich ocean, but terrestrial vertebrates needed to find a new source of calcium. This meant eating calcium-rich plants (or other vertebrates) and converting dietary calcium into bone, a process that required vitamin D.

Sunlight isn't just visible light; it's also ultraviolet radiation (UV). When certain wavelengths of UV hit the skin, vitamin D is created from a chemical precursor. Vitamin D isn't actually a vitamin in the literal sense of the word—a trace nutrient that the human body can't generate on its own and that must be ingested through the diet. Vitamin D is more akin to a multipurpose hormone that the body synthesizes itself with the help of sunshine (and cholesterol). Vitamin D is sufficiently important that cells throughout the body have the ability to generate it.

Given the widespread importance of vitamin D to vertebrates, it should come as no surprise that vitamin D deficiency causes similar health problems in zoo animals and humans. In 2005 Boston's Franklin Park Zoo celebrated the birth of Kimani, a western lowland gorilla. Kimani soon became sick and weak, showing "signs of the bone-softening disease rickets." Even suckling became a problem, and the inevitable malnutrition would only make matters worse.

The staff called Dr. Michael Holick, one of the world's leading vitamin D researchers. As a graduate student Holick discovered the major form of vitamin D that circulates in the bloodstream, which doctors now measure to check vitamin D status. The zoo staff had been administering 400 IU (international units) of vitamin D, double the recommended amount for human infants. Dr. Holick recommended 5,000 IU a day, more than ten times as much. Kimani recovered completely.

Unfortunately, vitamin D deficiency is a widespread problem at zoos. Many exotic species come from sunny equatorial climates, yet many of the world's top zoos are located at high latitudes and the animals spend significant time indoors, particularly during winter. For many of the same reasons, vitamin D deficiency is widespread among humans. One recent study found that 42% of Americans were deficient, with much higher rates for blacks (82%) and Hispanics (69%). Dr. Holick has advised both zoos and human organizations on how to avoid vitamin D deficiency via supplementation, but his preferred course is natural sunlight or synthetic lighting systems that mimic sunlight. It's now common practice for zoos (and even pet owners) to install UV-emitting lamps, particularly for species such as reptiles, which are adapted to high levels of sunshine.

Like Kimani, our hominin ancestors had a thick layer of black hair, but the underlying skin was only minimally pigmented and unaccustomed to direct sunlight. As our ancestors gradually became hairless, the intense, equatorial sunlight damaged their increasingly unprotected skin. Since early hominins and hunter-gatherers were forced to spend much of the day on the shadeless savannah, they benefited from a new form of sunblock: dark skin.

Dark skin is caused by high levels of melanin, a pigment that acts as a natural sunscreen. It's a trade-off: dark skin protects against skin damage, but people with dark skin need to spend more time in the sun in order for their bodies to generate vitamin D. Light skin makes it far easier for the body to generate vitamin D, but it's also more susceptible to skin damage. An analysis of the genes controlling skin pigmentation concluded that our hunter-gatherer ancestors became dark skinned a little over a million years ago. Trace any family tree far enough and everyone was black.

But at some point after humans left Africa, Europeans and Asians independently evolved lighter skin. For multiple groups to evolve lighter skin independently and for these mutations to spread so quickly through the local populations, lighter skin must have conferred a huge evolutionary advantage.

The most common explanation for the evolution of light skin is called the latitude hypothesis, which argues that as humans moved away from the equator to higher latitudes with weaker UV rays, they became vitamin D deficient. If vitamin D deficiency were sufficiently severe, it could cause a girl to grow up with a weak or deformed pelvis, increasing her chances of dying in childbirth. But recently the latitude hypothesis has been challenged as incomplete.

In a 2010 paper in *Medical Hypotheses,* Razib Khan pointed out that the latitude hypothesis doesn't adequately explain certain key facts. A number of indigenous peoples—such as the Inuit, Tasmanians, and Australian Aborigines—have been living far from the equator for thousands of years and still have dark skin (though the Inuit compensate for a lack of sun exposure with a diet rich in vitamin D, including fish livers, fish oil, and seal blubber). Another complication is that Amerindians in North and South America have fairly similar levels of pigmentation whereas there are dramatic differences between Eurasians and Africans. Furthermore, the genes that control light skin appear to have evolved less than 10,000 years ago, well after humans had left equatorial Africa.

Khan proposes that the Agricultural Revolution played a major role in the evolution of light skin. Vitamin D is critical to immune function, and the dramatic rise of infectious disease in agricultural societies placed enormous pressure on the immune system. While infectious disease ravaged early herder-farmers, their diet had taken a dramatic turn for the worse. A diverse and vitamin D–rich hunter-gatherer diet turned into a narrow, grain-based farmer diet deficient in micronutrients. At the very moment these early herder-farmers needed more vitamin D for their immune system they were getting less of it in their diet—so the body turned to its other source: sunlight. It shouldn't take long to see if this hypothesis holds up since many scholars are analyzing the genes that control skin pigmentation.

Clinical studies have confirmed the widespread importance of vitamin D to health, above and beyond bone conditions (rickets, osteomalacia, osteoporosis). Many studies indicate that vitamin D protects against internal cancers (colon, breast, prostate, ovarian); cardiovascular disease (hypertension, heart attack); and autoimmune disorders (multiple sclerosis, rheumatoid arthritis, type 1 diabetes). Sunlight is a common treatment for skin conditions such as psoriasis. Furthermore, vitamin D plays a direct role in the immune system's ability to mount a response to microbial infections.

The next big change in our relationship with the sun took place during the Industrial Age, when people started spending more and more time indoors. Rickets first emerged in Britain, which was at the forefront of the Industrial Revolution. Not only did Britain lead other countries in urbanization, but it is located at high latitude, is famously cloudy, and had terrible air pollution. Plus, Brits ate a nutrient deficient industrial diet full of refined flour, sugar, and alcohol. The movement indoors accelerated in the late nineteenth century with Thomas Edison's breakthrough incandescent lightbulb and the subsequent rise of electric lighting. Humans had finally severed their relationship with the sun.

But the pendulum had swung too far, and by the end of the Industrial Age, people began to realize the benefits of sunshine. Heliotherapy ("sun medicine") became popular, and many hospitals built sundecks for patients with rickets or tuberculosis. In 1903 the Nobel Prize in Medicine was awarded to Dr. Niels Finsen, who discovered the therapeutic value of UV radiation in treating lupus vulgaris, a form of tuberculosis that causes painful skin lesions. Scientists discovered dietary vitamin D, how the body generates vitamin D from UV light, and how to fortify milk through irradiation. The eventual fortification of foods with vitamin D helped people to avoid crippling conditions, such as rickets. This approach was typical of the Industrial Age: inadvertently removing something essential for human health, discovering it was essential for human health—and then developing an industrial method to add it back in.

In the mid-twentieth century, people started to spend more time in the sun seeking out a tan. Whereas the famously pale Queen Elizabeth caused a rash of blue blood imitators, an aspiring aristocrat made it socially acceptable to venture back into the sun: Coco Chanel. The French fashion designer and founder of the Chanel brand turned a tan into a status symbol—having a tan suggested that someone had the wealth and leisure time to vacation in warm, exotic locations. Tanning took off.

But as people rushed back into the sun, they got burned.

In 1938 a chemist named Dr. Franz Greiter invented the first modern sunscreen. Nearly twenty-five years later, Greiter also came up with the concept of "sun protection factor" (SPF), a measure of how well sunscreen blocks UVb, the type of rays that cause sunburns (and vitamin D synthesis). As SPF increased from 2 to 10 to 15 to 30 (which blocks about 97% of UVb rays), people became increasingly confident that they were protected from skin damage—but they weren't. Sunscreen manufacturers focused on preventing only the type of skin damage that people could easily feel: sunburn.

What few realized was that conventional sunscreens did not block *all* of the sun's rays—just the kind that causes sunburns (UVb). But sunlight also contains UVa, which causes skin damage even though it doesn't cause sunburn. In fact, there's more UVa in sunlight than UVb (twenty to forty times as much), and UVa penetrates the skin more deeply.

Over the course of human evolution, the body had never experienced a decoupling of UVa and UVb. But sunscreen decoupled the *signal* of damage (redness, sunburn from UVb) from one of the *sources* of damage (UVa). By using sunscreen that blocked only UVb, people incurred far more skin damage than they ever could have without it; they would have been better served by using no sunscreen at all, and getting out of the sun before their skin started to redden. Today sunscreen manufacturers make broad-spectrum sunscreens, which block both UVa and UVb—the best option for anyone expecting to be in the sun for an extended period of time.

But for more than half a century, pale people would emerge from a long winter of hibernation, travel to a latitude closer to the equator, lather on sunscreen, and go sit in the sun all day long—unwittingly incurring skin damage from intense UVa exposure. During this time, rates of skin cancer continued to rise. Garbage in, garbage out.

There are two main categories of skin cancer: non-melanoma and melanoma. Non-melanoma skin cancer (basal cell and squamous cell) are far more common but are easily treatable. Melanoma is rare (less than 5% of skin cancer cases) but accounts for the great majority of skin cancer deaths (more than 75%). Both types of skin cancer have been on the rise, whereas other major cancers have been steady or declining. Although excessive sun exposure plays a causal role in both types of cancer, there are many misconceptions about skin cancer too.

First of all, the risk of dying from melanoma is low, particularly if it is detected early. Unlike most other cancers, melanomas are visible—anyone can (and should) inspect their body for them. The absolute number of melanoma deaths is low. In the United States in 2001 there were an estimated 8,790 deaths due to melanoma—or just 1.5% of all cancer-related deaths. The most deadly cancers were lung (156,940 deaths); colon (49,380); breast (39,970); pancreas (37,660); prostate (33,720); liver (19,590); non-Hodgkin lymphoma (30,300); ovary (21,990); urinary bladder (17,230); esophagus (14,710); kidney (13,120); brain and nervous system (13,110); myeloma (10,610); stomach (10,340); acute myeloid leukemia (9,050)—and melanoma

(8,790). Furthermore, melanomas often appear on parts of the body that receive little sunlight (legs, back), and such malignancies usually don't carry the genetic mutations associated with UV damage. (Non-melanoma skin cancers are far more common, and they do tend to appear in areas—nose, face, ears—that have been exposed to the sun and sustained sun-related skin damage.)

The strongest risk factor for developing melanoma is having lots of moles—followed by fair skin, red hair, and sustaining severe sun-burns. While fair-skinned people are more likely to get sunburned, these risk factors (moles, fair skin, red hair) are still important inde-pendent of sun exposure.

A recent study published in *Nature* showed that "red-headed" mice developed malignant melanomas far more often than did dark-skinned or albino mice—in the complete absence of UV. (To make it more likely they would see melanomas develop, the researchers ge-netically altered the mice to make benign moles more common.) The authors suggested that oxidative damage due to the production of red pigmentation was causing the melanomas—sorry, Ginger, you're carcinogenic—and they cited evidence that such oxidative damage is amplified by exposure to UVa, the type of sunlight not blocked by conventional sunscreens.

Despite the excoriation of tanning beds in the press, there hadn't been clear scientific evidence that tanning bed usage caused mela-noma until 2010. The case-control study compared 1,167 melanoma patients with age- and gender-matched controls, all drawn from sun-starved Minnesota. The results showed a 74% increased risk of mela-noma for anyone who ever used a tanning bed, which increased with frequency ("50+ hours": 218%) and number of burns (">5": 212%). These are not small effects, and using a tanning bed does increase your risk of melanoma.

However, the subsequent media coverage lacked any indication that reporters had taken time to read the study. What many neglected to highlight was the increased risk of melanoma due to moles ("many": 1,281%), skin type ("very fair": 450%), and hair color ("red": 253%).

Having lots of moles carried roughly six times the risk of the highest frequency usage of tanning salons, and seventeen times the risk of the entire population who had ever used one. The paper also found that the risk of melanoma *decreased* with high levels of routine sun exposure, including that from outdoor activities or jobs. In contrast, the risk of melanoma *increased* with lifetime sunscreen usage(!), as well as by the number of sunburns. The headlines could just as easily have read: *"Avoid sunscreen! Regular sun exposure reduces risk of melanoma."*

Yet sunlight continues to be stigmatized: now it's officially a carcinogen. The International Agency for Research on Cancer, an offshoot of the World Health Organization, recently promoted ultraviolet radiation from Group 2A ("is probably carcinogenic") to Group 1 ("is carcinogenic")—joining tobacco, asbestos, benzene, radon gas, and plutonium. Yet none of these other carcinogens also reduces rates of colon, breast, and prostate cancer. If such a classification can't take into account the net impact on human health, it's a lousy classification. Protective benefits aside, the number of annual deaths due to melanoma (8,790) is comparable to deaths due to drowning (about 3,500). Stigmatizing sunlight as a carcinogen because some people get burned at the beach is like adding water to the list of controlled substances because some people drown in the ocean. People do drown—but that doesn't mean we stop drinking water; it means we teach kids how to swim.

The sun is not the problem; our love-hate relationship to the sun is. Most modern people have the same pattern of sun exposure: they get too little sun for much of the year (stuck in offices, classrooms, and homes), and then they lie out in the sun for too many hours in the summertime (often while on vacation closer to the equator). In fact, this pattern of sun exposure resembles those of astronauts in space: both too little and too much.

So how do we re-establish a healthy, balanced relationship with the sun? People worried about any type of skin damage should, first and foremost, avoid sunburns. Those most at risk of sunburn are fair-skinned people living or vacationing near the equator.

ASTRONAUTS AND THE SUN

Astronauts literally change their relationship to the sun: they leave Earth for outer space. As a result, they face extreme versions of every sun-related health problem faced by modern people, such as vitamin D deficiency, cancer, insomnia, and irritability.

Astronauts are at risk of "getting too much sun" because they are bombarded with solar radiation, typically blocked by Earth's atmosphere and magnetic field. They can suffer radiation poisoning, and they face limits on the cumulative time they can spend in space. Astronauts also avoid spacewalks during solar storms, periods of particularly intense solar radiation.

Astronauts are also at risk of "getting too little sun" because they are indoors all the time. They depend on vitamin D supplements to avoid a deficiency, which is a serious risk. Not only can a lack of vitamin D cause depression, but it compounds the stress on an astronaut's bone structure, which is already weakened due to zero gravity.

In space, night and day don't take place in twenty-four-hour cycles, and an astronaut's biological clock can easily drift without synthetic signals of night and day. Sleep can be difficult, with all the resulting problems. Needless to say, when astronauts return to Earth, they relish feeling the sun on their face— having physically re-established a healthier, more balanced relationship to the sun.

One of the best ways to avoid sunburns is to get sun on a regular basis. Regular exposure creates a base level of protection and generates plenty of vitamin D. Those most at risk of vitamin D deficiency are dark-skinned people living at high latitudes, who may even want to consider buying a UV lamp.

It's particularly important for children or young people to avoid sunburns, which raise the lifetime risk of skin cancer. However, when a kid is "growing like a weed," remember that a weed needs sunlight to grow. Sunshine is healthy for pregnant women and babies, who do not need to be kept in the shade every single moment of the day.

When not wearing sunscreen, the body is a reliable guide to safe sun exposure. Those first twenty minutes of sunshine usually feel amazing, which coincides with the body beginning to refill its vitamin D stores. That positive feeling usually fades to neutral at some point. Reddening skin is the body's signal that it's past time to get out of the sun. The pain of sunburn is a reminder of serious damage already done to the body. Remember that conventional sunscreen confuses the body, blocking the signal of damage (UVb) but not a source of damage (UVa). Your body is *not* a reliable guide to safe sun exposure when you are wearing conventional sunscreen.

For short periods in the sun, don't use sunscreen. For extended periods in the sun, use a broad-spectrum sunscreen, which protects against UVa and UVb. SPF 30 blocks 97% of UV, and higher SPF levels provide only a minuscule increase in protection; SPF 60 is not twice as good as SPF 30. At that point, the SPF level is far less important than how well and how often the sunscreen is applied. For those who want to avoid signs of aging, apply sunscreen to the face more frequently.

Artificial UV is not necessarily unhealthy, but the current high intensity tanning beds are. UV is UV, whether it comes from the sun or a lightbulb—what varies is the wavelength and intensity of UV. In principle, UV-emitting lights that replicate natural sunlight give the same benefits as real sunlight. Such lights make it possible for corals, used to the intense tropical sunshine, to be kept in home aquaria. Eventually it will become common to have indoor lights that emit UV calibrated to replicate natural sunlight.

The best way to add vitamin D to one's diet is through whole foods naturally rich in it (such as small oily fish) or fortified foods (such as milk or yogurt). Supplements are another option: cod-liver oil, fish oil, or vitamin D capsules—though supplements sometimes go bad. There are also multiple forms of vitamin D, and we have evolved to get the exact kind we need from sunshine. And unlike dietary supplements, sunshine is free.

Check for skin cancer every six months, but don't let the sun scare you. For non-melanoma skin cancer, look for any raised bumps that are red, firm, smooth, cracked, or irritated. For melanoma, look for any existing moles that change shape. Relative to benign moles, melanomas are asymmetrical, misshapen, larger, and have irregular borders or variation in color. If you have lots of moles, fair skin, or red hair, you are at risk of melanoma even if you stay out of the sun.

Night

Sleep affects just about everything in the human body, including mood, mental acuity, athletic performance, metabolism, immune function, and stress levels. Though the evolutionary function of sleep is still a bit of a puzzle, there's no question that sleep is profoundly important to good health.

The biggest changes in human sleep habits took place during the Industrial Age: gas lamps lit up the street; coffee and tea kept us up late (and became a crutch in the morning); mechanical clocks replaced the sun; and electric lights invaded the home and bedroom. People also started to sleep alone, on extremely soft mattresses, and in dedicated quiet spaces.

The evolutionary purpose of sleep is one of the longer running disputes in biology. One cause of the confusion, according to Dr. Jerome Siegel (head of the Center for Sleep Research at UCLA), is that sleep patterns vary considerably across species. Horses sleep only two hours a day, whereas the big brown bat sleeps twenty hours a day. Sleep is pervasive among birds and mammals, and as a result it seems to serve some essential physiological function—perhaps memory consolidation, repair of oxidative damage, or life extension. But for many species, sleep doesn't appear to be a biological necessity: after dolphins give birth, the mothers and calves are continuously awake and active for six or more weeks.

What's clear is that a species's sleep patterns have evolved to match the threats and opportunities it faces. Prey species sleep less than predators, particularly if they lack a safe space to sleep (burrows, nests). During extreme seasonal food shortages (winter), bears go into a sleep-like state: hibernation. Among sandpipers, the males will stay awake for three weeks straight during prime mating season. The key value to sleep, Siegel suggests, is energy conservation during times when food or mating opportunities are scarce. Since the brain uses roughly 20% of the body's energy, it shuts down too: the brain's energy usage drops considerably during sleep. Once sleep evolved, it probably was beneficial for the body to use that downtime in other ways (memory, oxidative repair).

Among hunter-gatherers, sleep patterns are quite a bit different compared to those typical of the Western world. First of all, hunter-gatherers usually didn't sleep in one uninterrupted block. Naps were common during daytime (particularly in tropical climates), and night-time sleep was broken up by tending the fire, keeping watch, talking, going to the bathroom, and sex. Sleep historian Dr. A. Roger Ekirch argues that until the Industrial Revolution, agriculturalists also practiced "segmented sleep" taking place in two parts: a "first sleep" and a "second sleep," each roughly four hours long. While it's not feasible to return to a segmented sleep pattern, it's a poignant illustration of how much human sleep has changed—and how little we realize it.

Our other sleeping habits have changed as well: what we sleep on, who we sleep with, the ambient noise level.

Modern people in the West tend to sleep on far softer surfaces than in the past. The instinct to build a comfortable place to sleep is nothing new: many species build nests, including gorillas, orangutans, and chimpanzees. Dogs and cats immediately know the purpose of their pet beds (even if they prefer yours). But the rise of super-soft mattress technology and enormous fluffy pillows goes quite a bit beyond how humans slept before. Hunter-gatherers are often comfortable sleeping on a soft patch of ground, animal skins, or thinly padded mats—without pillows. Our bedding may have become too soft for our own good. These days many doctors advise people with chronic back pain to use firmer mattresses, not softer ones.

In the past, sleeping was communal. Infants often slept in physical contact with their mother, a practice called co-sleeping, and young children often slept near their parents. Even after the days when people no longer had to crowd around a fire, multiple people would often share beds. In contrast, these days it's quite common for infants and young children to sleep by themselves in their own room. It's often difficult for young children to adjust to sleeping alone: the preverbal child's natural instinct is to be extremely afraid when alone, particularly at night. While the current arrangement may be more convenient for adults, it's a dramatic change from how children (and most young mammals) have always slept.

Communal, segmented sleep doesn't result in much silence. These days we have insulated ourselves from the sounds of other people and nature. From infancy we are training young children to expect near perfect silence, and it becomes harder for them to sleep without it. Again, by growing accustomed to comfort (softness, silence), we have made ourselves weaker and more dependent on those same conditions being present at all times.

Hunter-gatherers seem to fall asleep fairly easily, whereas today it seems like the only thing harder than winding down at the end of the day is waking up the next morning. The problem is that many different things affect sleep quality, including things in the daytime (sunlight, exercise, computer monitors, caffeine) and things in the nighttime (darkness, mattress firmness, other people, noise, alarm clocks).

The body's ability to wake up and fall asleep is controlled by our biological clock: circadian rhythm. Though circadian rhythm is regulated by internal mechanisms, it is continually reset by external cues of day and night. The sun is a reliable clock; it's no coincidence that the earliest clocks were sundials. In addition to light, our circadian rhythm also responds to eating and drinking, temperature, human interaction, and physical activity.

Our hunter-gatherer ancestors lived near the equator, where day and night alternate evenly over twenty-four-hour cycles. As a result, our circadian rhythm is closely tied to fairly even cycles of night and day. (When humans interbred with Neanderthals, we may have picked up some adaptations in circadian rhythm for living at higher latitudes.) By contrast, around the poles, six months of light follows six months of darkness. Researchers have found that some arctic species, such as reindeer, have a weaker circadian rhythm and are active during day or night. Their activity patterns tend to be driven by food availability and seasonal changes, not the sun.

Equatorial hunter-gatherers and arctic reindeer aside, anyone who has gone camping knows that humans have a built-in alarm clock that gets triggered by multiple factors: brightness, temperature, human chatter, and the smell of breakfast. After a day of hiking, a big meal, growing darkness, and no light but stars and a campfire, it's not uncommon for people to fall asleep hours before they would in the city. Our bodies operate in close synchronization with the rhythms of nature.

Today our bodies have become thoroughly confused by the artificial signals of modern life. Light is no longer a cyclical function of the sun, but of always-on indoor lights, TV screens, and computer monitors. Temperature no longer follows a dynamic cycle of cooling at night and warming during the day but sits at a static level set by the thermostat. Human chatter and social interaction used to follow a natural ebb and flow, but now we are more likely to live and sleep in isolation from real people, even while we have 24/7 access to artificial people (faces on TV, voices on the radio). Then, after utterly confusing our circadian rhythm, we try to take back control with stimulants (caffeine, nicotine) and depressants (alcohol, sleeping pills). Is it any wonder that a third of Americans are chronically sleep-deprived?

Many explorers have already faced extreme forms of these very same sleep issues. Dr. Jack Stuster is an adviser to NASA and author of *Bold Endeavors: Lessons from Polar and Space Exploration*, which he begins with a chapter on sleep. Sleep is one of the most challenging aspects of life among polar explorers, submarine personnel, and astronauts, all of whom live in habitats without a natural twenty-four-hour cycle alternating between day and night. Astronauts in low Earth orbit can experience more than a dozen sunrises and sunsets in one twenty-four-hour period. In such environments, sleep disorders are common, including insomnia (inability to sleep) and, to a lesser extent, hypersomnia (excessive sleep). It's also common to see a rise in irritability and a decline in motivation, mood, and performance on physical and mental tasks.

To improve performance, NASA and other agencies now create synthetic signals of day and night called *zeitgebers*. Essentially, zeit-gebers trick the body into thinking night and day are taking place in regular twenty-four-hour cycles.

One of the simplest and most effective zeitgebers is establishing a clear separation of light and dark. In 2010 NASA advised the rescue effort of the thirty-three Chilean miners who were trapped in a col-lapsed copper and gold mine. Initially the miners kept lights on at all times and didn't maintain a regular schedule. On NASA's advice the miners set up a separate dark room for sleeping and maintained a strict daily schedule. An American company called Lighting Science Group designed and donated a lighting system to help the miners maintain their circadian rhythm. The lights were made so that when they were on during the "day," they were brightened and shifted to the blue part of the color spectrum since blue and white light are prevalent in the morning. If lights had to be on during "night," then they were dimmed and shifted to the red part of the color spectrum. Unfortunately the lighting system got held up in customs and was never used.

Most modern people face a similar problem: light no longer dis-tinguishes between day and night. We get too little bright blue light in the morning since we're usually indoors and conventional light-bulbs are far dimmer than the sun. Then we get too much bright blue light in the evening from staring at our TVs and computer monitors.

Morning grogginess might be the new normal, but it doesn't

have to be. To get more light in the morning, one can either make a point to get actual sunshine or purchase a light box. A light box gives off much brighter light than a typical lightbulb. Turning it on when you're getting ready for the day (not even looking at it, but simply having it provide the light in the house) helps to wake up the body and set the circadian rhythm correctly. People like flight attendants, pilots, and nightshift workers often use light boxes to help their bodies adjust to jet lag or graveyard shifts.

Correcting circadian rhythm in the evening starts with dimming the computer monitor. Free software (f.lux is a good one) is easy to install and automatically adjusts monitor intensity and color depending on the time of day: brighter and bluer in the morning, dimmer and redder in the evening. After a few days the difference will hardly be noticeable—but it will be easier to get to sleep. It's also a good idea to cover any electronic devices in the bedroom, including tiny LEDs, and try not to use electronic devices in the hour before bed.

When a habitat lacks strong signals of daytime or nighttime, people tend to extend their waking hours a little bit, resulting in twenty-five- or twenty-six-hour days and a condition called "free-running." Dr. Stuster describes two informal experiments at Antarctic bases where the personnel were allowed to free-run: "The average advance was estimated to be about two hours per day, which offers the welcome illusion of a longer workday when there is much to be accomplished." Even though the researchers weren't actually working more hours when measured over a week or a month, they had the illusion of getting more done each day. For important missions, Stuster concluded that it's far better for personnel to stay synchronized with the actual twenty-four-hour day. That means astronauts and polar explorers have to get to bed on time, even if they consciously don't feel that they need to.

To help explorers get to bed, Stuster recommended avoiding scheduling tasks within one hour of the scheduled sleep period. This gave personnel time to relax before attempting to go to sleep. What's good advice for astronauts in high stress, high-pressure environments is good advice for all of us down here on Earth. Yet most of us have difficulty putting down the screens until right before we flip off the light—only to wake up exhausted.

Most people use electronic alarm clocks simply as a method to wake up in the morning. There are now a huge number of devices that improve upon the standard alarm clock to help people wake up more gently. Many measure sleep cycles and wake people at the optimal time in their sleep cycle. Some wake people with a vibrating arm band, which doesn't wake their partner. Some even shine UV on the skin. However, there is very little effort focused on the much harder problem of helping people get to sleep on time. Our biological clock helps us both wake up *and* go to sleep. Waking up is a lot easier after a good night's rest.

A useful technique is setting an alarm clock—not to wake up, but to get ready for bed. Set an alarm for an hour before bedtime. When it goes off, finish up any work on the computer, turn off the TV, turn off any unnecessary lights, and start to wind down for the day.

It's hard to wind down at the end of the day. But if getting a good night's rest is sufficiently important for high priority missions in outer space, it should also be important for all of us here on Earth.

Part Three

VISIONS

14

HUNTER

As an advocate of a hunter-gatherer diet, I found myself in a rather embarrassing situation: I had never hunted and killed an animal. Sure, I had shot guns before, and I had friends who hunted—but my father, uncles, and grandfathers didn't hunt, so I had never learned. If I wanted to truly re-engage with our Paleolithic food system, I had to learn how to hunt.

Hunting and fishing are in a decades long decline. The largest demographic driver has been increasing urbanization, but there are other dynamics at play. Since our days as hunter-gatherers, knowledge of hunting has been passed down by male relatives within extended families. But that also meant that once a family stopped hunting, it was unlikely that the younger generation would pick it up. More households headed by single mothers meant less chance of fathers passing on hunting knowledge. (This is in parallel to how the rise of hospital-based childbirth, dominated by male physicians, led to the loss of the accumulated wisdom of midwifery, typically passed down from one woman to the next.)

One bright spot in hunting statistics has been a rise in the number of female hunters. Guns tend to level the physical playing field between men and women, and we are approaching gender equality in hunting prowess for the first time in human history.

Over the last few years there has also been renewed interest in hunting among people who care about where their food comes from and have decided to become conscious meat-eaters. As urbanites have headed back into the woods, the result has been plenty of "city slicker" moments. Essays in *The Atlantic* and the *New York Times* about how hunting is the next big thing would be met with raised eyebrows by longtime hunters. The urbanite's first kill merits 5,000 words that explore childhood anxieties, moral anguish, and spiritual redemption in tortuous psychoanalytical detail; a rural twelve-year-old kid gets a picture and a pat on the back. It's not exactly a bold insight that hunting is deeply rooted in the human experience—or that killing a wild animal for the first time can be moving.

In early 2010 I attended a talk by Jackson Landers, a longtime vegetarian turned deer-hunting expert and "Locavore Hunter." After being raised a vegetarian, Landers decided to take up hunting as an adult, motivated in part by a lack of money for groceries. Just as there are "recession vegetarians" who cut back on store-bought meat to save money, there are also "recession hunters" who hunt to put food on the table. But Landers didn't have relatives who could teach him to hunt, so he taught himself—which is when he realized that many other people in the food movement were in the same position. So after years of learning and self-teaching, Landers wrote a book targeted to other novices: *The Beginner's Guide to Hunting Deer for Food.*

As someone who teaches beginners about hunting deer, Landers frequently runs into a phenomenon called the Bambi Effect—people getting squeamish about killing animals that are cute (deer, rabbits) but not about killing animals that are considered repellent (rats, pigeons). There's no reason to think that a rat values its life any less than a deer does, or feels less pain, yet most people instinctively treat them as separate cases.

If the Bambi Effect teaches us anything, it's that our moral intuitions don't necessarily line up with the moral consequences of our actions. When animal rights activists or moral philosophers try to draw moral judgments about wild animal populations, they often suffer from a bad case of "Bambi Ethics" or "Bambi Environmentalism."

They apply human morals to nature in a superficial way, without considering the actual ethical or environmental consequences of their actions. Nature is not a Disney movie.

Although *Bambi* is a lovely story about human emotions and morals, it doesn't teach us much about deer ecology. On the East Coast, humans killed off most natural predators of deer, such as wolves, mountain lions, and bears. Overpopulation inevitably resulted. Landers explains: "When food runs low it is infant mortality among deer that usually runs high. Remember that for the first six weeks or so of life, fawns are hidden away in brush where nobody sees them at all. If there isn't enough food around then the doe's body will reduce the volume or quality of milk available to the fawns. Fawn mortality spikes way up first, then if overpopulation weighed against available resources continues to be out of hand then you will have some older deer dying." So a shortage of predators—human or otherwise—means that lots of cute little Bambis are slowly and painfully starving to death. Even when abandoned fawns are found, rehabilated, and released, they tend to die particularly quickly.

Landers also points out the relatively minuscule "blood footprint" of deer hunting. Deer get to live in the wild, and then they die fairly quickly from a well-placed shot to the vitals. For a deer, the most likely alternatives are a slower and more painful death by a nonhuman predator (i.e., getting torn apart by a coyote), starvation, or disease. Being killed by a skilled human hunter may well be the least painful way for a deer to die. Even by the strict standards of someone who morally opposes killing animals, hunting is morally ambiguous at worst. One has to understand the dynamics of the species and habitat in question, and most armchair ethicists haven't the faintest clue.

To look at it from a holistic perspective, the health of a natural ecosystem is different from the health of any individual organism—and predators play an essential role in the health of wild habitats.

The long-term decline of hunting is now becoming an environmental problem, not all that different from the decline of any predator population. Though divided by class and culture, gun fearing environmentalists are waking up to the role that God fearing hunters have always played in conservation. State wildlife efforts are supported by sales of hunting licenses and taxes on hunting gear. Nonprofit conservation outfits live and die on the size of their membership rolls, often filled by the "hook and bullet" crowd. And, of course, hunters keep wildlife populations in check, which can otherwise devastate local habitats devoid of natural predators. Hunters are the best placed to understand this: predators have always had a deep knowledge of the ecology, life cycle, and behaviors of their prey.

It's difficult to trace cause and effect in complex systems like wild ecosystems or individual organisms, which are characterized by complicated feedback mechanisms. Unintended consequences are the rule, not the exception.

An unfortunately poignant example of Bambi Ethics took place in the United States in regard to the horse population. In 2006, having documented a variety of abuses—from living horses with missing limbs to others left to bleed to death—animal rights activists successfully lobbied for legislation that banned horse slaughtering. Yet the ban on slaughtering, driven in part by the provincial notion that My Little Pony shouldn't be eaten (honestly, I don't see why not), led to even more abuses. Responsible owners shipped horses to Mexico to be slaughtered, where conditions were far worse than at the American slaughterhouses. Others just abandoned their horses to die, unwilling to pay for humane euthanasia. Recognizing this, even PETA (People for the Ethical Treatment of Animals) argued for the re-legalization of horse slaughtering—and to their credit they pointed out that they never supported the ban in the first place. Horse slaughtering was quietly re-legalized in 2011.

When it comes to stewardship of animal populations, we have to start with things as they exist today. Humans have already altered wild habitats, typically wiping out other predators at the top of the food chain. Reintroducing predators has run into some problems: there's wavering local support for the growing wolf population in the Rockies, and there's not exactly anyone clamoring to reintroduce wolves along the Eastern Seaboard. At this point, the most ethical option is not to stop hunting animals, but to re-enter the food chain and replace the predators that we displaced. To be good stewards of such ecosystems, we have an ethical obligation to become surrogate predators.

The goal of hunting isn't to keep nature in some kind of unachievable stasis—it's always in a state of dynamic flux. The goal is to prevent a singularly invasive species from taking over and despoiling a habitat—which is exactly what most conservationists try to avoid when it comes to the human footprint. For example, Asian carp now clog up the Mississippi and threaten to do the same to the Great Lakes. Asian carp feed on tiny plankton, causing a collapse in other species that depend on the plankton (either directly or indirectly), reducing the overall diversity of the habitat. In Africa, the Nile perch has driven a majority of native species to extinction after being introduced at Lake Victoria, with a few lucky species only surviving on in captivity.

There's actually a straightforward solution to invasive species: *Eat 'em!*

For as long as humans have had projectile weapons, we have demonstrated our ability to eat species to extinction. We're good at it, we've done it before, and we know we can do it again (though we should stop short of extinction). How they taste is nothing that a little cooking technique and a lot of butter can't solve. Let's just turn this voracious talent of ours in a more productive direction—away from struggling species like Chilean sea bass (a more appetizing euphemism for the Patagonian toothfish) and toward invasive species that are overrunning their habitats.

It's time for us to become *invasivores.*

Some conservationists have concerns about harvesting invasive species for food, voiced in a paper published in *Conservation Letters.* The authors point out that turning an invasive species into an economic resource creates an incentive for people to maintain its population—and even expand it into new areas. Locals may even start to care about it. Seemingly without realizing it, the authors

RISE OF THE INVASIVORES

Asian carp: Native to China, Vietnam, and Russia, Asian carp
have spread through the Mississippi, threatening to enter
the Great Lakes. Asian carp eat continuously, sometimes
up to 40% of their body weight a day. Since they feed on
plankton, they are relatively free of pollutants. Great in
ceviche.

Feral pig: Typically a cross between wild boars and domesticated pigs, feral swine are estimated to number five million
in the United States, concentrated in the South and West.
They are voracious, smart, nocturnal, fast breeding—and
made of bacon. Yum!

Black spiny-tailed iguana: Native to Central and South America, these iguanas are overrunning parts of Florida. Though
mostly herbivorous, they also eat small vertebrates, including
eggs and hatchling sea turtles. Tasting like chicken but with
the texture of crab, they make great taco filler.

Lionfish: Native to the Indian Ocean, lionfish are destroying
reef fish populations in the Caribbean. Lionfish tastes like
a cross between lobster and Chilean sea bass.

Kudzu: Known as "the vine that ate the South," kudzu was
brought over from Japan in the late nineteenth century.
Kudzu grows over other plants, blocking their access to
light and killing them. Kudzu leaves can be eaten raw in a
salad or cooked like spinach. The purple blossoms can
be made into jelly, and the starchy roots can be eaten like
potatoes or ground up into a powder or paste.

made arguments that, when applied to endangered species, suggest
that turning them into an economic resource might be an excellent
way to ensure their survival.

In 2011 an Arizona restaurant announced that it would be serving lion tacos as a one-day promotion. The lion meat was to be legally

sourced from African lions that are bred and raised on a farm in California. Animal rights activists went berserk, sending death threats to the restaurant owner and his family, and he eventually withdrew the promotion. Now, it's not immediately clear why, from an ethical perspective, eating a lion raised on a farm in California is any different from, say, eating a cow—other than the Bambi Effect (or the Simba Effect?). According to the rationale laid out in *Conservation Letters,* raising endangered species as food would actually be an effective way to ensure the continuity of a species: create property rights, turn it into an economic resource, and let people pay to hunt it, eat it, or watch it. What we have to be careful about is that various species have different requirements for a decent life, so we may want to restrict this to only the most endangered species—the ones that stand to benefit most from greater numbers.

In fact, this is the exact same rationale used to justify eating heritage breeds. Heritage breeds are varieties of plants and animals that used to exist in far greater numbers but have been almost completely displaced by a tiny number of genetic variants. Popular among chefs and foodies, they often have more flavor than store-bought varieties, which were typically selected for their suitability to industrial agriculture, not for their taste. The farmers who raise heritage breeds desperately attempt to create space in the market, realizing that there is a clear path to those breeds' continued survival: people eating them. Species that hitch their wagon to humanity tend to hang around. It's not due to their hunting skills that there are more chickens than humans on earth.

If hunting is morally justified, in part, by environmental stewardship, then the flip side is a moral responsibility not to eat wild species into extinction. The closest many people come to participating in the Paleolithic food system is eating wild fish. Unfortunately, many wild fisheries are on the verge of collapse. Whereas the wild deer population is managed by local groups, the oceans are still one big commons. Overfishing predictably results when no individual or group has an incentive to maintain the resource over the long run.

So for me, the first question was "Which species to hunt?"

Noted hunter, author, and TV host Steven Rinella points out that in rural areas, children usually start with squirrel hunting (or shooting rats at the local landfill). Squirrels are abundant and easy to find; they can be shot with a low powered rifle or high powered pellet gun; hunting them doesn't require expensive specialty hunting gear; squirrel season is usually quite long; permits are inexpensive (or even unnecessary); and hunters are allowed to take many squirrels a day, thus offering more opportunities to practice. Plus, squirrel meat is perfect for stews.

Since I was not allowed to hunt squirrels in Central Park (or rats in the subway), the next most logical animal to hunt was deer. There are lots of them, they provide a fair bit of meat, and there is a large culture around deer hunting, so it would be easier to learn. When it came to choosing a method of hunting, I faced a catch-22. If a hunter uses a high powered rifle, critics of hunting say it's unfair—the animal never had a chance. Yet if a hunter uses traditional hunting methods, like a bow, the same critics say it's cruel—the animal could be wounded and suffer. Some people just can't be pleased, so it's pointless to try. Traditional forms of hunting put predator and prey on more equal footing and thus bring a greater unity with nature—but this kind of hunting is an acquired skill, and skills require a lot of time and practice to develop. As an unskilled hunter I chose to start with a gun and shooting at deer from a tree stand, which makes it easier to avoid the worst outcome: wounding but not killing the animal.

Joe, a family friend back in Michigan, heard that I was learning how to hunt, so he invited me to join him, his extended family, and close family friends at "Deer Camp." Each year around opening day, Deer Camp served as a reunion for all the men in the family—they had been doing it for decades. I jumped on the offer.

After Joe took me to pick up some hunting gear, we pulled into the farm where we would be hunting. It belonged to Joe's wife's uncle, Uncle Bob. There I met the whole hunting crew: Uncle Jay (Bob's brother), Josh (Bob's son), and Jim Sr., a close friend of Uncle Bob, who, along with his two adult sons—Jim Jr. and Chris—have hunted on his property for nearly twenty years. It was exactly the type of informal family tradition that I had lacked, and they welcomed me in. They did a great job as surrogate brothers and uncles, relentlessly making fun of me for every little thing I did wrong.

Uncle Jay lent me an old 12-gauge pump action shotgun, open sights (no scope), branded as Sears & Roebuck (made by Mossberg). I was shooting with slugs. (Unlike typical shotgun pellets, which spray at close range, a shotgun slug is a single lead projectile used at medium range. We were hunting in a populated area that requires hunters to use shotguns instead of longer-range rifles.) It had been a year since I had gone shooting, so Uncle Jay took me back into one of Uncle Bob's fields for a little target practice.

"I'm left-eye dominant, so I shoot left-handed," I told him.

"Nuts, if I knew you shot left-handed, I would have brought my left-handed shotgun," Jay deadpanned. It took me a few confused moments to realize he was making fun of me—shotguns work either way.

That was the first in a long series of gaffes. I forgot whether I was supposed to close one eye when looking down the sights of the shotgun (yes). They had binoculars with a range finder, and I looked through the wrong end. I would take a long time to line up a shot, pull the trigger, and hear a click—immediately followed by peals of laughter because I had forgotten to put a new shell in. After a little target practice we returned to Uncle Bob's for dinner and beers with the rest of the guys before turning in for a very short night's sleep.

We all woke up at 4:45 A.M. Joe drove me to the field where I had done target practice. The windshield was frosted over and the fog was thick, so Joe drove slowly through the darkness. Everybody had their favorite spots, and Uncle Jay gave me his lucky tree stand, located just inside the tree line on the edge of a soybean field. The sun hadn't risen yet, the fog hadn't lifted, and it was hard to see ten feet in front of me. We found the stand, I clambered up a metal ladder to a platform thirty feet up in a tree, and Uncle Jay left for his own spot.

It was just me, the darkness, and the fog.

My first impression of hunting had nothing to do with being a hunter-gatherer, but of being an animal. A hunter must hide: quiet his voice, mask his scent, and camouflage himself as plants and dirt. Not only is this difficult, it's disorienting. I completely lacked the senses that I needed (smell), and the ones I had were calibrated to an urban lifestyle (sight, hearing).

At the start I was completely paranoid. Every tiny movement seemed like a signal flare revealing my location, every rustle a fog-horn announcing my whereabouts to all the animals in the forest. Hypersensitized, I held my breath and basically didn't move a muscle for the first two and a half hours, intensely focusing on the fog in front of me. Eventually I realized that it was probably all right to shift in my seat. Looking for prey became less a matter of constant intense focus and more of a wandering gaze looking for flashes of movement interspersed with systematic scans of the terrain.

More than just blending into the background, a good hunter takes on the mindset of his prey. He must experience the world as his prey does. For example, deer hunters know that deer have far superior senses of hearing and smell than humans do. Hunters quickly learn the importance of quiet, slow, and steady movements, scent-less soaps and deodorant, and staying downwind. Hunters wear a combination of camouflage matching the color and pattern of their hunting environment, and blaze orange for safety. It's not just a fashion statement—it's the ideal color to be invisible to deer (which have poor vision in the orange part of the color spectrum) and highly visible to humans.

Oddly, the two groups of people who most often put themselves in the mind of another species are hunters and animal rights activists. But while animal rights activists seem to focus only on the pain of animals, good hunters experience a broader spectrum of their prey's conscious experience—not just fear and pain. As a result, hunters tend to be a pretty humane bunch. Like the bias for violent, negative stories on the nightly news, all the attention goes to the rare hunter who indiscriminately poaches, wounds, and butchers animals—and not to the millions who don't.

There's actually very little shooting in hunting. This may come as a surprise to people whose only experience with hunting is the video game *Big Buck Hunter*. Among hunters, not only is it frowned upon to wound (and not kill) an animal, but it's also considered an indication of skill to make a clean kill with one shot, dropping the animal where it stands. Most hunters are models of patience and restraint, passing up many more shots than they end up taking. There can be any number of reasons: an obstructed view, a bad angle, the range, too much movement, poor visibility, or simply because it's a hunting partner's turn to shoot. Deer hunting is less like paintball and more like bird-watching. Perhaps it's no surprise that the current generation of teenagers is more excited by video games.

The first morning passed and I didn't see a deer. Dawn and dusk are the two best times to hunt, since deer are largely nocturnal. Late in the morning I climbed down, met up with Uncle Jay, and joined the other guys for lunch. I returned to the stand a few hours later, but the afternoon was just as slow as the morning. Hours of nothing.

Then I saw one.

A doe was about twenty yards away, in front of me to my left, at about ten o'clock. She had wandered a couple of feet into the harvested soybean field and was nibbling on some of the leftovers. Her location happened to be the one exact spot where branches obstructed my view. I knew I couldn't get a clean shot off. Even so, it was my first look at a deer and I wanted to see if I could get my gun around and into position without startling her. I slowly maneuvered into place.

Actually, there were two deer. The doe was accompanied by a buck fawn, which was still hanging back behind the tree line. Unable to get a clean look at the doe's vitals, I just sat there and watched. After a couple of minutes they turned around and started walking back into the woods. I stood up in my tree stand, which was facing toward the soybean field, and turned around. They were moving too quickly between the trees, and I didn't think to use my deer call to make them pause. Once again, I couldn't get a clean look. They disappeared into the deep woods.

Maybe they would come back, I thought, so I remained standing and scanned the underbrush. It was dusk, and light was fading fast. Sure enough, a few minutes later, one of the deer came out of the deep woods. It stopped about thirty yards away. I leaned against the tree with my shoulder to steady myself, took aim, exhaled slowly, and pulled the trigger. Over three and a half days of hunting, I only took one shot—but it was one *good* shot.

The deer fell where it stood. I quickly chambered a new shell, preparing to take a second shot if necessary. It wasn't. The deer moved its limbs for a few seconds then was motionless. Shot or stunned deer will sometimes play dead and then bound away upon one's approach, so I remained in the stand for a few more minutes with my sights on the deer. Then I climbed down out of the stand and approached the body. My hunting partner, Uncle Jay, left his stand and joined me.

"Keep your gun trained on the deer," he said.

It was long dead. The slug had entered through the spine above the front shoulder, moving through the vitals, exiting at a lower point on the far shoulder—a clean kill.

"Nice shot," Uncle Jay said. "Congrats on your first deer. Looks like a buck fawn."

And then it dawned on me. Bambi was a buck fawn: I had just shot Bambi.

For me—and more important, for the buck fawn I just shot—the Bambi Effect wasn't just a philosophical exercise. I felt exhilaration, pride, respect, gratitude. There was no chorus of angels or sulfur and brimstone. I had shot a deer. Uncle Jay gave me a pat on the back.

We put the safeties on, set down our guns, and Uncle Jay talked me through skinning and gutting it. For someone unaccustomed to touching a dead animal, much less skinning one, even placing my hand on the dead deer was a little gross. I started at the breastbone and carefully cut down the center of the stomach, being careful to avoid puncturing the gut. An ill-placed nick of the blade can release a morass of bile and half-digested plant matter. It stinks terribly, even to seasoned hunters, and dressing a gut shot deer is the most unpleasant task in hunting.

After successfully moving past the gut, I continued in a delicate manner, almost as if I could somehow kill, dress, butcher, and eat the entire animal without getting blood on my hands. Uncle Jay stopped me, laughed, and looked me in the eye. "Not gonna be able to do this without getting your hands dirty," he said. I took up the blade and stuck my hands inside the deer's body. My hands were cold, and the deer's body warmed them. It's an odd feeling to warm yourself in another animal's dead body: I didn't have to eat it for energy; I absorbed its heat directly.

The best way to field dress (and butcher) a deer is to cut along natural joints and seams; deceptively, this makes it appear as if the animal was made to be butchered. After cutting down the belly, I had cut around each side of the penis and down to the anus. Uncle Jay had mercy on me, pulling out the anus himself and tying it off to prevent poop from coming out. Then I went back inside the groin to detach the lower digestive tract. Because I had cut the esophagus, the upper digestive tract was also detached. Then, using only my hands, I separated the entire gut from the inside of the deer's rib cage, pulled it out of the chest cavity, and dropped it onto the grass.

That's what it means to "gut" a deer.

Then I moved on to the remaining internal organs. My shot had destroyed the spine and part of the lungs but had left the edible organ meats intact: heart, kidneys, and liver. I removed those and put them each in a plastic Ziploc bag, which Uncle Jay then placed in a small cooler.

It was just about dark at this point. We left the deer where it lay, walked half a mile to the truck, drove it back through the field, and stopped near to where the deer carcass lay. He took the two hind legs, I took the two forelegs, and we carried it out of the woods. Then

I dragged the body to the truck, loaded it in the back, and drove off to see how everyone else had fared.

There are few better feelings than returning from a successful hunt. When we got back, all the guys had already gathered in one of the big barns. We cracked open some cold ones. Joe had scored a 12 point buck, a beast of an animal—the Great Prince of the Forest to my Bambi. My deer carcass looked small hanging from a hook in the big barn.

"That's a pretty big dog you shot there," Uncle Bob said with a barely disguised grin.

It definitely was no trophy, but I consoled myself with the fact that natural predators target the young or sickly. Plus, young deer have more tender meat, so it would be good to eat.

"Wait for an older buck or doe next time," Uncle Bob said. "It gives them a chance to grow, and you'll get more meat."

Jim Jr. helped me skin the rest of the deer as it hung in the barn. There was a distinct but hard to place moment when it stopped looking like a deer and started looking like venison. Jim then showed me how to remove the tenderloins, in order to get those refrigerated quickly.

After dinner we drove the deer carcasses to the home of Joe's father-in-law, who runs a small butchering operation during deer season. He has a refrigerated room that can hold a dozen or so deer carcasses waiting to be butchered, and a separate room to break them down into cuts. A few days later I pulled out of Uncle Bob's driveway with a (small) cooler full of delicious venison.

One of the most satisfying aspects of a successful hunt is sharing the meat with others. Eating big game always has been a communal activity for hunter-gatherers. Not only did we hunt in packs, but successful hunts often involved an element of luck; sharing reduces the risk of going home empty-handed. And since meat quickly spoils without refrigeration, there's no way for one person to hoard it. Even though we now have deep freezers, there's still no reason not to share.

I cooked the liver for a paleo potluck at a local CrossFit box. Most people make the mistake of cooking liver for too long, which actually gives it a stronger, more "iron-y" taste. I just cut it into small strips, cooked it in grass-fed butter for a minute or so on each side, and served it with onions sautéed in butter. I made some of the tenderloin for Thanksgiving dinner. Again, the big danger is over-cooking it. Wild game contains less fat than beef, and that means it cooks faster. I just added a few herbs, salt, and pepper.

Delicious.

Vegetables you've grown in your own garden just taste better. Meals that you've cooked yourself just taste better. And yes, animals that you've killed yourself just taste better.

15

GATHERER

There is an annoying aspect to eating paleo: many people mistakenly believe that I eat an exclusively carnivorous diet—all meat, all raw, all the time. As delicious as that sounds, it's not actually true. But my persona as a modern hunter-gatherer is perceived as a pure "hunter"—and my foil was a pure "gatherer": vegans and vegetarians.

Even though this is somewhat of a false dichotomy, we live in a time when meat-eating has come under fire, especially from advocates of a plant-based diet, animal rights activists, and environmentalists. I was forced to confront a barrage of uncomfortable questions: Is it ethical to eat meat, particularly if it were sourced from factory farms? Is a meat-based diet environmentally sustainable? Should I date vegetarian women?

It may come as a surprise that I found important common ground: there *are* serious environmental and ethical problems with the industrial food system.

Without question, the industrial food system has some major environmental drawbacks: fertilizer runoff creates coastal dead zones; monocrop farming depletes the topsoil of nutrients; overuse of antibiotics breeds antibiotic-resistant bacteria; eating meat requires more land devoted to growing feed for animals. Many of these negative consequences of industrial agriculture go unseen by the average person, who has little day-to-day knowledge of where food comes from. I have to give credit to those who were at the forefront of pointing out these problems, especially since I wasn't among them.

At the same time, traditional agriculture is not exactly a vegetarian utopia. A traditional "organic" farm is a complicated and productive synergism of species. Animal manure fertilizes the soil. Crop rotation harnesses the power of cover crops (usually nitrogen-fixing legumes) to renew soil fertility. Pigs can convert just about any inedible waste into delicious bacon. Sheep, goats, cows, and other ruminants can graze on land unsuitable for crops. Genetic diversity among both plants and animals provides diversification against insects and pests and maintains the overall stock of genetic diversity in the food system. Domesticated animals have always been inseparable from traditional farming at scale: it is possible to herd without domesticated plants, but it is next to impossible to farm without domesticated animals.

Animals bring a great deal of value to a farm: they provide food (turning inedible grasses into highly nutritious meat, milk, and eggs), produce fertilizer (manure), and generate horsepower (plowing, transportation). The people who actually farm, not just opine on it, depend on animals as both a source of income and a source of sustenance. No traditional farmers, no traditional farming.

As the Industrial Revolution uprooted traditional agriculture, industrial machines displaced beasts of burden. Horses had it rough: tractors replaced the plow horse, trucks replaced the cart horse, and chemical fertilizers replaced horse manure. The only thing that animals could do more efficiently than machines, in the short run, was convert grass and grain into meat, milk, and eggs. Large industrial farms increasingly specialized in growing one species of plant (soybeans, corn, wheat), and large factory farms specialized in raising one species of animal (chickens, cows, pigs). The traditional farm's interconnectedness of species—plant, animal, human—came to an end.

Industrial agriculture increased yields, lowered the cost of food, and led to greater urbanization (wealth creating and eco-friendly)—but it also changed our relationship with domesticated species. As industrial methods were applied to raising and slaughtering animals, efficiency was ruthless; the warm flesh of biology stood no chance against the cold steel of the factory. The fiercest critics of this new industrial paradigm were vegans, vegetarians, and animal rights activists.

There are two main philosophies of animal activism: animal *welfare* and animal *rights*. Advocates of animal welfare are primarily interested in reducing animal suffering. Most vegetarians fall into this category. Their stance boils down to a fairly straightforward utilitarian calculus that, at some point, animal suffering trumps human needs and wants. This is a logic that most non-vegetarians accept at some level, given widespread disapproval of puppy mills, cockfighting, and general animal cruelty.

Advocates of animal rights—who think of themselves as "abolitionists"—consider using animals in any way to be wrong, and a reduction in animal suffering is just a distraction that perpetuates an inherently unethical system of exploitation. They believe that animals have an inalienable right to their own lives, and that therefore it's not permissible to eat animals if there are other sources of food. ("Because they taste good" doesn't count.)

Regardless of how animal suffering factors in to anyone's moral calculus, factory farms are undeniably unpleasant and painful for the animals. One problem is severe overcrowding. Animals don't have room to move or sometimes even turn around. Chickens can't stretch their wings and alternate between extreme discomfort and outright pain. Living in a confined space with so many other members of their species is extremely stressful. Left to their own devices, they often wound or kill each other. The tips of bird beaks have to be cauterized off so the birds don't peck each other to death. Gestation crates are designed to prevent mother pigs from fighting and crushing their babies due to overcrowded conditions.

Not only are their physical spaces constrained, but the animals' natural life cycles are completely disrupted. Animals are kept indoors, experience no natural cycles of day or night, seasons, or mating cycles. Young are taken from their mothers, and mothers can't rear or nurse their own babies. Dairy production requires only nursing females, which means a lot of male calves become veal. Male chickens don't produce eggs or desirable meat—and because they are considered economically worthless, they are killed soon after they hatch, sometimes by being ground up alive.

Factory farms don't even live up to the hunter's ethic: a natural life and a swift death.

Leading a natural life can be a theoretical proposition for species that have been heavily genetically modified. Industrial chickens have breasts so heavy they can barely walk. Some of this is undoubtedly beneficial to humans without doing major harm to animals—a cow that specializes in milk production, not meat production, is not necessarily a bad thing.

Disease is another problematic aspect of factory farming. Similar to the rise of infectious disease in early cities, crowded factory farms are exceedingly filthy and conducive to germs. One troubling possibility is what would happen when such a disease jumps to *Homo sapiens*. Furthermore, farmers routinely use antibiotics to keep animals from dying from infections. The consistent overuse of antibiotics is leading to resistant strains of bacteria that do not respond to known medications. In one study in Boston, nearly 20% of *E. coli* patients carried strains with multidrug resistance, up from 2% only four years prior.

Yet if vegetarianism's strength has been unearthing these problems, its weakness has been creating practical solutions to them. Sometimes it sounds like the entire vegetarian movement is a one-drum orchestra—*Less meat!*—and supporters just keep banging it over and over. Factory farming hasn't appreciably slowed in the United States and is quickly spreading to China and other parts of the developing world. Global meat consumption is up, not down. When vegetarians tried to popularize the notion of "Meatless Mondays" among meat-eaters, they were implicitly acknowledging the limited appeal of full-on vegetarianism.

If asked, many vegetarians report that they chose their diet for philosophical, ethical, and moral reasons, in addition to health reasons. Though moral philosophers provide arguments in defense of vegetarianism, heady arguments can't possibly explain vegetarianism's gut level appeal to millions of people.

There are many paths to vegetarianism, but the most well trodden one follows three steps: (1) greater empathy for animals; (2) visceral disgust with eating meat; and (3) a starkly moralistic outlook on the issues surrounding meat.

First, many eventual vegetarians grow up humanizing animals. This attitude is fostered by lots of exposure to pets, stuffed animals, and Disney movies; little exposure to hunting, fishing, or working farms; and only ever eating meat that is sold and served in ways that mask its animal origin. At some point they have an epiphany that meat actually comes from an animal. Since animals are humanized, they have greater empathy for them, and they can't bring themselves to eat meat anymore.

Second, vegetarians often use disgust to create and reinforce an aversion to eating meat. Since most people grow up enjoying meat, the disgust mechanism is necessary to make meat seem distasteful and revolting. Due to their lack of exposure to the origins of Paleolithic meat (hunting, fishing) or Agricultural meat (working farms), many people already have a disgust reflex with a hair trigger. Knowledge of the origins of Industrial meat (factory farms) triggers extreme disgust and all meat becomes viscerally revolting.

Third, due to the close ties between disgust and moral judgments, eating meat becomes not just a question of health or a cool utilitarian calculus, but of stark, black-and-white morality. Abstaining from animal products becomes a moralized act of physical purity and cleansing.

So who follows this path to vegetarianism?

In theory, vegetarianism is a lifestyle that anyone might adopt. In practice, vegetarianism is popular among a very specific slice of the general population in the Western world: young urban women. Studies of vegetarians generally find that 65 to 75% of vegetarians are female—in other words, two to three times as many women as men. Given the common path to vegetarianism, this skew starts to make sense.

A look at the General Social Survey reveals which characteristics correlate with empathy toward animals. In 2008, 1,400 people were asked their level of agreement with the following statement: "Scientists should be allowed to do research that causes pain and injury to animals like dogs and chimpanzees if it produces new information about human health problems." A person's sex was more important in determining the response than were political views, religious views, education, intelligence, race, or age. Half of men (52%) agreed or strongly agreed with the statement on animal testing, nearly twice the number of women (27%) who agreed. A third of women strongly disagreed (31%), more than double the number of men (14%). American women appear to have greater empathy toward animals than American men do.

Nature and nurture both play a role in this, and it's tricky to untangle their contribution. Men tend to be innately more violent than women, and culture often reinforces this tendency. Men and boys are supposed to toughen up, deal with the cruel world, take violence and dish it out when necessary, and not be wimpy or cry. Some male vegetarians have described how their rejection of meat felt emasculating, since they were also rejecting the ancient male role of killer and griller. Vegetarians frequently try to counteract this feminine connotation by touting all the manly men who are vegetarian (*Mike Tyson!*). One article even profiled a few masculine kale-loving "hegans." At the very least, the protestations to the contrary show that the perception exists.

Whether male or female, a person is understandably traumatized if they learn that the meat on their plate used to be a cute, cuddly friend—and the result is often a moment of intense aversion or disgust.

The sense of disgust is an increasingly well-understood phenomenon. Steven Pinker describes disgust as an "intuitive microbiology," a capacity that keeps us away from potential sources of infection. Drs. Paul Rozin, Jonathan Haidt, and Clark McCauley—three of the preeminent scholars on the subject of disgust—have found that around the world disgust is triggered by the same nine categories: "food, body products, animals, sexual behaviors, contact with death or corpses, violations of the exterior envelope of the body (including gore and deformity), poor hygiene, interpersonal contamination (contact with unsavory human beings), and certain moral offenses." To the extent that there is a common denominator, it is that all of these categories are potential vectors for disease (recall chapter 4).

Studies have repeatedly shown that women have a much more sensitive disgust reflex than men. Evolutionarily, this tendency makes a lot of sense. Women used to spend much of their lives in close contact with children, whether pregnant, nursing, or beyond. Pregnant women and infants are particularly susceptible to infection, and it would have been a matter of life and death to stay away from sources of contamination. It's not that women have "weak stomachs"; they just have discriminating tastes. The fact that vegetarianism ends up attracting a lot of women isn't necessarily a coincidence; it may be their evolved psychology playing out in a modern context.

If this hypothesis is true, one would predict that women would be particularly susceptible to the disgust-based tactics used by advocates of vegetarianism. For example, advocates of vegetarianism often depict meat-eating as an inherently disgusting act. A common tactic is to refer to meat as a "corpse," "carcass," or "decomposing flesh"—all of which are potential disease vectors that can trigger disgust. Many books that attempt to persuade people to be vegan have copious references to most of the nine categories related to disgust. They're a veritable shit show of corpses, feces, blood, urine, and spit—subtly (or not so subtly) playing up the specter of contamination, disease, and moral and physical impurity.

Skinny Bitch, a bestselling vegan diet book that targets young urban women, tries to gross out readers: "Pretend you are eating 'perfect meat.' Great. But what exactly are you eating? 'Meat' is the decomposing, decaying, rotting flesh of a dead animal." The authors also summon a sense of physical contamination from ingesting meat: "You want to put a dead animal corpse—that has been rotting away for months—in your mouth? In your body?" Foods that are "gross" are so self-evidently unhealthy that any scientific discussion becomes superfluous.

Even highbrow treatments of veganism use the same tactics. Jonathan Safran Foer, author of the bestselling *Eating Animals*, marshals his considerable writing talents to gross out his readers: "[H]ow good could a drug-stuffed, disease-ridden, shit-contaminated animal possibly taste?" However, it doesn't require much literary talent to turn people's stomachs with descriptions of factory farms; they are, in fact, quite disgusting and are hotbeds of pathogens.

Animal rights activists decry that modern consumers don't know where their food comes from, yet their disgust-based tactics actually *depend* on people not knowing where their food comes from. People familiar with farms, hunting, or butchering animals don't get disgusted as easily. The contemporary trend of ethical meat-eating—permaculture farming, locavore hunting, specialty butchers—has been excoriated by animal rights activists such as Foer, who see it as a way for so-called ethical omnivores to clear their conscience while still eating plenty of factory farmed meat. Both sides seem to realize that participation in humane animal slaughter is one of the antidotes to the "gross out" tactics used by vegans and animal rights activists.

But disgust isn't just about being "grossed out"; it's also intimately tied to our moral judgments. Humans move surprisingly easily from physical disgust to moral revulsion. In *The Righteous Mind*, Jonathan Haidt describes the role of disgust in separating one group of people from another. Throughout history, disgust has been harnessed to achieve in-group purity and cleanliness at the expense of filthy, inhuman outsiders. The problem is that these moral intuitions can easily be used to justify the persecution of others. The disgust reflex is powerful, and thus potentially dangerous. For that reason alone, using disgust in a sociopolitical context merits caution.

PETA—not a group that anyone would describe as cautious—understands the power of disgust and how it can drive moral judgments. In 2003 PETA released an exhibition called "Holocaust on Your Plate," featuring giant panels that juxtaposed images of animals crammed into factory farms and Jews crammed into concentration camps. Though PETA funded the project with money from a Jewish donor, the exhibition unsurprisingly caused uproar in the wider Jewish community and invited a harsh condemnation from the Anti-Defamation League. More than just trivializing the Holocaust, this intentionally provocative tactic showed a stunning lack of historical awareness of the role that disgust played in the persecution of the Jewish people.

Historically, vegetarianism has been swept up in various moral and ideological crusades, which seem to alternate between legitimate moral advances and those of more dubious merit.

Vegetarianism was a popular plank of the Progressive Era's "Clean Living Movement," which also championed alcohol prohibition and antismoking laws. Dr. John Harvey Kellogg—inventor of Kellogg's Corn Flakes, a prominent member of the Seventh-day Adventist Church and noted advocate of vegetarianism—believed that eating meat increased the sexual appetite (which he regarded as a very bad thing). He waged a campaign against masturbation, even undertaking the sexual mutilation of boys (by sewing closed the foreskin to prevent an erection) and girls (by applying acid to the clitoris).

Acting only out of their desire for the betterment of mankind, Progressives also championed another way to purify humanity by purging it of unclean elements: eugenics. Advocates of eugenics defended forced sterilization of "undesirables" as a cleansing purge for the greater health of society.

Modern vegetarians show surprisingly little self-awareness of the historical role of disgust in the rise of their own belief system, and how disgust has the potential to drive dangerously ideological viewpoints.

HITLER THE VEGETARIAN

In any argument over the merits of vegetarianism someone inevitably mentions Adolf Hitler. In a 1937 profile of Hitler in the *New York Times* the author observed that it was "well known that Hitler is a vegetarian," but also indicated he ate milk, eggs, and occasionally meat. According to the diary of Joseph Goebbels, Nazi minister of propaganda, Hitler had hopes of imposing vegetarianism within Germany after winning the war: "He believes more than ever that meat-eating is harmful to humanity. Of course he knows that during the war we cannot completely upset our food system. After the war, however, he intends to tackle this problem also." Nazi Germany even instituted the most stringent animal welfare laws of its era, including restrictions on hunting, trapping, and vivisection.

Many have struggled to explain the apparent paradox between Hitler's attitude toward animals and his extermination of the Jews, but there is no paradox to explain. Hitler had an extreme sense of disgust, which litters his writings and speeches when he was referring to "undesirable" elements of society. Hitler the vegetarian would also use terminology similar to that of modern vegans, describing meat-eaters as "corpse-eaters" (*leichenfresser*).

This heightened sense of disgust contributed to an extreme ideology of moral and physical purity—which is great if you're a member of the in-group, but horrific if you're a member of an out-group. Purification of the body could be brought about only through purging it of "unclean" elements (meat, alcohol, tobacco), and the same was true of purifying the in-group of contamination from "unclean" elements (Jews, Gypsies, the disabled, homosexuals).

More recently, another area where vegetarianism has become stridently moralized is in feminist ideology. The seminal piece linking feminism and vegetarianism is Carol Adams's 1990 book *The Sexual*

Politics of Meat: A Feminist-Vegetarian Critical Theory, which the *New York Times* has described as "a bible of the vegan community." This vegan holy book asserts that meat-eating is a mechanism to enforce "patriarchy," a state of affairs where men are the primary authority figures in society (and thus can be blamed for anything and everything wrong in society).

Adams's path to vegetarianism should sound familiar. After returning home from her first year at Yale Divinity School, she learned that her family's pony had been shot in a hunting accident. Running to the site, she witnessed "the dead body of a pony I had loved." That night she took a bite out of a hamburger—and realized she could never look at meat in the same way again. Eventually she developed a stronger aversion to meat and gave it up entirely. Over time she began to view meat-eating in starkly ideological terms—as a symbol of male oppression—and wrote her influential book on the subject.

As just one example of her ideological viewpoint, Adams makes the dubious yet incendiary claim that meat-eating encourages rape. Adams's meat-hating, man-hating mantra—"Eat Rice Have Faith in Women"—is intended to undermine the male culture of meat-eating, thus undermining male power, thus reducing rape.

Rapists deserve lengthy jail sentences—and rape victims deserve serious scholarship, not feminist illogic.

Adams seems unaware that rape (or rape-like behavior) has been observed in species with all manner of diets, such as chimpanzees, dolphins, birds, and spiders. Adams's claim also runs aground on the observation that hunting has been an enduring source of male sex appeal for millions of years—that is to say, heterosexual women have generally rewarded great hunters with *consensual* sex. When CBS News correspondent Bob Simon asked a young Masai man why the tribe continues to hunt increasingly endangered lions, he answered, "It makes you famous. You get the whole community to know you, because you killed a lion . . . If you had one girlfriend, you get twenty more." Among large-scale contemporary cultures, Adams would be hard-pressed to find one that is more rice-loving and vegetarian-friendly than India—which also happens to have an atrocious record on sexual violence toward women. The best way to prevent rape is to understand what causes it, and that requires clear-eyed scientific research unsullied by ideology—in much the same way scientists study other destructive phenomena, such as hurricanes or earthquakes.

Adams's ideological advocacy of vegetarianism is also hard to square with a tolerant and inclusive vision of female empowerment that is unprejudiced toward women who choose to bear children. Pregnancy is a particularly risky time to eat a vegan diet. Women who would like control over their own reproductive system would be wise to ignore feminist dietary dogma.

Adams is correct that meat has long been associated with masculinity for as long as men have been hunters—and that association with men seems to drive her negative attitude toward meat-eating. Yet the hierarchical patriarchy that Adams so despises sprang out of the Agricultural Revolution. Our pre-agricultural days weren't a feminist utopia, but hunter-gatherer tribes were characterized by fewer power imbalances and relatively more equality between the sexes. To the extent that our diet is to blame for patriarchy, then Adams has it exactly backward: it was the shift from an animal-based Paleolithic diet to a plant-based Agricultural diet that led to patriarchy.

Wheat is a better symbol of oppression than meat.

Given that hunter-gatherer women did more gathering than men did, it's entirely plausible that women's initiative and ingenuity were responsible for the inadvertent then purposeful domestication of plants—which led to the Agricultural Revolution, which led to patriarchy. I'm fairly certain that men would have been perfectly content to spend all day hunting game, barbecuing ribs, taking naps, making weapons, planning raids, and having sex.

NONE OF what I have written detracts from the realities of the factory farm system—nor from the fact that vegetarians and animal rights activists have been the driving force behind unearthing abuses in factory farming, abuses that are quite shocking even to unsquea-mish meat-loving hunters. But the strident and self-evident moral superiority of vegetarianism should give us pause, and perhaps we should question whether ideology is blinding people to the harm that vegetarianism may be perpetuating among some of its adherents, and whether this movement is actually advancing its stated ethical and environmental goals.

Vegetarianism's strengths and weaknesses derive from these same three qualities: empathy for animals, a sensitive disgust reflex, and viewing meat-eating in starkly moralistic terms.

First, vegetarians' greater empathy for animals has clearly sensi-tized them to the plight of animal suffering, much of which is very real and very legitimate. On the other hand, this view can lead to Bambi Ethics or Bambi Environmentalism—human morality applied to nature in a superficial way. It's impossible to live on this planet without indirectly killing animals, whether through eating soybeans or using airplane fuel. Crop farming kills thousands of small animals, either directly via pesticides, trapping, or harvesting machines, or in-directly through displacement. Eating one hunted deer or pastured cow, nose to tail, creates a smaller blood footprint than does eat-ing meal after meal made from industrial soybeans. Hunting invasive species is clearly healthy for humans *and* beneficial for the environ-ment; raising domesticated animals is inseparable from traditional agriculture.

Second, a visceral disgust regarding conditions at factory farms is appropriate, since they often *are* disgusting. At the same time vege-tarians haven't shown a stomach for ethical and environmentally friendly substitutes for meat, such as oysters or insects. If artificial meat is eventually grown in a laboratory, then the more closely it actually resembles meat, the less likely that vegetarians will actually eat it. It will be a real vegetarian dilemma if lab grown meat turns out to be more environmentally friendly than soybeans.

Third, the power of vegetarian ideology has motivated millions to speak out against the factory farm system. On the other hand,

EATING INSECTS

Eating insects sounds disgusting to Westerners, but not to the Chinese (scorpions on a stick), Cambodians (deep-fried tarantulas), Mexicans (toasted grasshoppers), or Ghanaians (winged termite bread). Locusts are widely eaten in the Middle East and have been for a long time: they were a dietary staple of John the Baptist (he paired them with locally sourced organic honey), and certain species were acceptable to eat under the Jewish and Islamic dietary codes. Insect eating is common in 80% of countries in the world, and more than a thousand species of insects are eaten.

There are a number of advantages to eating insects. Nutritionally, they're a rich source of protein and other nutrients. Environmentally, they convert feed and water into edible nutrients far more efficiently than does livestock and they require far less space. To vegans and vegetarians, a good case can be made that insects can be harvested more humanely than can many vegetarian crops, which often require huge swaths of land, harvesting machines that kill lots of animals, and insecticides that eradicate lots of . . . insects.

Most people have eaten insects without realizing it. The USDA knows it's impossible to keep insects entirely out of food and thus the agency sets a maximum allowable limit. The upper limit for wheat flour is an "average of 75 or more insect fragments per 50 grams" (685 insect fragments per pound). Americans also enjoy eating a number of insect-like species—invertebrates with an exoskeleton—and even treat them as delicacies, dipping them in butter: lobster, crab, crayfish, and shrimp.

ideological rigidity has limited their available options to actually change the factory farm system. Vegetarians have been resistant to financially supporting an alternative food system based on ethically raised meat. Since they ideologically oppose buying any type of meat, they refuse to buy ethically raised meat from entrepreneurs who are trying to create an alternative to the factory farm system and thereby alleviate the suffering of domesticated animals.

For decades, vegetarians—by definition—have been staging an economic boycott against meat. Yet it is far from clear that this preferred form of vegetarian advocacy has been successful at advancing its major goals. The problem with boycotts is that they tend to work only under certain conditions. Successful boycotts occur when a large number of consumers join the boycott. Small groups can wage a successful boycott by damaging a company's reputation—but in order for this to work, many people have to be sympathetic to the cause.

Boycotts don't work very well when organized by small groups whose views aren't shared by the general population, and who make unrealistic demands. For small groups with limited resources and goals outside the mainstream, prizes work better than boycotts.

If, say, 5% of the population is vegetarian, that means that the market for factory farmed meat is 5% smaller. To any of the big agribusinesses, that 5% hit isn't going to put them out of business. They can further identify vegetarians as a consumer segment and then turn around and sell them Boca Burgers made with industrial soybeans.

However, that same 5% would have a huge impact on the sales of entrepreneurial, ethical farms that are experimenting with alternative food systems. Talk to any entrepreneur about the importance of that first dollar of revenue, breaking even, and finally getting to cash flow positive—all are major milestones. That means in terms of "starting up" a more humane food system, one can have a far greater impact by contributing money to start-ups that are doing it right than by abstaining from buying products from established players that are doing it wrong. Here's the kicker: once the big guys see that there's money to be made by being ethical, they'll get into the game themselves.

But the very people who clamor the loudest about animal suffering won't actually pay for meat that has been ethically slaughtered. If 5% of the population had been insisting on ethically raised meat for the last two decades, a lot more progress would have been made in satisfying that demand. The relatively tiny Jewish community has been willing to pay a small premium for kosher slaughter for millennia, and they've been *getting* kosher slaughter for millennia.

In 2008 PETA switched from boycotts to prizes when it offered a $1 million prize to "the first laboratory to use chicken cells to create in vitro (test-tube) meat if the product were commercially viable by June 30, 2012." At the time this book was going to press, no one had won the prize—but two labs were close to announcing test-tube hamburgers, and PETA decided to extend the deadline. That $1 million prize money makes a much bigger impact as a carrot enticing innovation than it does as a stick punishing large agribusiness, to which $1 million is a rounding error.

The entire vegetarian movement could be modeled on the same principle—but that would entail eating meat, a moral sin so great that it can't be contemplated even as part of a practical solution.

There is another ideological blind spot to vegetarianism: the fervent insistence that a vegetarian diet is necessarily or optimally healthy. Vegetarians do tend to smoke less, drink less, exercise more, and probably do a number of other things right. Given the importance of disgust in vegetarianism, it should be no surprise that vegetarians are highly selective about what they put in their body. However, when it comes to mental health, the picture grows less favorable.

In 2012 a landmark German study found that vegetarians are considerably more likely to have mental disorders than people who eat meat. A number of smaller studies had suggested that might be the case, but this larger effort followed several thousand people and used a more rigorous methodology. Of 4,181 people randomly selected from the German population, 1.3% were completely vegetarian ($n=54$) and 4.5% were predominantly vegetarian ($n=190$). Psychological assessments didn't just come from a self-reported paper survey—each person in the study was assessed by "clinically trained interviewers (psychologists and physicians) with an average interview duration of 65 minutes." The interviewers inquired about depressive disorders, anxiety disorders, somatoform disorders (symptoms of illness unexplained by a medical diagnosis), and eating disorders—as well as their prevalence over one-month, twelve-month, and lifetime intervals. Because vegetarians have socio-demographic skews that are known to correlate with mental disorders (female, young, highly educated, single, urban), the study authors created a matched control group out of the meat-eaters based on those five characteristics.

The differences were significant. Not only did the vegetarians have higher rates of every type of mental disorder than did the meat-eaters, but these effects held steady—or even grew larger—when compared with the demographically similar controls. Furthermore, the frequency of depressive, anxiety, and eating disorders (though not somatoform) was even higher among complete vegetarians than predominant vegetarians. Even among meat-eaters, the people with mental disorders ate less meat.

Based on the reported onset of these disorders and the age of starting to eat vegetarian, the paper concluded that vegetarianism did *not* cause mental disorders. However, it was abundantly clear that people with mental disorders were being attracted to vegetarianism. Why?

One possibility is that vegetarianism perpetuates (or even exacerbates) mental disorders. Socially, vegetarianism provides a reason to restrict food intake and avoid eating in public, and it offers an ostensibly principled rationale that is hard for others to challenge. Physiologically, there are clear mechanisms by which a vegetarian diet might worsen brain function, such as deficiencies in omega-3 fatty acids (which are commonly found in fish) and vitamin B12 (which is almost entirely absent from plant foods). This is also in line with anecdotal evidence from former vegans who have reported an improvement in mental health upon adopting an omnivorous diet. Most people forget that the brain is an organ like the others, and a lack of proper nutrition must necessarily lead to a weakening of its function.

In some cases, vegetarianism itself may be a sign of an underlying disorder. As noted, many advocates of vegetarianism try to elicit an aversion to meat by using tried-and-true triggers of disgust, such as bodily fluids, corpses, rotting flesh, and the specter of infection. However, since the risk of infection from eating a well-done steak is actually quite low (in fact, veggies are often to blame for modern foodborne illnesses), the immune system is, in essence, responding to an imaginary threat. Thus, an overly sensitive disgust reflex that leads to vegetarianism may be akin to an obsessive-compulsive disorder in which someone washes their hands hundreds of times a day (or someone who thinks they become "unclean" by touching a menstruating woman).

If true, a hypersensitive disgust reflex would manifest itself in ways besides an aversion to meat. A general wariness of ingesting "unclean" substances may create an aversion to alcohol, tobacco, pesticides, "toxins," or anything that has come in contact with meat. An eagerness to purge "impurities" may explain the popularity of juice fasts and cleanses, which allegedly rid the body of contaminants. It may even explain why some vegetarians develop a decidedly peculiar interest in laxatives and colon cleanses; even the shit in their own bodies becomes a source of physical contamination.

These efforts at "detoxification" share a focus—or fixation—on avoiding mysterious impurities (often called "toxins"), which happen to be *everywhere*. While there are such things as toxins, practitioners of alternative medicine often use the term broadly and amorphously, with little or no attention paid to the scientific definition of toxicity. If disgust is the driver, that may explain why "toxins" are treated a lot like germs: invisible, lurking in bodily fluids, easily transmissible, and deadly. To the extent a hypersensitive disgust reflex results in destructive behaviors, vegetarianism might fairly be described as a symptom of an underlying immunological disorder.

On the other hand, vegetarianism can act as a palliative against eating disorders. It doesn't take too many conversations with vegetarians to find a history of anorexia, bulimia, orthorexia (extreme avoidance of foods perceived to be unhealthy), and yo-yo dieting. A

LET THEM EAT MEAT

Rhys Southan is a former vegan, now a meat-eater, who critiques vegan arguments on his blog *Let Them Eat Meat* (LetThemEatMeat.com). Here are his tips for vegans and vegetarians who are ready to eat meat again but still feel weird about taking that first bite.

- Don't believe the horror stories. Ex-vegans and vegetarians getting sick the first time they eat meat again is largely a myth. Part of the confusion comes from how it feels to accidentally ingest meat as a true-believing vegetarian. This can indeed lead to severe queasiness, but most likely this is psychosomatic: emotion and cognitive dissonance instead of actual intolerance.
- Ease into it. Try eating a little bit of meat with tons of vegetables. Sushi is a good choice—the protective barrier of rice and seaweed is like training wheels.
- Eat the meat you're craving, or the meat that seems least intimidating. Some go straight for red meat or bacon, because they're obsessing about juicy steaks and they've heard bacon is "the gateway meat." For others, fish makes for a smoother transition.

number of current vegetarians came to their diet as a healthier alternative to the eating disorders that plague so many young women. Dig into these stories and a similar theme emerges: body image issues during high school and college, repeated attempts to control calories by eating a low-fat diet and exercising, repeated failure. For better or worse, the rise of vegetarianism owes much to the absurdly destructive advice from the media and conventional health authorities to eat a low-fat diet, counting calories all the way, and a lack of a healthy relationship to food.

- Certain animals, like bivalves and jellyfish, don't seem to experience life any more than plants do. Unfortunately, a lot of vegetarians are particularly disgusted by these slimy things, which is why you don't see too many "bivalvegans" enjoying this guilt-free option.
- Eating less popular meats, like organs, makes sense for ex-veggies who want to minimize their impact on animals, but it's not easy to leap straight from soy cutlets to liver. The best tasting offals are arguably sweetbreads, bones (marrow and broth), with heart coming in third, so kick off your nose-to-tail career with those.
- One reason it's easy for some to give up meat is that they haven't been exposed to a large variety of animal foods, so they don't realize how big a sacrifice they're making. For many aspiring ex-vegans, their favorite animal product will end up being one they've never tried before. Rather than returning to meat with an old reliable, like Grandma's chicken and carrots, consider starting with something new. Duck confit, perhaps?
- In the "freegan" ethic, you don't have to take responsibility for what you eat, so long as it will otherwise go to waste. If you're feeling more ethical conflict than disgust, you could try that steak your friend can't finish. Or if you're even more adventurous, there's always dumpsters or road kill.

Given that our entire nation has employed this failed strategy, it should come as no surprise if it seems that America has a national eating disorder. More people feel squeamish about eating meat. We are told that it is bad for us. We are more easily grossed out than ever before. Fewer and fewer people grow up on working farms, hunting, or keeping chickens in their backyard. Grocery stores and food corporations go to great lengths to remove any cue that the meat we eat actually used to be a living animal. For many people, their disgust reflex can be triggered by a chicken with the feet still attached, or a little bit of blood in a steak. We are witnessing the secular rise of soft vegetarianism.

Vegetarianism aside, parents have the responsibility to raise children with a healthy relationship to food. Without minimizing the constant challenge of feeding finicky children, we cannot allow kids to subsist on a diet of Tater Tots, buttered noodles, and pizza. America has completely re-engineered itself around the whiny demands of toddlers and children, but a hungry child *will* eventually eat. Believe it or not, countless generations of children finished their supper before the advent of Kraft Mac & Cheese and ice-cream sandwiches.

Furthermore, we can't raise our children without ever teaching them that chicken tenders actually come from . . . *a chicken*. But to teach our children where our food comes from, we can't be ashamed of the truth.

My personal opposition to the worst aspects of factory farming isn't motivated by feeling animals' pain. Put a wounded animal directly in front of me and I feel its pain. Remove it from view and I sleep soundly. As Adam Smith pointed out long ago (in reference to an earthquake in China), humans have difficulty feeling the pain of other humans, much less animals.

My opposition to the mistreatment of animals is honor-based. What we do to many factory farm animals is dishonorable in the same way that carelessly wounding an animal while hunting is dishonorable. In combat, respected adversaries have always merited a quick and painless death. There is every reason to extend that honor to the animals that give us our strength.

And yes, I still intend to hunt, kill, gut, skin, butcher, cook, and eat animals.

How, then, to create a more ethical food system?

To begin with, a large swath of humanity is never going to stop eating meat. It's healthy, it tastes good, and it's been "what's for dinner" since before we were human. The persistence of meat in our meals seems especially likely given that even vegetarians consume meat-like substances such as tofu burgers and soy bacon. We can expect meat to remain in the human diet for the foreseeable future.

The question therefore becomes: how can we improve animal welfare?

An improvement in animal welfare is more likely to occur if it doesn't depend solely—or even primarily—on extending empathy or honor to animals. As Adam Smith observed, "It is not from the benevolence of the butcher, the brewer, or the baker that we expect our dinner, but from their regard to their own interest." Vegetarians take note: trying to inspire benevolence in the butcher is the definitive example of a failed strategy in a market economy. Better to bribe the butcher and pay a small premium for ethical slaughter.

The virtue of this approach is that it incentivizes incremental improvements to the existing factory farm system. Dr. Temple Grandin's pioneering designs of more humane slaughterhouses are now used in slaughterhouses across the country. She has arguably done more for animal welfare than all other efforts combined—ever. But this means being willing to work with those oh so evil corporations—even, horrors, *McDonald's!*—a notion that is anathema to so many in the food movement. Elements of the environmental movement have wised up to this, and realized that rather than demonizing WalMart (or only demonizing it), cooperating with it to make small tweaks in the supply chain can result in enormous efficiency gains. To the extent that humane animal slaughter doesn't result in greater efficiency, this means we have to be willing to pay a little bit more for humanely slaughtered meat. To do this we need to support entrepreneurs who are innovating in the food space, and criticize the existing paradigm by creating the alternatives. The goal isn't to feed the world but to spark innovation and incentivize incremental improvements by established players.

Another reason to alter the factory farm system is a purely selfish one: preventing antibiotic resistant strains of bacteria is a matter of human welfare. At the very moment when antibiotics are losing their effectiveness in human populations and the discovery of new ones has slowed to a crawl, we are squandering their potency on *livestock*. Effective antibiotics are a linchpin of modern medicine; without them, it all falls apart. We are financing the creation of virulent biological weapons that one day may be turned against us. This alone should be sufficient reason to create more hygienic conditions for animals. Doing what is required for better hygiene—more space, cleaner conditions—would go a long way to improving animal welfare.

In the end, vegetarianism is a laudable choice for many people. Most vegetarians have no wish to impose their eating choices on anyone else, nor do they agree with the radical ideology of a small coterie of animal rights extremists and feminists. They just want to eat in a way that they find meaningful and healthy—*and there's nothing wrong with that*.

But given that vegetarianism is essentially a pure "gatherer" strategy, it should come as no surprise that vegetarianism doesn't appeal to many hunters. But the food movement needs people who can do the dirty work: hunt wild boar, gut deer, eat invasive species, try insects, raise animals the right way, and pay for ethically raised meat.

That role falls to us.

Conclusion

HABITATS, OLD AND NEW

Several decades ago, an architecture student named Jon Coe paid a visit to Boston's Franklin Park Zoo to sketch elephants for an art assignment. He entered the Elephant House to find a small, dingy space with three elephants chained to the ground. They were fighting with each other.

"Why are they chained?" Coe asked one of the keepers.

"Because they're fighting."

"Why are they fighting?"

"Because they're chained."

The experience opened Coe's eyes to the power of habitat design. The ill-conceived Elephant House was eliciting destructive behavior from the elephants, and the elephants' destructive behavior seemed to justify concrete walls and steel chains. That was the moment he was inspired to create habitats for animals, not people.

Coe left the "respectable" path of architecture and wandered into the wilderness of his own profession. Yet when he arrived at the zoo, he found architects firmly ensconced.

When a zoo goes through the effort of a capital campaign or a public levy, the donors want something impressive and iconic to show for it. That usually means bringing in a famous architect to design a structure that satisfies human sensibilities, rather than the sensibilities of whichever species actually has to live there. It's why zoo directors have a long-running joke about the most dangerous animal in the zoo: the architect. At their best, architects ignored biology; at their worst, they spurned it.

In 1932 the London Zoo commissioned a new penguin pool from modernist architect Berthold Lubetkin, who took full advantage of what was still a novel building material: reinforced concrete. It was praised by art and architecture critics for its radical simplicity; one professor even aspired to live in a similar structure, forcing him to simplify his needs. David Hancocks, the widely respected former director of Seattle's Woodland Park Zoo, looks back in horror: "No one asked the penguins how they enjoyed having to simplify their needs to live each day in their minimalist pit." The structure was even designated a national landmark, perpetuating its use until 2003, long after it should have been retired. It now stands empty, having achieved an even more perfect minimalism without any penguins in residence.

In 2011 the London Zoo opened Penguin Beach. It is large enough to sustain an entire breeding colony while deep enough to allow extensive diving and swimming. It uses textures that mimic Antarctic surfaces, with both rocky and sandy beaches for the breeding grounds preferred by respective penguin species. Visitors have underwater viewing stations, so children can see the penguins up close as they so effortlessly dive and swim, inspiring awe and appreciation.

In the intervening years between the two exhibits, Coe and his generation of landscape architects had led a quiet revolution. Their motto: "Nature is the model."

Coe wanted to design habitats that respected the nature of each animal. Rather than concrete and steel—materials that a wild animal would never experience—why not use wood and dirt? Instead of a complete absence of plant life (or artificial plants), why not grow real trees and shrubs? And why not use plant species that actually grow in the animal's natural habitat?

This ethos—*Nature is the model*—is applicable to the health of all species. A holistic, habitat-based approach to human health is long overdue.

A "habitat" is any physical environment: home, car, school, office. A habitat is the food choices available in the grocery store, and the limitations of a budget. A habitat is the social environment: family, friends, neighbors, and co-workers. A habitat is culture: customs, laws, and technology. *Everyone lives in a habitat.*

Habitat has an enormous influence on each person's past development, current decisions, and future direction. A person who lives his entire life in the city will likely never learn to hunt and thus never be exposed to the role that hunters play in environmental stewardship. Social perceptions of what is "normal" cause a parent to put shoes on a young child's feet—even indoors, in the backyard, or on a grassy field—which makes it more likely a child will develop flat feet. A bacterial infection doesn't respond to antibiotics due to the actions of distant people and animals.

Habitats influence behavior, but our behavior can alter our habitat—and more than any other species, humans have the ability to do so.

It's never been easier to modify one's personal habitat. Choose different foods at the grocery store. Join a gym with a motivating and fun atmosphere. Surround yourself with people who maintain healthy habits. Switch from a sitting desk to a standing desk. It won't be long before all the lights in a house will brighten and dim with the time of day, helping to re-establish a more natural circadian rhythm. Temperature too: the next generation of thermostats is already available, dynamically changing temperature throughout the day (warmer) and night (cooler). Rather than using a jarring alarm to wake up, there are now "sunrise" clocks that use UV exposure to gently awaken you.

Initial efforts at habitat design don't always get it right. Jon Coe is the first to admit that the early efforts of naturalistic habitat design in zoos were a bit amateurish. "Sometimes researching an animal's habitat meant leafing through the pages of *National Geographic*," he recalled. "Some of the early habitat design features were simply intended to create the right spirit." These entrepreneurial amateurs didn't wait for expert approval to start experimenting. As better information became available, they simply integrated it into their thinking. It was an act of wisdom and humility to use nature as the starting point, rather than attempting to impose an anthropocentric vision of how things ought to be.

"It's not just that we don't know all the answers," said Coe. "It's that we don't even know the right questions to ask."

SOME OF the most important questions bear on not only our local, personal habitats, but also on that of the one we all share: Earth. How do all seven billion people on the planet eat a diet that allows them not only to survive, but to thrive?

The burgeoning food movement is a backlash against industrial farming and has offered up one answer to getting back in touch with food: eating local. The last decade has witnessed the rise of "locavorism," a diet based on obtaining food from local sources, such as farmers markets, directly from farmers, or from one's own backyard.

There are many benefits to using local sources of food. It helps people understand where food comes from. It creates a sense of community and connection, lacking in the depersonalized mass market. It supports food entrepreneurs who are innovating not only in agricultural methods, but also in ethical slaughter of animals. Local food is fresh and often tastes better than the store-bought alternative. By eating heritage breeds, people support the continued existence of living agricultural history and maintain genetic variety in the food supply. Growing one's own herbs and vegetables is satisfying and relaxing. All these things can add both health and meaning to life.

Yet it's not clear whether locavorism is a viable, scalable strategy. At the core of locavorism is the concept of "food miles," a standard that measures the sustainability of a food based on the distance it travels from farm to plate. The fewer food miles, the thinking goes, the better—as if the pure distance a food must travel determines its overall environmental impact. This concept is deeply flawed, as some leading locavores have acknowledged.

A complete tally of the environmental cost of any food must also include its suitability to the climate, the natural fertility of the soil, nutrients extracted from the soil, fertilizer usage, irrigation, greenhouse heating, and refrigeration (as well as any number of other factors). When all these issues are taken into account, transportation costs dramatically recede in importance. Large container ships are remarkably efficient at transporting goods, for example, and therefore ocean shipping accounts for only a small percentage of the resources used to produce food. "Food miles" is an alluring concept, but a profoundly incomplete one.

If everyone were to eat locally, it would mean that people should no longer live in nations with poor agricultural productivity, such as Japan, Canada, and Hong Kong. Yet it somehow seems unlikely that people are going to uproot and cluster around the world's most fertile areas, such as California's Central Valley, the Argentinian Pampas, and the Ukraine. "Living close to the earth" sounds enticing, but it's actually big cities, which so violently mar the natural landscape, that are the most resource efficient and thus, the most sustainable.

In *The Locavore's Dilemma: In Praise of the 10,000-Mile Diet*, Canadian economists Pierre Desrochers and Hiriko Shimizu question what it means to eat "locally." Does it mean only eating food grown within a hundred miles? Ten miles? One mile? Does it mean eating only food that you grew yourself? Taken to its logical conclusion, locavorism for everyone on the planet is a recipe for poverty. Not only do some voices in the food movement recommend the Poor Farmer Diet, but they also seem to want us to go back to literally being poor farmers.

The part of the world with the most people engaged in local, small-scale, organic, non-GMO agriculture is Africa. Africans need to use every method at their disposal to improve crop yields—high-yielding seeds, chemical fertilizers, crop rotations, farm technology—that will help them break out of the cycle of rural poverty. Only at that point will they be wealthy enough to afford . . . local, organic farming.

The wealth of advanced nations was enabled, in part, by improvements in agricultural productivity. Fewer farmers could grow more food at lower cost, enabling more people to congregate in cities, leading eco-friendly lives. The growth of Asian economies in the twentieth century was preceded by gains in agricultural productivity, enabled by the Green Revolution and Dr. Norman Borlaug (who won a Nobel Peace Prize in 1970 for breeding higher-yield crop varieties). In fact, major cities would not be possible at all without the *original* Agricultural Revolution: genetic modification through breeding.

In the same way that humanity grew beyond what a hunter-gatherer food system could support, we have now grown beyond what a purely agricultural food system can support. It is nearly as naïve to think that organic agriculture can feed the world as it is to think that hunting and gathering can. Given that we are locked into an industrial food system for the foreseeable future—advantages and disadvantages both—where should we go from here?

For decades, one favored solution has been to turn back the clock to a pre-industrial agricultural diet and food system (i.e., local, organic, whole). Part of this is motivated legitimate problems with the industrial food system, but part also seems motivated by a visceral distaste with the Industrial Revolution and nostalgia for our allegedly happier agricultural days. But those happy times never actually existed. Farmwork is grindingly hard and often delivers meager yields outside of naturally fertile areas. (In a way, not acknowledging the drawbacks to agricultural life is less defensible than idealizing a hunter-gatherer existence, our memory of which is shrouded by a much longer period of time and an absence of written records.)

Given that there isn't enough productive farmland to grow organic produce for everyone, there are two ways the "pre-industrial" approach can play out. First, organic agriculture could be enjoyed only by the rich, akin to a monarch hunting in the Royal Forest. In twelfth- and thirteenth-century England, approximately one-third of southern England was set aside for use by royalty—preserving their access to a pristine Paleolithic food system at the expense of agricultural land for peasants. The second alternative is that we would have to downsize in every way: have fewer babies, eat less meat, buy less stuff. In other words, less humanity.

This second option has long been popular with many intellectuals, and a general distaste for humanity was never far below the surface. In fact, that's often the explicit goal of environmentalism: to reduce the human footprint on the earth. A common line of thinking is that humanity is akin to an invasive species, so much kudzu devouring everything in its path, growing out of control—until the habitat is destroyed, ensuring our own destruction in the process. And there's some truth to that: seven billion people is a lot of people.

But what would a truly sustainable lifestyle look like?

The entire world population can't and certainly won't "return" to a mythical agricultural existence like hobbits in the Shire. So far, the evidence shows that the most sustainable mode of existence for mankind seems to be a Paleolithic lifestyle, living in small-scale roving bands using Stone Age technology. It worked for a few million years, far longer than our Agricultural or Industrial paradigms. At the same time, it's not clear that a Paleolithic lifestyle is actually sustainable (or at the very least, stable) over the long term; after all, it led us to where we are now.

Agriculture didn't change everything, *we* changed everything.

To return to a long-term sustainable mode of living, we would have to go back not only before agriculture and before the technology of the Upper Paleolithic (projectile weapons, complex culture), but also before whatever cognitive developments made those advances possible. We'd have to go back to a time before we were big-brained humans—a time before we were *us*.

Though turning back the clock isn't a viable solution, there is a simple, seemingly unassailable logic to the "less stuff" calculus of sustainability. When looking at the industrial food system, eating less meat *does* result in lower land and resource use than eating rice and beans. Having fewer babies *does* result in fewer mouths to feed. Buying less stuff *does* result in using less stuff rather than buying more stuff. In the short run, simply cutting back on our use of resources *does* bring environmental gains—and those gains are sometimes the difference between complete habitat destruction or preservation. So it matters.

But in the long run, simply using "less stuff"—*within our current Industrial paradigm*—will not be sufficient to markedly reduce humanity's footprint on Earth. Attempts to turn back the clock are likely to prove futile. Also any approach that precludes large-scale civilization and human flourishing isn't much of a solution.

The path to sustainability doesn't lie in our past, but in our future. Rather than trying to turn the clock back, we have to turn the hands forward, faster. Instead of shrinking, we need to *grow*—to innovate and create. And we need to grow faster than we've ever grown before.

The developing world is mostly just playing catch-up to a standard of living afforded by an Industrial paradigm. While this initially brings environmental degradation, the simple truth is that poor people can't afford to care about the environment. Once countries reach a certain level of material prosperity, people start to pay attention to things like air quality, water quality, and wildlife conservation.

Today, people get agitated about emissions of various particulates, but the air quality in, say, London hasn't been this good for hundreds of years, since before the Industrial Revolution. In modern times, the worst environmental degradation and disasters have taken place in the Soviet Union and Communist China. The air is shockingly filthy in Beijing today, but it will be filthy for a far shorter period of time than the London air was during Britain's two hundred years of industrialization.

Once people are more prosperous, they voluntarily have fewer children. In fact, the end of population growth is in sight: peak population will hit in a few decades. It won't be long before we run into problems associated with population *decline* since many of our political institutions were set up with the implicit expectation of consistent growth and demographic expansion. In fact, those problems are already coming to the fore in aging, stagnant countries like Japan—and Europe isn't far behind.

The question is whether we can grow our way out of the problem or whether a dimmer future will take hold: a period of relative stagnation that won't appreciably reduce the human footprint on the planet, any deterioration of which will only motivate more extreme measures, further slowing economic growth and thus sowing seeds of conflict between great powers who see themselves in an increasingly zero-sum world. A downward spiral will not be good for the environment.

Our future depends on the next paradigm in human existence: the Information Age.

Biology is an information technology, and we are finally learning how to hack it. Scientists are using a patient's own stem cells to grow organs that won't be rejected during transplantation. Unborn children can be screened for rare genetic abnormalities that might eventually be fixed with gene therapy.

We are even bridging the gap between biology and computers, man and machine. Millions of people are already "cyborgs." Some people who are deaf can hear again due to cochlear implants. War veterans with missing limbs are now able to control prosthetic devices with their minds. Pacemakers may eventually be replaced with completely artificial hearts.

Bio-engineers are designing bacteria that could generate energy from industrial waste. And yes, companies are genetically modifying our food.

Not all of these changes will be good ones—and those should be resisted. But without being too fatalistic, all prior growth revolutions—Paleolithic, Agricultural, Industrial—took place without planning or coordinated control. So far, the Digital Revolution is no different. The danger, of course, is that we engineer our way into disaster—but that's why our design solutions should hew closely to those in the natural world. Nature *must* be the model.

The uncertainty of the future is all the more reason to conserve traditional ways of living—and when it comes to food, preserving our traditional food systems. Just because everyone on the planet can't survive on our Paleolithic food system doesn't mean that human-ity should stop hunting. There are good reasons to continue hunt-ing, just as there are many reasons to continue traditional forms of agriculture—as any locavore, chef, or backyard gardener can attest.

When it comes to our food systems, we should be taking an "all of the above" approach, incorporating the best from the Paleolithic and Agricultural, while addressing the worst of the Industrial.

For our Paleolithic food system, its strength is also its weakness: wild spaces are generally not under direct human ownership or con-trol. This is good for the health of wild ecosystems, but there just aren't enough wild animals to feed seven billion people.

So it's definitely not going to feed the world.

Our Agricultural food system serves as the baseline by which we measure the successes and failures of our Industrial food system. Traditional agriculture offers a standard of humane treatment of do-mesticated animals, as well as what good agricultural foods actually taste like. It also shows that conventional agriculture is hard, usually with lower yields. We need to support local agriculture to maintain a stock of genetic diversity in our food supply (heirloom seeds, heri-tage breeds), to provide a fallback food system, to put pressure on the industrial food system to become more humane in its treatment of animals, and to continue innovating with traditional techniques to increase yields.

But it's probably not going to feed the world.

Our Industrial food system currently feeds the world, but has some serious health, ethical, and environmental drawbacks. While curbing the worst abuses and problems, we also need to realize that industrial agriculture is here for the time being. Higher levels of agri-cultural productivity are key to global development, which will make people prosperous enough to afford to care about the environment and ethical treatment of animals.

If we are to maintain each of these food systems, that means we need advocates for each of them. We need people who fiercely defend the right to hunt—and who actually hunt. We *need* hunter-gatherers.

We need people who fiercely defend traditional farming, buy local, raise heritage breeds—and who actually farm. We *need* herder-farmers.

We need people who fiercely defend the benefits of the industrial food system, its ability to lower the cost of food, encourage economic development, and lift people out of poverty.

And we need responsible people who care about the future of humanity, the food system, and the environment to be involved in applying Information Age technology in a wise and responsible way. As eco-pragmatist Stewart Brand has said, "We are as gods and have to get good at it."

When it comes to the future of the planet—distinct from human-ity—it's also worth pondering the wisdom of the late great philoso-pher (and comedian) George Carlin:

"The planet will be here for a long, long, LONG time after we're gone, and it will heal itself, it will cleanse itself, 'cause that's what it does. It's a self-correcting system. The air and the water will recover, the Earth will be renewed, and if it's true that plastic is not degrad-able, well, the planet will simply incorporate plastic into a new para-digm: the Earth plus plastic. The Earth doesn't share our prejudice towards plastic. Plastic came out of the Earth. The Earth probably sees plastic as just another one of its children. Could be the only reason the Earth allowed us to be spawned from it in the first place. It wanted plastic for itself. Didn't know how to make it. Needed us. Could be the answer to our age-old egocentric philosophical ques-tion, 'Why are we here?' Plastic . . . *assholes*."

It's a conceit to think humanity can destroy the planet. We can very well destroy ourselves, but cockroaches and cyanobacteria aren't going extinct anytime soon. If we screw up and destroy ourselves, the Earth will, as Carlin said, "shake us off like a bad case of fleas. A surface nuisance."

What exactly is the point of humanity living in some boring, utopian, supposedly sustainable stasis? Human beings are not fun-damentally different from other species in our ability to experience pleasure or pain. What makes humanity so unique is what we are capable of accomplishing: culture, technology, exploration, creation.

The situation calls for more conservation *and* more risk taking: more conservation of old habitats here on Earth, more risk taking as we push beyond Earth into new habitats.

The challenge may seem daunting, but we can do what our ancestors did: take one small step after another until we arrive in a very different place. Risen apes or fallen angels, we walk tall with eyes forward—one foot firmly planted on the ground of what we are, the other reaching into the future of what we can become.

Resources

- Visit **HunterGatherer.com/Resources** for a complete set of resources, including a shopping guide, recipes, tips for getting started, and vendors. Also available are resources for fasting, movement, standing desks, barefoot running, hot and cold exposure, sun, and sleep.

- Visit **HunterGatherer.com/Stand** to submit a photo of you and your standing desk and be featured as an "Upstanding Citizen."

- Visit **HunterGatherer.com/NYC** for a free paleo guide to New York City, including restaurants, Russian baths, events, deals, and more.

Recommendations

1. What to Eat: *Mimic a Hunter-Gatherer (or Herder) Diet*
Stop counting calories. Eat the right foods: meat, seafood, roots and tubers, leafy vegetables, eggs, fruit, and nuts. Experiment with full-fat fermented dairy. Aim for a diet where the bulk of calories comes from seafood and animals, but the physical bulk comes from plants. Don't be afraid of fat, eat nose to tail, and eat a variety of plants.

2. How to Eat: *Follow Ancient Culinary Traditions*

Respect ancient culinary wisdom. Follow traditional recipes. Eat fermented foods (sauerkraut, kimchi). Eat raw foods (sashimi, ceviche, tartare). Make broths and stocks. Cook at low heat, using traditional fats and oils (coconut oil, beef tallow, butter, ghee, olive oil). Eat your colors. Eat time-honored "superfoods": liver, eggs, seaweed, cold water fish. Enjoy real butter. Salt to taste. Drink tea.

3. What Not to Eat: *Avoid Industrial Foods, Sugars, and Seeds*

Avoid processed foods of the Industrial Age, including sugar (sweetened foods, table sugar, dried fruit, plus artificial sweeteners) and vegetable oils (canola oil, soybean oil, corn oil, peanut oil). Avoid eating large, concentrated quantities of the seed-based crops of the Agricultural Age, such as grains (wheat, corn, barley, oats) and legumes (soy, beans, peanuts). If grains are eaten, go with rice.

BEVERAGES: Drink water as thirsty. Drink traditional beverages in moderation, if desired (tea, coffee, wine, alcohol, milk). Avoid industrial beverages (soda, energy drinks, skim milk).

4. Make It Meaningful: *Experiment, Customize, Enjoy*

Use these guidelines as a starting point for your own experimentation. Modify according to your own health, goals, tastes and preferences, background, and budget. Make your diet meaningful (family recipes, ethnic cuisine). Be comfortable breaking away from it to enjoy life (celebrations, unique experiences).

5. Lead a Healthy Lifestyle

Sleep as much as possible. Move and exercise regularly. Stay on your feet (stand, walk, run). Get regular, moderate sun. Try some intermittent fasting. Try some hot and cold exposure. Make it meaningful in order to make it an ongoing lifestyle.

Notes

Additional notes can be found at HunterGatherer.com/Notes.

1. Becoming the Caveman

1 **my first ever TV appearance** John Durant, interview by Stephen Colbert, *The Colbert Report,* February 3, 2010. http://www.colbertnation.com/the-colbert-report-videos/263270/february-03-2010/john-durant (accessed December 21, 2012).

3 **"Nothing in biology makes sense except"** Dobzhansky, 1973.

3 **an innate fear of snakes** Öhman & Mineka, 2001.

3 **Evolutionary psychology can also explain some of our moral intuitions** Lieberman, Tooby, and Cosmides, 2003.

5 **a twenty-six-page essay by Dr. Art De Vany** A. De Vany, "Evolutionary Fitness," December 11, 2000. It is no longer available on his website: http://artdevanyonline.com.

6 **The general mismatch hypothesis** With respect to nutrition, see Eaton and Konner, 1985.

10 **a feature on our group** J. Goldstein, "The New Age Caveman and the City," *New York Times,* January 8, 2010.

Part One: Origins

13 **Origins** The name for Part One comes from Kelly, 2010.

2. Know Thy Species *(Animal Age)*

15 **530 million years ago** The date of the Cambrian Explosion, the rapid appearance (on a geological scale) of most animal phyla in the fossil record. Valentine, Jablonski, and Erwin, 1999.

16 **his actual name is Mokolo** "Gorillas Go Green: Apes Shed Pounds While Doubling Calories on Leafy Diet, Researcher Finds," *ScienceDaily,* February 21, 2011. http://www.sciencedaily.com/releases/2011/02/110217091130.htm (accessed December 16, 2012).

16 **fed according to the official guidelines** National Research Council, 2003.

16 **the number one killer of male gorillas in captivity** Meehan and Lowenstine, 1994.

16   the number one killer of male humans in civilization World Health Organization, 2012.

16   Median life expectancy for male gorillas in zoos Kristen Lukas, personal communication, July 9, 2012.

17   her dissertation on body fat and obesity in captive gorillas Less, 2012.

17   Gorilla Species Survival Plan The Gorilla SSP home page can be found at http://www.clemetzoo.com/gorillassp (accessed December 15, 2012).

19   cholesterol levels tend to be higher among captive gorillas Schmidt et al., 2006.

22   Gorilla "Diets" Cousins, 1976.

22   loaves of bread, candy, and even alcohol Hancocks, 2001, pp. 1, 55.

25   *things got worse before they got better* Coe, 1995.

25   inaugural games of the Roman Colosseum See Dio's description here: http://penelope.uchicago.edu/Thayer/E/Roman/Texts/Cassius_Dio/66*.html#25 (accessed December 23, 2012). Dio, 1925, book 66, par. 25.

25   "The creatures have a rank smell" J. Stuart, "The Polar Bear Who Lived at the Tower . . . Along with a Grumpy Lion and a Baboon Who Threw Cannon Balls: Britain's First (and Most Bizarre) Zoo," *Daily Mail Online,* September 21, 2010. http://www.dailymail.co.uk/news/article-1313816/The-polar-bear-lived-Tower—grumpy-lion-baboon-threw-cannon-balls-Britains-bizarre-zoo.html (accessed December 21, 2012).

26   In the 1850s a gorilla could expect to live about six months in captivity Jon Coe, personal communication, February 21, 2011.

26   chronic ailments came to the fore Kitchener and Macdonald, 2005.

27   antidepressants J. Laidman, "Zoos Using Drugs to Help Manage Anxious Animals," *Toledo Blade,* September 12, 2005.

27   A 2001 survey of U.S. and Canadian zoos Murphy and Mufson, 2001.

27   In 1978 Seattle's Woodland Park Zoo opened its new gorilla habitat To appreciate the revolutionary shift to landscape immersion, see Hancocks, 2001, pp. 111–48.

27   the gorillas had chronic diarrhea, but it went away Jon Coe, personal communication, February 21, 2011.

27   "Know thy species" comes from Dr. Jonas Salk Salk, 1972, p. 102.

FURTHER READING David Hancocks is the former director of Seattle's Woodland Park Zoo, and his lucid book is the single best treatment of the past, present, and future of zoos: Hancocks, 2001, *A Different Nature.* Just another metaphysical vision quest with a telepathic gorilla: Quinn (1995),

Ishmael. This book explores the concept of civilization as a zoo: Morris (2009), *The Human Zoo.* A textbook on the management of zoo animals: Hosey, Melfi, and Pankhurst (2009), *Zoo Animals.* A textbook on evolution and animal behavior: Alcock (2009), *Animal Behavior.*

3. Rise and Fall *(Paleolithic Age)*

29   **2.6 million years ago** The date of the earliest stone tools (Oldowan), which were found in East Africa. Roche, Blumenschine, and Shea, 2009.

31   **brain size more than doubled** Lee and Wolpoff, 2003.

31   **endurance running** Bramble and Lieberman, 2004.

31   **bones that bear the distinct markings of an animal having been butchered** Semaw, 2000.

31   **Changes in diet played an important role** Leonard et al., 2003.

31   **2% of our body mass but consumes roughly 20% of our energy** Mink, Blumenschine, and Adams, 1981.

32   **the role of cooking on the expansion of the brain** Wrangham, 2010.

32   **The earliest evidence of cooking** "Million-year-old Ash Hints at Origins of Cooking," *Nature News,* April 2, 2012. http://www.nature.com/news/million-year-old-ash-hints-at-origins-of-cooking-1.10372 (accessed December 23, 2012).

32   **energy constraints on brain size** Fonseca-Azevedo and Herculano-Houzel, 2012.

34   **Evolution hasn't stopped** Hawks et al., 2007.

36   **"what happened to the early farmers who started eating a starchier diet"** Larsen, 1995.

36   **"Smaller jaws"** Von Cramon-Taubadel, 2011.

37   **Early farming populations lost as much as five inches of height** Mummert et al., 2011.

37   **"Contemporary hunter-gatherers regularly live well into their sixties and seventies"** Gurven and Kaplan, 2007.

37   **a longer childhood before puberty** Kaplan et al., 2000.

37   **life expectancy initially *dropped* after the Agricultural Revolution** Galor and Moav, 2007.

40   **"from a distance they look like giants"** Vaca, 1993, p. 44.

41   **what an ancestral human lifestyle might have looked like** For a good summary of the ethnographic record on hunter-gatherers (and references to more in-depth treatments), see Marlowe, 2005.

42   **Cancer was less common** It's hard to ascertain cancer incidence in the Paleolithic, but there are good reasons to think it was lower. Given the importance of infectious agents in causing cancer and the increase in infectious disease during the Agricultural Revolution, it's highly likely that cancer became more prevalent too. Also, cancers of the female reproductive system (breast, endometrium, ovary) have been tied to modern lifestyle changes. For example, see Eaton et al., 1994.

42 **considerable violence** Pinker, 2011, pp. 36–58.

43 **urban farmers eating plant-based diets** I am not in a position to assess Gnostic or anagrammatic interpretations of the Bible, but I found Hatfield's analysis of biblical diets to be thought-provoking: Hatfield, 2009, pp. 23–29.

FURTHER READING See Lieberman (2013), *The Story of the Human Body.*

4. Moses the Microbiologist *(Agricultural Age)*

44 **Moses the Microbiologist** This chapter title comes from Hart, 2007, p. 54.

44 **8,000 B.C.** The approximate date of the earliest continuously inhabited city, Jericho. Though settled by pre-agricultural Natufians even earlier, farmers started living there around 8350 B.C.; see Bar-Yosef, 1986.

46 **Pathogens are responsible for far more health conditions than is generally appreciated** Cochran, Ewald, and Cochran, 2000.

46 **at least one in six cases of cancer** De Martel et al., 2012.

46 **a major risk factor for schizophrenia** Brown, 2008.

46 **it starts out virulent then becomes less dangerous over time** On factors that influence virulence of infectious diseases, see Ewald, 1994.

47 **spices have antimicrobial properties** Billing and Sherman, 1998.

47 **meat dishes tend to call for more spices than do vegetable dishes** Sherman and Hash, 2001.

47 **"toothbrushes"** Hyson, 2003.

50 **"Cleanliness is next to godliness"** In a 1791 sermon called "On Dress," Protestant pastor John Wesley said, "Cleanliness is, indeed, next to godliness." The phrase is often mistakenly presumed to appear in the Bible, but it likely derives from a passage in the Talmud by Rabbi Phinehas ben Yair (Abodah Zarah 20b: 10-12): http://www.come-and-hear.com/zarah/zarah_20.html (accessed December 11, 2012).

51 **a generalized obsession with potential routes of infection** Curtis and Biran, 2001.

52 **cannibalism** Diamond, 2000.

52 **inflated the lungs and submerged them in water to look for any leaks—a telltale sign of tuberculosis** Hart, 2007, pp. 67–68, 143–72.

53 **a valuable service in the local ecology: devouring common**

carriers of disease I found Ben Hobrink's book on science in the Bible to be insightful, particularly the chapters on the ecological logic of kashrut (though I do not agree with all his examples or conclusions). See Hobrink, 2011, chapter 4.

54   borrowed from Zoroastrianism, or vice versa Noting that biblical scholarship has advanced over the past century, see the 1906 *Jewish Encyclopedia*'s entry on Zoroastrianism, particularly "Resemblances Between Zoroastrianism and Judaism." Found online at http://www.jewishencyclopedia .com/articles/15283-zoroastrianism (accessed December 23, 2012).

55   they may carry a greater disease risk More than eight hundred years ago Maimonides believed that there were health reasons for avoiding pork. For a more modern take on the issue, I recommend Paul Jaminet's three-part series on the relationship between pork consumption and liver cirrhosis, liver cancer, multiple sclerosis, and hepatitis see P. Jaminet, "Pork: Did Leviticus 11:7 Have It Right?" perfecthealthdiet.com, February 8, 2012. http://perfecthealthdiet.com/2012/02/pork-did-leviticus-117-have-it-right (accessed December 12, 2012).

55   Anthropologist Dr. Marvin Harris Harris, 1998, p. 71.

57   The Nobel-worthy commandment to wash your hands Allegranzi et al., 2009. Table 1 contains a list of hand washing practices in religions around the world. It's worth noting that such cultures often develop customs of washing their hands in more circumstances than explicitly called for in Scripture.

57   washing without soap is better than nothing Burton et al., 2011. See also Luby et al., 2011.

57   Jews have been avid bathers for millennia The Essenes, an ancient sect of Judaism, were building ritual baths (mikveh) in the second century B.C. and were probably bathing in streams for far longer. Taylor, 2004.

58   All Jews had to come clean, so to speak, on the Sabbath The Essenes took cleanliness seriously. According to Taylor, the Jewish historian "Josephus writes that the Essenes do not defecate on the Sabbath." Quoted in Taylor, 2004.

59   Parsis The similarity between the Parsis and the Jews was noted as early as 1563. The Portuguese physician Garcia de Orta wrote, "We Portuguese call them Jews, but they are not so. They are Gentios who came from Persia." De Orta should know: he was Jewish. Orta, 1903, pp. 445–46. Cochran, Hardy, and Harpending's paper on Ashkenazi IQ also contains a paragraph on similarities between Jews and Parsis: Cochran, Hardy, and Harpending, 2006.

59   India India arrived at a different solution to infectious disease:

the caste system. India's lowest caste is known as the Untouchables, a social class whose members performed unclean jobs, such as waste disposal, butchering, tanning hides, and burying corpses. Everyone from higher castes treated Untouchables as literally untouchable—and if they did come in contact with an Untouchable they had to wash thoroughly. Untouchables had to drink from different wells and live in different parts of the city. They were treated as contagious. Given the nature of their professions, they probably were more likely to be ill or carriers of infection. Similar "untouchable" castes existed throughout South Asia, Japan, and parts of Africa. The growth of these societies may have depended on social stratification. The Untouchables were immuno-slaves, acting as a biological bulwark against infectious disease. For evidence that different castes have different genetic signatures in relation to immune function, see Pitchappan, 2002.

60   fingernails trimmed to less than a quarter of an inch Centers for Disease Control and Prevention, 2002, p. 33 (Recommendation 6B).

60   gonorrhea can cause infertility Centers for Disease Control and Prevention, 2012a.

60   more permissive sexual practices began to emerge in the late 1950s, soon after the discovery of penicillin in 1943 Francis, 2013.

61   sex between men Diep et al., 2008. Also see Bolan, Sparling, and Wasserheit, 2012.

61   bestiality Zequi et al., 2012.

61   Jewish women have particularly low rates of cervical cancer Menczer, 2003.

61   common among prostitutes Wattleworth, 2011.

61   some aspect of Jewish sexual practices Drain et al., 2006.

61   a review of the costs and benefits of male circumcision American Academy of Pediatrics, Task Force on Circumcision, 2012.

64   Pope Clement VI tried to quell the massacres Byrne, 2008, p. 68.

64   But what if the Jewish people actually *were* less afflicted by the Black Death? One of the infamous forced confessions came from Balavignus, a fourteenth-century Jewish physician from Strasbourg, France, who was subsequently executed. The forced confession itself is well documented, but I've also come across modern sources relating a backstory that I've been unable to corroborate. Supposedly, when the Black Death broke out, Balavignus led a cleanup of the Jewish ghetto and urged strict adherence to the Mosaic Law. The rats decided they'd rather live in the Christian part of town—and when Christians saw that

Jews were dying less often, Balavignus was blamed. If anyone knows of historical sources that shed light on this story, I'd love to hear about it (john@huntergatherer.com). For the story, search online or see Atkinson, 1958, pp. 57–62.

65 **Dr. Ignaz Semmelweis** Semmelweis, 1983.

65 **statistics on Jewish mortality rates** Fishberg, 1901.

65 **"unprecedented tenacity of life"** Fishberg, 1901

66 **New York City's Lower East Side** Dwork, 1981, pp. 1–40.

66 **mortality in the Jewish and Catholic population of Gibraltar** Sawchuk, Tripp, and Melnychenko, 2012.

FURTHER READING Much of the best biblical scholarship is written in German or Hebrew, languages that I don't read. The most comprehensive text in English (that I know of) analyzing the scientific basis of rules found in the Bible and Talmud is Preuss (1978), *Biblical and Talmudic Medicine*. Also see the excellent bibliography (and content) in Hart (2007), *The Healthy Jew*. For a profile of Maurice Fishberg and his work, see the first chapter of Ostrer (2012), *Legacy*. Separately, for a discussion of Ashkenazi Jewish intelligence, see chapter 7 of Cochran and Harpending (2010), *The 10,000 Year Explosion*. Prior to the time period discussed, I would argue that a scientifically sound hygiene code gave Jews (and Parsis) an initial advantage in urban, commercial, and dirty professions. On the relationship between infectious disease and religion, see the many interesting papers by Randy Thornhill and Corey Fincher, such as Fincher and Thornhill, 2012, "Parasite-stress Promotes In-group Assortative Sociality: The Cases of Strong Family Ties and Heightened Religiosity."

5. Homo Invictus *(Industrial Age)*

68 **1769** The date of James Watt's patent on a dramatically improved steam engine that would power the Industrial Revolution. His last name would become the standard unit of power: the watt.

68 **James Glaisher and Henry Coxwell** Coxwell, 1889, pp. 130–50.

71 **During the Seven Years' War (1756–1763)** Available online at http://books.google.com/books?id=K0RMAAAAMAAJ&pgis=1 (accessed December 23, 2012). "Scurvy." 1892, *Chamber's Encyclopaedia: a Dictionary of Universal Knowledge*, W. & R. Chambers: 270.

73 **"not a man escaped the repeated attacks of rheumatism and cold"** U.S. Navy, 1999, pp. 1–6.

74 **large amounts of refined sugar in their diet** Sheridan, 1974, pp. 18–35.

74 "In London, mostly 1800 onwards, they have absolutely dreadful teeth" Gibbons, 2012.

74 the first popular "diet book" Banting, 1863.

75 *rickets,* an "absolutely new disease" Dunn, 1998.

76 supplemental oxygen systems weighing twenty-two pounds Windsor, McMorrow, and Rodway, 2008.

77 Worries include "low sensory input, lack of motivation" "Shuttle-Mir Background—Long-Duration Spaceflight," *NASA*, April 4, 2004. http://spaceflight.nasa.gov/history/shuttle-mir/history/to-h-b-long .htm (accessed December 16, 2012).

78 If one had to categorize all these habitat features My approach to categorizing habitat features was inspired by Nassim Taleb's afterword to De Vany, 2010, pp. 148–57.

82 "the ability to perceive meaning in seemingly random events" Suedfeld, 1997.

82 "Homo Invictus" Suedfeld and Henley, 2012.

FURTHER READING A NASA adviser synthesizes lessons from interviews with polar personnel and astronauts, debriefing reports, explorers' diaries and ships' logs, and historical accounts of expeditions: Stuster (2011), *Bold Endeavors*. Also see Suedfeld (1987), "Extreme and Unusual Environments."

6. Biohackers *(Information Age)*

84 1946 The date of the unveiling of ENIAC, a giant computer used by the U.S. military to calculate artillery firing tables. Digital age historian George Dyson says, "It is impossible to predict where the digital universe is going, but it is possible to understand how it began. The origin of the first fully electronic random-access storage matrix, and the propagation of the codes that it engendered, is as close to a point source as any approximation can get." Dyson, 2012, pp. ix–xi.

84 "We have found the secret of life" I. Noble, " 'Secret of Life' Discovery Turns 50," *BBC News*, February 27, 2003. http://news.bbc.co.uk/2/hi/ science/nature/2804545.stm (accessed December 16, 2012).

85 5,386 base pairs The original paper sequenced 5,375 base pairs: Sanger et al., 1977.

85 "Human DNA is like a computer program" Gates, Myhrvold, and Rinearson, 1996, p. 228.

85 biology is an information technology Hood and Galas, 2003.

86 "To qualify as a hack" Levy, 2010, p. 8. For the origins of hacking at MIT and elsewhere, see pp. 3–106.

86   **"tools"** On the differences between hackers and tools, see the web-page of Brian Harvey, University of California, Berkeley: http://www.eecs .berkeley.edu/~bh/hacker.html (accessed May 4, 2013). Also, see Levy, 2010, p. 8.

86   **"a door opened to a world"** The Mentor, "Hacker's Manifesto," *Phrack* 1 (7), September 25, 1986. See online at: http://www.phrack.org/ issues.html?issue=7&id=3#article (accessed May 4, 2013).

86   **This hacker philosophy** See Levy, 2010, pp. 23–32.

87   **"Move fast and break things"** See "Mark Zuckerberg's Letter to Investors: 'The Hacker Way,'" online at: http://www.wired.com/business/ 2012/02/zuck-letter (accessed May 4, 2013).

87   **Coca-Cola was originally concocted** H. Edwards, "6 Hugely Successful Products Originally Invented for Something Else," Mental Floss, January 26, 2012. http://mentalfloss.com/article/29840/6-hugely -successful-products-originally-invented-something-else (accessed May 4, 2013).

87   **Programmer Eric Raymond described** Raymond, 2008. Available online at: http://www.catb.org/~esr/writings/cathedral-bazaar (accessed May 4, 2013).

88   **Paul Graham likes to invest in** Levy, 2010, p. 392.

88   **Quantified Self** See online at: http://quantifiedself.com (accessed May 4, 2013).

89   **"Science advances one funeral at a time"** Planck doesn't appear to have coined this exact phrase, but it's derived from him: http://en.wikiquote .org/wiki/Max_Planck (accessed May 4, 2013).

89   **"Any living cell carries with it"** Delbruck quoted in Hood and Galas, 2003.

90   **"Nature is a tinkerer, not an engineer"** The point is made in Jacob, 1977.

90   **morning sickness has a biological function** Flaxman and Sherman, 2008.

91   **"The hydraulic model"** Pinker, 2003, p. 65.

93   ***"information transfer* in living material"** "The Nobel Prize in Physiology or Medicine 1962: Francis Crick, James Watson, Maurice Wilkins." NobelPrize.org. http://www.nobelprize.org/nobel_prizes/medicine/ laureates/1962 (accessed December 16, 2012).

FURTHER READING On the history and philosophy of hackers, see Levy, 2010, and Raymond, 2008. For a history of the Information Age, see Dyson, 2012. On the future of technology, see Kelly, 2010.

Part Two: Here and Now

7. Food: The Conventional Wisdom

97 "Convenience Store Diet" M. Park, "Twinkie Diet Helps Nutrition Professor Lose 27 Pounds," CNN, November 8, 2010. http://www.cnn .com/2010/HEALTH/11/08/twinkie.diet.professor/index.html (accessed October 15, 2012).

98 As science journalist Gary Taubes has written Taubes, 2010, pp. 80–86.

99 even babies born on the early side of normal Noble et al., 2012.

100 molecules that feed beneficial bacteria in the baby's stomach Zhang et al., 2012.

101 Dr. Oz Roizen and Oz, 2009.

101 the Mayo Clinic Mayo Foundation for Medical Education and Research, 2010.

103 Cheez Whiz D. Hevesi, "Edwin Traisman, 91, Dies; Helped Create Iconic Foods," *New York Times,* June 9, 2007.

103 35.7% of adult Americans were obese Ogden et al., 2012.

106 "calories in, calories out" "Three potato chips" comes from Taubes, 2010, p. 58. For an extended discussion on calories, see pp. 15–86.

107 chaired by Senator George McGovern U.S. Senate Select Committee on Nutrition and Human Needs, 1977.

107 the body needs cholesterol Lecerf and De Lorgeril, 2011.

108 egg intake and cardiovascular disease Zazpe et al., 2011.

108 statins Wierzbicki, Poston, and Ferro, 2003.

108 Roughly 40% of fats in human breast milk are saturated Jensen, 1999.

108 A recent Dutch study examined reports from three leading U.S. and European advisory committees Hoenselaar, 2012.

109 a meta-analysis on the link between saturated fat and heart disease Siri-Tarino et al., 2010.

109 French Paradox Ferrières, 2004.

109 "Israeli Paradox" Yam, Eliraz, and Berry, 1996.

109 a new study scares people about eating red meat Pan et al., 2012.

111 McDonald's cooked its French fries in beef tallow This paper gives the history of trans fats being adopted as a substitute for saturated fats, as well as CSPI's role in the switch: Schleifer, 2012.

113 chimpanzees, our closest primate relatives, eat some meat According to primatologist Craig Stanford, "[I]t seems clear that chimpanzees value fat above all else in the carcasses of their prey. We infer this from their preference for the brain and the bone marrow, two of the most fat-rich body parts" (Stanford, 2001, p. 152).

113   By 2.6 million years ago Semaw, 2000.

113   Stable isotope analyses of some Paleolithic hominin remains Katzenberg et al., 2010.

113   Of contemporary hunter-gatherer societies studied, most have gotten more than 50% of their calories from animal products Cordain, 2007. Also see Kaplan et al., 2000.

114   Of five major studies conducted on vegetarians Key et al., 1999.

114   Mormons, who are similar except for eating meat, are also healthier For a few comparisons with Seventh-day Adventists, see Lyon and Nelson, 1979. For more on Mormon health, also see Enstrom and Breslow, 2008.

114   lower bone mineral density Smith, 2006.

114   consumption of animal protein has been shown to reduce osteo-porosis and hip fractures Munger, Cerhan, and Chiu, 1999. Also see Promislow, 2002.

114   more likely to lose their period (amenorrhea) or become tempo-rarily infertile Griffith and Omar, 2003.

114   *The China Study* Campbell, 2005.

115   studies of contemporary herders show low rates of cardiovascu-lar disease Little, 1989.

116   What did that grandmother recognize as food? Cordain, 2007. See also Kaplan et al., 2000.

116   only a handful of small, short clinical trials testing approxima-tions of Paleolithic diets For example, see Jönsson et al., 2009; Jönsson et al., 2010; Osterdahl et al., 2008; Frassetto et al., 2009.

8. Food: Principles for a Healthy Diet

119   a 2012 study of the Hadza tribe in Tanzania Pontzer et al., 2012.

120   A review of the diets of 229 foraging societies Cordain, 2007.

120   In another study of nine contemporary hunter-gatherer tribes Kaplan et al., 2000.

120   the Kitavans, a tribe of Pacific Islanders Lindeberg et al., 2003.

121   cannibalism Diamond, 2000.

122   10–20% of calories in the form of protein Bilsborough and Mann, 2006.

122   Protein is the most satiating of the macronutrients Bertenshaw, Lluch, and Yeomans, 2008.

123   the Inuit had very specific methods of dividing carcasses
Stefansson, 1960, pp. 25–39.

124   Eating nose to tail is the ultimate nutritional supplement
Vucetich, Vucetich, and Peterson, 2011.

125   Ancient culinary traditions Pollan's book is a good source on
ancient culinary traditions, though I don't think his skepticism of meat is
justified on health grounds: Pollan, 2009.

126   humans have been boiling bones Wu et al., 2012.

128   The blackened part of heavily cooked meat Daniel et al., 2011.

129   "An egg is superior" For this verse in the Talmud, see http://
www.come-and-hear.com/berakoth/berakoth_44.html (accessed December 14, 2012).

129   the most nutritious part of the egg: the yolk C. Masterjohn,
"The Incredible, Edible Egg Yolk," July 2005. http://www.cholesterol-and
-health.com/Egg_Yolk.html (accessed December 26, 2012).

129   eating eggs has not been shown to cause cardiovascular disease
Zazpe et al., 2011.

129   When Inuit hunters kill a seal Borre, 1991. See also Stefansson,
1960, pp. 33, 104, 130.

131   "As much as meat loves salt" D. L. Ashliman, " 'Love Like Salt':
Folktales of Types 923 and 510." http://www.pitt.edu/~dash/salt.html
(accessed December 25, 2012).

132   "the world's oldest medicine" Johns, 1991.

132   Geophagy Young, 2012.

133   Despite all the hysteria over the sodium added to industrial
food M. W. Moyer, "It's Time to End the War on Salt," *Scientific American,*
July 2011.

133   *Avoid Industrial Foods, Sugars, and Seeds* A more in-depth discussion
of the scientific literature surrounding sugar, grains, legumes, and vegetable
oils can be found here: Jaminet and Jaminet, 2012.

134   Fructose For the most critical view of sugar, particularly fructose,
see Robert Lustig's popular lecture on the topic: "Sugar: The Bitter Truth."
http://www.youtube.com/watch?v=dBnniua6-oM (accessed December 28,
2012).

135   excessive omega-6 consumption has been associated with higher
rates of obesity Dayton et al., 1966.

135   mental illness Su et al., 2003.

135   violence Hibbeln, Nieminen, and Lands, 2004.

135   allergies, asthma Chilton et al., 2008.

135   and cancer Lloyd et al., 2010.

136   laboratory experiments on mice, diets excessively high in PUFAs You et al., 2005. See also Rivera et al., 2010.

136   nearly 70% of global agricultural crops by weight Jaminet and Jaminet, 2012, p. 196.

136   gut inflammation in over 80% of people Bernardo et al., 2007.

136   lupus, type 1 diabetes, and multiple sclerosis Fasano, 2006.

137   Consumption of wheat has been associated with . . . cardiovascular disease P. Jaminet, "The China Study: Evidence for the Perfect Health Diet." July 9, 2010. http://perfecthealthdiet.com/2010/07/the-china-study -evidence-for-the-perfect-health-diet (accessed December 28, 2012).

137   and cancer Hoggan, 1997.

137   female sheep that eat too many of certain pasture legumes Croker, Barbetti, and Adams, 2005. See also Adams, 1995.

9. Fasting

146   the Topeka Zoo had five overweight lions Altman, Gross, and Lowry, 2005.

147   The !Kung Bushmen Thomas, 2007.

148   The only food that they'll stop to gather is honey Hill et al., 1987.

149   Eastern Orthodox The statistics on Eastern Orthodox fasting were calculated from the official 2013 calendar (http://www.goarch.org/chapel/ chapel/calendar) in conjunction with rules stipulated here: http://home .wavecable.com/~photios/fasting.htm (accessed December 23, 2012).

150   air or spirit swallowing (*fuqi*) Eskildsen, 1998, p. 45.

151   wild animals often just stop eating altogether when facing an acute infection Hart, 1988.

151   Many pathogens are dependent on specific amino acids for their metabolism, such as tryptophan Brown et al., 1991.

151   *autophagy* Rabinowitz and White, 2010.

151   targeting "the biggest polluters" Hirota, Kang, and Kanki, 2012.

151   a study of Kenyan children Wander, Shell-Duncan, and McDade, 2009.

152   Studies on rabbits Kluger and Rothenburg, 1979.

152   and hamsters Held et al., 2006.

152   "we had healthier gums than ever before" Frankl, 2006, p. 30.

152   This is not to say that all methods of religious fasting were equally effective This paper reviews fasting in Islam, Eastern Orthodox

Christianity, and the biblical Daniel Fast: Trepanowski and Bloomer, 2010. It's easy to see how different fasting customs could produce different results.

153 activating ancient starvation defenses Lee, Raffaghello, and Longo, 2012.

153 In an intriguing 2008 study, two groups of mice Raffaghello et al., 2008.

153 Additional work has shown that fasting kills tumor cells Lee et al., 2012.

154 Uncontrolled case studies in ten human cancer patients Safdie et al., 2009.

154 Mormons have notably lower rates of coronary artery disease Horne et al., 2008.

154 A *ketogenic diet* Barañano and Hartman, 2008.

156 Women should keep a closer eye on the effects of intermittent fasting This is an overview of the limited research that has been conducted on women and fasting: S. Ruper, "A Review of Female-Specific Responses to Fasting in the Literature," June 4, 2012. http://www.paleoforwomen.com/shattering-the-myth-of-fasting-for-women-a-review-of-female-specific-responses-to-fasting-in-the-literature (accessed December 23, 2012).

158 fasting and food intake are also tied to circadian rhythm Fuller, Lu, and Saper, 2008.

159 Argonne Anti–Jet Lag Diet Reynolds and Montgomery, 2002.

159 Dr. Clifford Saper, a neuroscience researcher P. J. Skerrett, "A 'Fast' Solution to Jet Lag," May 12, 2009. http://blogs.hbr.org/health-and-well-being/2009/05/a-fast-solution-to-jet-lag.html (accessed December 23, 2012).

10. Movement

164 Consider the Paraguayan Aché tribe O'Keefe et al., 2011.

169 subsistence agriculture requires even higher levels of physical activity than foraging Pontzer et al., 2012.

169 CrossFit was founded S. Cooperman, "Getting Fit, Even if It Kills You," *New York Times,* December 22, 2005.

169 philosophy of fitness "What Is Fitness?" *The Crossfit Journal,* October 2002. http://library.crossfit.com/free/pdf/CFJ_Trial_04_2012.pdf (accessed December 15, 2012).

175 the race we call the marathon R. James, "A Brief History of the Marathon," *Time,* October 30, 2009. http://www.time.com/time/nation/article/0,8599,1933342,00.html (accessed December 23, 2012).

176 "Spartan Race, Tough Mudder, Warrior Dash, and Muddy

Buddy" N. Heil, "American Gladiators," *Outside*, November 30, 2011. http://www.outsideonline.com/outdoor-adventure/first-look/American -Gladiators.html (accessed October 30, 2012).

177 **MMA largely sprang out of the Gracie family** T. P. Grant, "MMA Origins: The Gracie Era in the UFC," *Bloody Elbow*, April 8, 2012. http://www.bloodyelbow.com/2012/4/8/2926660/mma-origins-Royce-Gracie -UFC-MMA-History-Dan-Severn-Ken-Shamrock-ninjutsu (accessed December 23, 2012).

179 **positioning yoga as a competitive sport** S. Beck, "National Yoga Competition Tests Even the Audience," *New York Times*, March 4, 2012.

179 **high-profile sex scandals** W. J. Broad, "Yoga and Sex Scandals: No Surprise Here," *New York Times*, February 27, 2012.

181 **cheetah cubs practice on actual prey** Caro and Hauser, 1992. I came across this work in a post by Dr. Peter Gray, an expert in play: http://www.psychologytoday.com/blog/freedom-learn/201104/the-human-nature -teaching-i-ways-teaching-we-share-other-animals (accessed December 23, 2012).

181 **a re-introduction program: captive-born tamarins** Stoinski and Beck, 2004.

182 **"But start to plan a playground for kids"** Jon Coe, personal communication, February 21, 2011.

11. Bipedalism: Stand, Walk, Run

186 **shaped the entire human body from head to toe** Bramble and Lieberman, 2004.

187 **hunter-gatherer women traveled about 6 miles per day** Marlowe, 2005.

187 **the average American travels about 1.5 miles on foot each day** O'Keefe et al., 2011.

188 **Scottish epidemiologist Dr. Jerry Morris** Morris et al., 1953.

188 **"inactivity physiology"** For an overview of inactivity physiology and specifics on lipoprotein lipase, see Hamilton, Hamilton, and Zderic, 2007. For evidence that time spent sitting is harmful independent of vigorous exercise, see Healy et al., 2008. This Canadian study showed a dose-response relationship between sitting and all-cause mortality, independent of vigorous activity: Katzmarzyk et al., 2009. For how physical inactivity may contribute to general inflammation and metabolic deterioration, see Pedersen, 2009.

188 **An Australian study showed that after every twenty minutes of sitting** Dunstan et al., 2012.

189   **Dr. James Levine** Levine et al., 2006.

189   **Video games and books also contain natural breaks** T. Klosowski, "How Sitting All Day Is Damaging Your Body and How You Can Counteract It," *Lifehacker,* January 26, 2012. http://lifehacker.com/5879536/how-sitting -all-day-is-damaging-your-body-and-how-you-can-counteract-it (accessed December 23, 2012).

190   **Victor Hugo** Nichol, 1893, p. 73.

190   **Nathaniel Hawthorne** Bruce, 2010, pp. 168–170.

190   **Henry Wadsworth Longfellow** Ward, 1882, p. 459.

190   **Charles Dickens** Slater, 2009, p. 290.

191   **Friedrich Nietzsche** Nietzsche and Kaufmann, 1954, p. 471.

191   **Virginia Woolf** Bruce, 2010, pp. 168–170.

191   **Ernest Hemingway** Hemingway, 1917, p. 700.

191   **Vladimir Nabokov** Harper, 2008, p. 32.

191   **August Wilson** Bruce, 2010, pp. 168–170.

191   **Other upstanding citizens include** For Thomas Jefferson, Benjamin Franklin, Winston Churchill, Oliver Wendell Holmes, Lewis Carroll, E. B. White, and Philip Roth, see Bruce, 2010, pp. 168–170.

191   **Otto von Bismarck** "Alike in summer and winter the Emperor rises early, and by five o'clock he is occupied at his standing desk. He examines all proposals laid before him, particularly such as relate to military or foreign affairs" (Fournier, 1896, p. 214).

191   **Richard Wagner** "during composition he often paced to and fro, sometimes going to the grand piano in the next room to play single chords or phrases, which he then wrote down at his standing-desk" (Glasenapp and Ellis, 1908, p. 290).

192   **"However, I stand for 8–10 hours a day"** "Memo from the Department of Defense Summarizing Approved Methods of Interrogation, with Annotation from Secretary of Defense Donald Rumsfeld," *NSA,* December 2, 2002. See online at http://www.gwu.edu/~nsarchiv/NSAEBB/NSAEBB127/ 02.12.02.pdf (accessed December 23, 2012).

192   **Dr. Seth Roberts** S. Roberts, "Effect of One-Legged Standing on Sleep," March 22, 2011. http://blog.sethroberts.net/2011/03/22/effect-of -one-legged-standing-on-sleep (accessed December 24, 2012).

194   **"stands in a pair of his oversized loafers on the worn skin of a lesser kudu"** This interview can also be read online at http://www.the parisreview.org/interviews/4825/the-art-of-fiction-no-21-ernest-hemingway (accessed December 23, 2012). Plimpton, 1958.

194   **"If I sit down, I write a long opinion"** Bruce, 2010, pp. 168–170.

194   "a simple standing desk which would not have fetched more than two shillings" Boughton-Wilby, 1903, p. 585.

194   The State Department displays one of Jefferson's drafting desks The display on Jefferson's desk reads: "This architectural style American table-desk is said to have been designed and used by Thomas Jefferson for drafting many important documents, possibly including portions of the Declaration of Independence. It was in his apartment at 7th and Market Streets, Philadelphia, 1775–1776" ("Thomas Jefferson's Desk," Washington, D.C.: The Diplomatic Reception Rooms, U.S. Department of State).

195   confident, strong posture Carney, Cuddy, and Yap, 2010.

196   a third or more of runners sustain some sort of injury each year Van Gent et al., 2007.

196   Running with a forefoot strike Lieberman et al., 2010.

196   In a study of runners on the Harvard track team Daoud et al., 2012.

197   "If barefoot running is a fad" Saxton and Wallack, 2011, p. 229.

200   Shoes even change the very shape of our feet D'Aout et al., 2009.

200   80% of women had a foot deformity Frey et al., 1993.

201   wearing thin socks causes worse balance than going barefoot Shinohara and Gribble, 2009.

202   Barefoot Horses Saxton and Wallack, 2011, pp. 48–49.

203   "Though human ingenuity may make various inventions" Da Vinci, 1970, p. 126.

FURTHER READING   Howell, 2010, The Barefoot Book.

12. Thermoregulation

208   our ancestors lost their fur Rogers, Iltis, and Wooding, 2004.

209   "In the sauna one must conduct himself" Aaland, 1978, p. 75.

210   Sweat Baths Around the World Aaland's book Sweat (1978) contains information on all major types of sweat bathing traditions listed in this sidebar. Much of the same information can be found on Aaland's website: http://cyberbohemia.com/Pages/sweat.htm (accessed December 14, 2012).

210   "Many Indians, men and women, stark naked" Aaland, 1978, p. 177.

211   Mayan ruins dating to 2,500 years ago J. N. Wilford, "Before Rome's Baths, There Was the Maya Sweat House," New York Times, March 20, 2001.

211   "the temazcalli is still so common" Groark, 1997.

211   more than two million saunas "Statistics Finland: Housing," Statistikcentralen. http://www.stat.fi/tup/suoluk/suoluk_asuminen_en.html (accessed December 15, 2012).

211   African *sifutu* Harrison, 2004, p. 63.

211   Karo (Indonesian) *oukup* A. Gunawan, " 'Mandi Oukup' Is More Than Just a Bath," *Jakarta Post,* July 1, 2001.

211   Indian *swedana* Douillard, 2004, pp. 281–86.

211   Celtic *teach alluis* Killanin and Duignan, 1967, p. 311.

212   Herodotus wrote about the use of sweat baths Herodotus, 1889, book IV, par. 73–75.

212   Finnish women actually used to give birth in a sauna Pentikäinen, 2001, p. 31.

212   Russian women used to give birth in saunas too Aaland, 1978, p. 118.

212   After childbirth, Mesoamerican women Groark, 2005.

212   George Catlin described the "vapour bath" of the Mandan Catlin, 1842, pp. 98–99.

213   an intense cooling-off may be a more effective treatment Kukkonen-Harjula and Kauppinen, 2006.

213   A study of winter swimmers found they were slower to shiver Vybíral et al., 2000.

213   one study found reductions in the initial shock of entering cold water persisted Tipton, Mekjavic, and Eglin, 2000.

214   "The idea is not to have the best sauna on the block" Aaland, 1978, p. 17.

214   few risks Kukkonen-Harjula and Kauppinen, 2006. See also Hannuksela and Ellahham, 2001.

215   Tim Ferriss features a story about Ray Cronise Ferriss, 2010, pp. 122–27.

216   starvation victims have lower than normal body temperatures Keys et al., 1950.

218   a fever is a natural immune response to infection Nesse and Williams, 2012, pp. 27–29. See also Kluger, 1986.

218   Dr. Matthew Kluger infected thirteen iguanas with bacteria Bernheim and Kluger, 1976a.

218   When he injected more iguanas with bacteria and gave them a fever suppressant Bernheim and Kluger, 1976b.

218   an inverse relationship between fever and mortality Kluger et al., 1998.

218   people with aquariums have long used the trick of heating up their tanks Haname, "Using Heat to Treat Ich in Freshwater Tropical Fish." http://www.aquahobby.com/articles/e_ich2.php (accessed December 13, 2012).

218 "Give me a chance to create a fever" American Cancer Society, 2012a.

218 Dr. Julius Wagner-Jauregg "The Nobel Prize in Physiology or Medicine 1927: Julius Wagner-Jauregg," NobelPrize.org. http://www.nobelprize.org/nobel_prizes/medicine/laureates/1927 (accessed December 15, 2012).

218 take about a day longer to recover from chicken pox Doran et al., 1989.

218 the common cold lasts about a day longer too Sugimura et al., 1994.

219 one in six cases of cancer are caused by infection De Martel et al., 2012.

219 a field called immunotherapy American Cancer Society, 2012b.

219 "We have listened to nature" Cann, Van Netten, and Van Netten, 2003.

FURTHER READING Gluckman, Beedle, and Hanson, 2009. See also Nesse and Williams, 2012.

13. Sunrise, Sunset

222 phytoplankton and zooplankton Holick, Holick, and Guillard, 1982.

222 This meant eating calcium-rich plants Holick, 1989.

222 Boston's Franklin Park Zoo celebrated the birth of Kimani See the introduction of Holick, 2010.

223 42% of Americans were deficient Forrest and Stuhldreher, 2011.

223 our hominin ancestors had a thick layer of black hair Jablonski, 2004.

224 An analysis of the genes controlling skin pigmentation Rogers, Iltis, and Wooding, 2004.

224 Razib Khan pointed out Khan and Khan, 2010.

225 Many studies indicate that vitamin D protects against internal cancers Garland et al., 2006; Holick, 2004; Giovannucci et al., 2008.

225 the immune system's ability to mount a response to microbial infections Liu et al., 2006.

226 there's more UVa in sunlight than UVb Kollias, Ruvolo, and Sayre, 2011.

227 The most deadly cancers were Siegel et al., 2011.

228 the genetic mutations associated with UV damage Curtin et al., 2005.

228 The strongest risk factor for developing melanoma Lazovich et al., 2010.

228 "red-headed" mice developed malignant melanomas Mitra et al., 2012.

228 scientific evidence that tanning bed usage caused melanoma Lazovich et al., 2010.

229 now it's officially a carcinogen El Ghissassi, Baan, and Straif, 2009.

229 deaths due to drowning Centers for Disease Control and Prevention, 2012c.

232 Dr. Jerome Siegel Siegel, 2012.

233 Among hunter-gatherers, sleep patterns are quite a bit different J. Warren, "How to Sleep Like a Hunter-Gatherer," *Discover,* December, 2007.

233 "segmented sleep" Ekirch, 2005, pp. 300–323.

235 When humans interbred with Neanderthals Sankararaman et al., 2012.

235 some arctic species, such as reindeer, have a weaker circadian rhythm Van Oort et al., 2005. See also Lu et al., 2010.

235 a third of Americans are chronically sleep-deprived Centers for Disease Control and Prevention, 2012b.

235 Sleep is one of the most challenging aspects Stuster, 2011, pp. 44–55.

236 NASA advised the rescue effort R. Wright, "NASA Chilean Miners Rescue Oral History Project: Interview with Albert W. Holland," *NASA,* April 25, 2011. http://www.jsc.nasa.gov/history/oral_histories/CMR/HollandAW/HollandAW_4-25-11.htm (accessed December 16, 2012).

237 jet lag Vosko, Colwell, and Avidan, 2010.

237 "free-running" Stuster, 2011, p. 47.

Part Three: Visions

14. Hunter

241 Hunting and fishing are in a decades long decline D. Nelson, "The Vanishing Hunter Part I: Hunting Participation in Long-Term Retreat," *Delta Waterfowl Magazine,* Spring 2008. http://www.deltawaterfowl.org/media/magazine/archive/vanishinghunter/part1.php (accessed December 21, 2012). See also Leonard, 2007.

242 Essays . . . about how hunting is the next big thing For example, see: Garner, D. "A New Breed of Hunter Shoots, Eats and Tells," *New York Times,* October 1, 2012.

242 *The Beginner's Guide to Hunting Deer for Food* Landers, 2011.

243 "When food runs low it is infant mortality among deer that usually runs high" Jackson Landers, personal communication, April 7, 2011.

243 Even when abandoned fawns are found, rehabilitated, and released This study showed particularly high mortality rates among captured fawns that were released back into the wild in Missouri: Beringer et al., 2004. Those that survived tended to live near human settlements.

243 the least painful way for a deer to die In this Pennsylvania study, 218 deer fawns were captured, radio tagged, and monitored. Roughly half died over the following thirty-four weeks. The top causes of death were predation (46.2%, mostly from black bears and coyotes) and natural causes excluding predation (27.4%, mostly starvation and disease). Human-related causes of death (vehicles, hunting) constituted the bulk of the rest. Vreeland, Diefenbach, and Wallingford, 2004.

244 even PETA . . . argued for the re-legalization of horse slaughtering P. Jonsson, "Lifting Horse Slaughter Ban: Why PETA Says It's a Good Idea," *Christian Science Monitor,* November 30, 2011. http://www.csmonitor.com/USA/2011/1130/Lifting-horse-slaughter-ban-Why-PETA-says-it-s-a-good-idea (accessed December 13, 2012).

245 Some conservationists have concerns about harvesting invasive species for food Nuñez et al., 2012.

246 Rise of the Invasivores Landers, 2012.

246 Asian carp T. Lam, "Carp Can Be Harvested—But Who Will Eat It?" *Detroit Free Press,* July 21, 2011.

246 Feral pig L. W. Foderaro, "Wily, Elusive Foragers Invade Upstate New York," *New York Times,* March 11, 2012.

246 lion tacos R. Goldman, "Arizona Restaurant Scraps Lion Tacos from Menu," *ABC News,* January 25, 2011. http://abcnews.go.com/Travel/lion-taco-plan-scrapped-arizona-restaurant-threats/story?id=12756798 (accessed December 13, 2012).

15. Gatherer

258 factory farms are undeniably unpleasant and painful Mench et al., 2008.

259 ground up alive "Chicken Culling." Wikipedia. http://en.wikipedia.org/wiki/Chick_culling (accessed December 13, 2012).

259 Disease is another problematic aspect of factory farming Silbergeld, Graham, and Price, 2008.

259 nearly 20% of *E. coli* patients carried strains with multidrug resistance Pop-Vicas and D'Agata, 2005.

259 the limited appeal of full-on vegetarianism K. Johnson, "Meatless Mondays Catch On, Even with Carnivores," *New York Times,* June 16, 2011.

260 Abstaining from animal products becomes a moralized act Rozin, Markwith, and Stoess, 1997.

260 65 to 75% of vegetarians are female 74.2% female among completely or predominantly vegetarian (Germany, general population, 1998–1999): Michalak, Zhang, and Jacobi, 2012; 72.5% female (Sweden and Norway, age 15–16, 2002): Larsson et al., 2002; about 77% female (Australia, teenagers, 1998): Worsley and Skrzypiec, 1998; about 65% female based on my own calculations from reported numbers (U.S.A., general population, 2012): F. Newport, "In U.S., 5% Consider Themselves Vegetarian," Gallup, July 26, 2012. http://www.gallup.com/poll/156215/consider-themselves-vegetarians.aspx (accessed December 13, 2012).

261 which characteristics correlate with empathy toward animals Razib Khan, "Who Objects to Painful Tests on Animals?" July 13, 2012. http://blogs.discovermagazine.com/gnxp/2012/07/who-objects-to-painful-tests-on-animals (accessed December 16, 2012).

261 a few masculine kale-loving "hegans" K. Pierce, "Men Leave Their Own Mark on Veganism," *Boston Globe,* March 24, 2010.

261 "intuitive microbiology" Pinker, 2003, p. 383.

262 disgust is triggered by the same nine categories Rozin, Haidt, and McCauley, 2008.

262 women have a much more sensitive disgust reflex than men Curtis, de Barra, and Aunger, 2011.

262 "Pretend you are eating 'perfect meat.' Great" Freedman and Barnouin, 2005, pp. 78–79.

263 Foods that are "gross" are so self-evidently unhealthy For just a few examples explicitly using the word "gross," see Freedman and Barnouin, 2005, pp. 11, 64, 78, 120, 124.

263 "a drug-stuffed, disease-ridden, shit-contaminated animal" Foer, 2009, p. 127.

263 Jonathan Haidt describes the role of disgust Haidt, 2012.

264 a harsh condemnation from the Anti-Defamation League "ADL Denounces PETA for Its 'Holocaust on Your Plate' Campaign; Calls Appeal for Jewish Community Support 'The Height Of Chutzpah,'" February 24, 2003. http://www.adl.org/PresRele/HolNa_52/4235_52.htm (accessed November 3, 2012).

264 Vegetarianism was a popular plank of the Progressive Era's "Clean Living Movement" Engs, 2003, p. 344.

264 sexual mutilation Kellogg, 1891, pp. 295–96.

264 eugenics Engs, 2001, pp. 137–49.

265 Hitler the Vegetarian A. Frangos, "Carni-Fuhrer," *Slate,* February 26, 2004. http://www.slate.com/articles/life/food/2004/02/carnifuhrer.html (accessed December 13, 2012).

265 "well known that Hitler is a vegetarian" O. D. Tolischus, "Where Hitler Dreams and Plans," *New York Times,* May 30, 1937.

265 "He believes more than ever that meat-eating is harmful to humanity" Goebbels, 1948, p. 188.

265 the most stringent animal welfare laws of its era Arluke, 1996, pp. 132–66.

265 "corpse-eaters" (*leichenfresser*) Gilbert, 1947, p. 129.

266 "a bible of the vegan community" K. Jesella, "The Carrot Some Vegans Deplore," *New York Times,* March 27, 2008.

266 "the dead body of a pony I had loved" Adams, 2010, p. 10.

266 the dubious yet incendiary claim that meat-eating encourages rape That's pretty much the thesis of the entire book, but see chapter 2, "The Rape of Animals, the Butchering of Women," particularly the subsection "Sexual Violence and Meat Eating" in Adams, 2010, pp. 64–91.

266 "If you had one girlfriend, you get twenty more" "Poison Takes Toll on Africa's Lions," *CBS News,* March 29, 2009. http://www.cbsnews .com/8301-18560_162-4894945.html (accessed November 3, 2012).

267 Pregnancy is a particularly risky time to eat a vegan diet The CDC cites a variety of studies on vitamin B12 deficiency (http://www.cdc .gov/ncbddd/b12/manifestations.html). For example, see Black, 2008.

269 "insect fragments per 50 grams" U.S. Food and Drug Administration, 2011.

271 PETA switched from boycotts to prizes People for the Ethical Treatment of Animals, "PETA Offers $1 Million Reward to First to Make In Vitro Meat." http://www.peta.org/features/in-vitro-meat-contest.aspx (accessed March 11, 2012).

271 a landmark German study Michalak, Zhang, and Jacobi, 2012.

273 the scientific definition of toxicity D. Gorski, "Fashionably Toxic," May 23, 2011. http://www.sciencebasedmedicine.org/index.php/fashionable -toxins (accessed December 21, 2012).

276 an earthquake in China Smith, 1767, pp. 211–12.

277 "It is not from the benevolence of the butcher" Smith, 1896, p. 15.

Conclusion: Habitats, Old and New

279 "Why are they chained?" Jon Coe, personal communication, February 21, 2011.

280 a long-running joke about the most dangerous animal in the zoo Hancocks, 2001, p. 138.

280 "No one asked the penguins" Hancocks, 2001, p. 76.

280   Penguin Beach D. Derbyshire, "London Zoo Unveils Lavish New £2m Pool for P-p-p-pampered Penguins," *Daily Mail Online,* May 27, 2011. http://www.dailymail.co.uk/travel/article-1391458/London-Zoo-unveils-new-penguin-pool.html (accessed December 31, 2012).

283   If everyone were to eat locally Desrochers and Shimizu, 2012.

289   "We are as gods" Brand, 2009, p. 1.

289   "The planet will be here for a long, long, LONG time" G. Carlin, "Saving the Planet." http://youtu.be/7W33HRc1A6c (accessed December 31, 2012).

290   Risen apes or fallen angels Those evocative terms, used in a different context, were originally used in Ardrey, 1963, p. 354.

Bibliography

Aaland, M. 1978. *Sweat: The Illustrated History and Description of the Finnish Sauna, Russian Bania, Islamic Hammam, Japanese Mushi-buro, Mexican Temescal, and American Indian and Eskimo Sweat Lodge.* Santa Barbara, CA: Capra Press.

Adams, C. J. 2010. *The Sexual Politics of Meat: A Feminist-Vegetarian Critical Theory.* 20th Anniversary Edition. New York: Continuum.

Adams, N. 1995. "Detection of the Effects of Phytoestrogens on Sheep and Cattle." *Animal Science* 73: 1509–15.

Alcock, J. 2009. *Animal Behavior: An Evolutionary Approach.* Sunderland, MA: Sinauer Associates.

Allegranzi, B., Z. A. Memish, L. Donaldson, and D. Pittet. 2009. "Religion and Culture: Potential Undercurrents Influencing Hand Hygiene Promotion in Health Care." *American Journal of Infection Control* 37 (1): 28–34.

Altman, J. D., K. L. Gross, and S. R. Lowry. 2005. "Nutritional and Behavioral Effects of Gorge and Fast Feeding in Captive Lions." *Journal of Applied Animal Welfare Science* 8 (1): 47–57.

American Academy of Pediatrics' Task Force on Circumcision. 2012. "Male Circumcision." *Pediatrics* 130 (3): e756–85.

American Cancer Society. 2012a. "Heat Therapy." http://www.cancer.org/treatment/treatmentsandsideeffects/complementaryandalternativemedicine/manualhealingandphysicaltouch/heat-therapy (accessed December 15, 2012).

———. 2012b. "Immunotherapy." http://www.cancer.org/treatment/treatmentsandsideeffects/treatmenttypes/immunotherapy/index (accessed December 15, 2012).

Ardrey, R. 1963. *African Genesis: A Personal Investigation into the Animal Origins and Nature of Man.* Montreal: McGill-Queen's Press.

Arluke, A. 1996. *Regarding Animals.* Philadelphia: Temple University Press.

Atkinson, D. T. 1958. *Magic, Myth and Medicine.* Greenwich, CT: Fawcett Publications.

Banting, W. 1863. *Letter on Corpulence, Addressed to the Public.* London: Harrison and Sons.

Bar-Yosef, O. 1986. "The Walls of Jericho: An Alternative Interpretation." *Current Anthropology* 27 (2): 157–62.

Barañano, K. W., and A. L. Hartman. 2008. "The Ketogenic Diet: Uses in Epilepsy and Other Neurologic Illnesses." *Current Treatment Options in Neurology* 10 (6): 410–19.

Berbesque, J. C., F. W. Marlowe, and A. N. Crittenden. 2011. "Sex Differences in Hadza Eating Frequency by Food Type." *American Journal of Human Biology the Official Journal of the Human Biology Council* 23 (3): 339–45.

Beringer, J., T. Meyer, M. Wallendorf, P. Mabry, and W. R. Eddleman. 2004. "Post-release Survival of Rehabilitated White-tailed Deer Fawns in Missouri." *Wildlife Society Bulletin* 32 (3): 732–38.

Bernardo, D., J. A. Garrote, L. Fernández-Salazar, S. Riestra, and E. Arranz. 2007. "Is Gliadin Really Safe for Non-coeliac Individuals? Production of Interleukin 15 in Biopsy Culture from Non-coeliac Individuals Challenged with Gliadin Peptides." *Gut* 56 (6): 889–90.

Bernheim, H. A., and M. J. Kluger. 1976a. "Fever and Antipyresis in the Lizard Dipsosaurus Dorsalis." *American Journal of Physiology* 231 (1): 198–203.

Bernheim, H. A., and M. J. Kluger. 1976b. "Fever: Effect of Drug-induced Antipyresis on Survival." *Science* 193 (4249): 237–39.

Bertenshaw, E. J., A. Lluch, and M. R. Yeomans. 2008. "Satiating Effects of Protein but Not Carbohydrate Consumed in a Between-meal Beverage Context." *Physiology and Behavior* 93 (3): 427–36.

Billing, J., and P. W. Sherman. 1998. "Antimicrobial Functions of Spices: Why Some Like It Hot." *The Quarterly Review of Biology* 73 (1): 3–49.

Bilsborough, S., and N. Mann. 2006. "A Review of Issues of Dietary Protein Intake in Humans." *International Journal of Sport Nutrition and Exercise Metabolism* 16 (2): 129–52.

Black, M. M. 2008. "Effects of Vitamin B12 and Folate Deficiency on Brain Development in Children." *Food and Nutrition Bulletin* 29 (2 Suppl): S126–S131.

Bolan, G. A., P. F. Sparling, and J. N. Wasserheit. 2012. "The Emerging Threat of Untreatable Gonococcal Infection." *New England Journal of Medicine* 366 (6): 485–87.

Borre, K. 1991. "Seal Blood, Inuit Blood, and Diet: A Biocultural Model of Physiology and Cultural Identity." *Medical Anthropology Quarterly* 5 (1): 48–62.

Boughton-Wilby, T. 1903. "Odd Corners of Musical Vienna." *The Windsor Magazine* 17: 580–86.

Bramble, D. M., and D. E. Lieberman. 2004. "Endurance Running and the Evolution of Homo." *Nature* 432 (7015): 345–52.

Brand, S. 2009. *Whole Earth Discipline: An Ecopragmatist Manifesto.* New York: Viking.

Brown, A. S. 2008. "The Risk for Schizophrenia from Childhood and Adult Infections." *The American Journal of Psychiatry* 165 (1): 7–10.

Brown, R. R., Y. Ozaki, S. P. Datta, E. C. Borden, P. M. Sondel, and D. G. Malone. 1991. "Implications of Interferon-induced Tryptophan Catabolism in Cancer, Auto-immune Diseases and AIDS." *Advances in Experimental Medicine and Biology* 294: 425–35.

Bruce, H. 2010. *Page Fright: Foibles and Fetishes of Famous Writers.* Toronto: McClelland and Stewart.

Burton, M., E. Cobb, P. Donachie, G. Judah, V. Curtis, and W.-P. Schmidt. 2011. "The Effect of Handwashing with Water or Soap on Bacterial Contamination of Hands." *International Journal of Environmental Research and Public Health* 8 (1): 97–104.

Byrne, J. P. 2008. *Encyclopedia of Pestilence, Pandemics, and Plagues, Volume 1.* Santa Barbara, CA: ABC-CLIO.

Campbell, T. C. 2005. *The China Study: The Most Comprehensive Study of Nutrition Ever Conducted and the Startling Implications for Diet, Weight Loss, and Long-Term Health.* Dallas: BenBella Books.

Cann, S. A. H., J. P. Van Netten, and C. Van Netten. 2003. "Dr. William Coley and Tumour Regression: A Place in History or in the Future." *Postgraduate Medical Journal* 79 (938): 672–80.

Carney, D. R., A. J. C. Cuddy, and A. J. Yap. 2010. "Power Posing: Brief Nonverbal Displays Affect Neuroendocrine Levels and Risk Tolerance." *Psychological Science* 21 (10): 1363–68.

Caro, T. M., and M. D. Hauser. 1992. "Is There Teaching in Nonhuman Animals?" *The Quarterly Review of Biology* 67 (2): 151–74.

Catlin, G. 1842. *Letters and Notes on the Manners, Customs, and Condition of the North American Indians.* London: George Catlin.

Centers for Disease Control and Prevention. 2002. "Guideline for Hand Hygiene in Health-Care Settings." *Morbidity and Mortality Weekly Report* 51 (Rr-16): 33 (Recommendation 6B).

———. 2012a. "Detailed STD Facts—Gonorrhea." http://www.cdc.gov/std/gonorrhea/STDFact-gonorrhea-detailed.htm (accessed November 7, 2012).

———. 2012b. "Insufficient Sleep Is a Public Health Epidemic." http://www.cdc.gov/features/dssleep (accessed December 16, 2012).

———. 2012c. "Unintentional Drowning: Get the Facts." http://www.cdc

.gov/homeandrecreationalsafety/water-safety/waterinjuries-factsheet
.html (accessed December 16, 2012).

Chilton, F. H., L. L. Rudel, J. S. Parks, J. P. Arm, and M. C. Seeds. 2008.
"Mechanisms by Which Botanical Lipids Affect Inflammatory
Disorders." *The American Journal of Clinical Nutrition* 87 (2): 498S–503S.

Cochran, G., J. Hardy, and H. Harpending. 2006. "Natural History of
Ashkenazi Intelligence." *Journal of Biosocial Science* 38 (5): 659–93.

Cochran, G., and H. Harpending. 2010. *The 10,000 Year Explosion: How
Civilization Accelerated Human Evolution.* New York: Basic Books.

Cochran, G., P. W. Ewald, and K. D. Cochran. 2000. "Infectious Causation
of Disease." *Perspectives in Biology and Medicine* 43 (3): 406–48.

Coe, J. C. 1995. "The Evolution of Zoo Animal Exhibits." In *The Ark Evolving,
Zoos and Aquariums in Transition,* edited by C. W. Wimmer, 95–128. Front
Royal, VA: Smithsonian Institution Conservation and Research Center.

Cordain, L. 2007. "Implications of Plio-Pleistocene Hominin Diets for
Modern Humans." In *Evolution of the Human Diet. The Known, the
Unknown, and the Unknowable,* edited by P. S. Ungar, 363–83. Oxford, UK:
Oxford University Press.

Cousins, D. 1976. "A Review of the Diets of Captive Gorillas (Gorilla
Gorilla)." *Acta Zoologica et Pathologica Antverpiensia* (66): 91–100.

Coxwell, H. T. 1889. *My Life and Balloon Experiences.* London: W. H. Allen.

Croker, K., M. Barbetti, and N. Adams. 2005. "Sheep Infertility from Pasture
Legumes." *Department of Agriculture Western Australia, Farmnote* 41.

Curtin, J. A., J. Fridlyand, T. Kageshita, H. N. Patel, K. J. Busam, H. Kutzner,
K.-H. Cho, S. Aiba, E.-B. Bröcker, P. E. LeBoit, D. Pinkel, and B. C.
Bastian. 2005. "Distinct Sets of Genetic Alterations in Melanoma." *New
England Journal of Medicine* 353 (20): 2135–47.

Curtis, V., and A. Biran. 2001. "Dirt, Disgust, and Disease: Is Hygiene in
Our Genes?" *Perspectives in Biology and Medicine* 44 (1): 17–31.

Curtis, V., M. de Barra, and R. Aunger. 2011. "Disgust as an Adaptive
System for Disease Avoidance Behaviour." *Philosophical Transactions of the
Royal Society of London. Series B, Biological Sciences* 366 (1563): 389–401.

Da Vinci, L. 1970. *The Notebooks of Leonardo Da Vinci.* Vol 2. Edited by
J. P. Richter. New York: Dover Publications.

Daniel, C. R., K. L. Schwartz, J. S. Colt, L. M. Dong, J. J. Ruterbusch,
M. P. Purdue, A. J. Cross, N. Rothman, F. G. Davis, S. Wacholder,
B. I. Graubard, W. H. Chow, and R. Sinha. 2011. "Meat-cooking
Mutagens and Risk of Renal Cell Carcinoma." *British Journal of Cancer*
105 (7): 1096–1104.

Daoud, A. I., G. J. Geissler, F. Wang, J. Saretsky, Y. A. Daoud, and D. E.

Lieberman. 2012. "Foot Strike and Injury Rates in Endurance Runners: A Retrospective Study." *Medicine & Science in Sports & Exercise* 44 (7): 1325–34.

D'Aout, K., T. C. Pataky, D. De Clercq, and P. Aerts. 2009. "The Effects of Habitual Footwear Use: Foot Shape and Function in Native Barefoot Walkers." *Footwear Science* 1 (2): 81–94.

Dayton, S., S. Hashimoto, W. Dixon, and M. L. Pearce. 1966. "Composition of Lipids in Human Serum and Adipose Tissue During Prolonged Feeding of a Diet High in Unsaturated Fat." *Journal of Lipid Research* 7 (1): 103–11.

De Martel, C., J. Ferlay, S. Franceschi, J. Vignat, F. Bray, D. Forman, and M. Plummer. 2012. "Global Burden of Cancers Attributable to Infections in 2008: A Review and Synthetic Analysis." *The Lancet Oncology* 2045 (12): 1–9.

De Vany, A. 2010. *The New Evolution Diet: What Our Paleolithic Ancestors Can Teach Us About Weight Loss, Fitness, and Aging.* New York: Rodale.

Desrochers, P., and H. Shimizu. 2012. *The Locavore's Dilemma: In Praise of the 10,000-Mile Diet.* New York: PublicAffairs.

Diamond, J. M. 2000. "Talk of Cannibalism." *Nature* 407: 25–26.

Diep, B. A., H. F. Chambers, C. J. Graber, J. D. Szumowski, L. G. Miller, L. L. Han, J. H. Chen, F. Lin, J. Lin, T. H. Phan, H. A. Carleton, L. K. McDougal, F. C. Tenover, D. E. Cohen, K. H. Mayer, G. F. Sensabaugh, and F. Perdreau-Remington. 2008. "Emergence of Multidrug-resistant, Community-associated, Methicillin-resistant Staphylococcus Aureus Clone USA300 in Men Who Have Sex with Men." *Annals of Internal Medicine* 148 (4): 249–57.

Dio, C. 1925. *Roman History.* Cambridge, MA: Harvard University Press, Loeb Classical Library.

Dobzhansky, T. 1973. "Nothing in Biology Makes Sense Except in the Light of Evolution." *American Biology Teacher* 35: 125–29.

Doran, T. F., C. De Angelis, R. A. Baumgardner, and E. D. Mellits. 1989. "Acetaminophen: More Harm Than Good for Chickenpox?" *Journal of Pediatrics* 114 (6): 1045–48.

Douillard, J. 2004. *The Encyclopedia of Ayurvedic Massage.* Berkeley, CA: North Atlantic Books.

Drain, P. K., D. T. Halperin, J. P. Hughes, J. D. Klausner, and R. C. Bailey. 2006. "Male Circumcision, Religion, and Infectious Diseases: An Ecologic Analysis of 118 Developing Countries." *BMC Infectious Diseases* 6 (1): 172.

Dunn, P. M. 1998. "Francis Glisson (1597–1677) and the 'Discovery' of

Rickets." *Archives of Disease in Childhood—Fetal and Neonatal Edition* 78 (2): F154–F155.

Dunstan, D. W., B. A. Kingwell, R. Larsen, G. N. Healy, E. Cerin, M. T. Hamilton, J. E. Shaw, D. A. Bertovic, P. Z. Zimmet, J. Salmon, and N. Owen. 2012. "Breaking Up Prolonged Sitting Reduces Postprandial Glucose and Insulin Responses." *Diabetes Care* 35 (5): 976–83.

Dwork, D. 1981. "Health Conditions of Immigrant Jews on the Lower East Side of New York: 1880–1914." *Medical History* 25 (1): 1–40.

Dyson, G. 2012. *Turing's Cathedral: The Origins of the Digital Universe.* New York: Pantheon.

Eaton, S. B., and M. Konner. 1985. "Paleolithic Nutrition: A Consideration of Its Nature and Current Implications." *The New England Journal of Medicine* 312: 283–89.

Eaton, S. B., M. C. Pike, R. V. Short, N. C. Lee, J. Trussell, R. A. Hatcher, J. W. Wood, C. M. Worthman, N. G. Jones, and M. J. Konner. 1994. "Women's Reproductive Cancers in Evolutionary Context." *The Quarterly Review of Biology* 69 (3): 353–67.

Ekirch, A. R. 2005. *At Day's Close: Night in Times Past.* New York: W. W. Norton.

El Ghissassi, F., R. Baan, and K. Straif. 2009. "A Review of Human Carcinogens—Part D: Radiation." *IARC Working Group on the Evaluation of Carcinogenic Risks to Humansgenic Risks to Humans.*

Engs, R. C. 2001. *Clean Living Movements: American Cycles of Health Reform.* Westport, CT: Praeger Publishers.

———. 2003. *The Progressive Era's Health Reform Movement: A Historical Dictionary.* Westport, CT: Praeger Publishers.

Enstrom, J. E., and L. Breslow. 2008. "Lifestyle and Reduced Mortality Among Active California Mormons, 1980–2004." *Preventive Medicine* 46 (2): 133–36.

Eskildsen, S. 1998. *Asceticism in Early Taoist Religion.* SUNY Press.

Ewald, P. W. 1994. *Evolution of Infectious Disease.* Oxford, U.K.: Oxford University Press.

Fasano, A. 2006. "Systemic Autoimmune Disorders in Celiac Disease." *Current Opinion in Gastroenterology* 22 (6): 674–79.

Ferrières, J. 2004. "The French Paradox: Lessons for Other Countries." *Heart British Cardiac Society* 90 (1): 107–111.

Ferriss, T. 2010. *The 4-Hour Body: An Uncommon Guide to Rapid Fat-Loss, Incredible Sex, and Becoming Superhuman.* New York: Crown Publishing Group.

Fincher, C. L., and R. Thornhill. 2012. "Parasite-stress Promotes In-group

Assortative Sociality: The Cases of Strong Family Ties and Heightened Religiosity." *Behavioral and Brain Sciences* 35 (2): 61–79.

Fishberg, M. 1901. "The Comparative Pathology of the Jews." *New York Medical Journal* 73: 537–43, 576–82. In *Jews and Race: Writings on Identity & Difference, 1880–1940*, edited by M. B. Hart. Waltham: Brandeis University Press, 2011.

Flaxman, S. M., and P. W. Sherman. 2008. "Morning Sickness: Adaptive Cause or Nonadaptive Consequence of Embryo Viability?" *The American Naturalist* 172 (1): 54–62.

Foer, J. S. 2009. *Eating Animals*. New York: Little, Brown.

Fonseca-Azevedo, K., and S. Herculano-Houzel. 2012. "Metabolic Constraint Imposes Tradeoff Between Body Size and Number of Brain Neurons in Human Evolution." *Proceedings of the National Academy of Sciences of the United States of America* 109 (45): 18571–76.

Forrest, K. Y. Z., and W. L. Stuhldreher. 2011. "Prevalence and Correlates of Vitamin D Deficiency in US Adults." *Nutrition Research* 31 (1): 48–54.

Fournier, A. 1896. "Francis Joseph and His Realm." In *The Forum*, 21:214. New York: The Forum Publishing Company.

Francis, A. M. 2013. "The Wages of Sin: How the Discovery of Penicillin Reshaped Modern Sexuality." *Archives of Sexual Behavior* 42 (1): 5–13.

Frankl, V. 2006. *Man's Search for Meaning*. Boston, MA: Beacon Press.

Frassetto, L. A., M. Schloetter, M. Mietus-Synder, R. C. Morris, and A. Sebastian. 2009. "Metabolic and Physiologic Improvements from Consuming a Paleolithic, Hunter-gatherer Type Diet." *European Journal of Clinical Nutrition* 63 (8): 947–55.

Freedman, R., and K. Barnouin. 2005. *Skinny Bitch*. Philadelphia: Running Press.

Frey, C., F. Thompson, J. Smith, M. Sanders, and H. Horstman. 1993. "American Orthopaedic Foot and Ankle Society Women's Shoe Survey." *Foot & Ankle* 14 (2): 78–81.

Fuller, P. M., J. Lu, and C. B. Saper. 2008. "Differential Rescue of Light- and Food-entrainable Circadian Rhythms." *Science* 320 (5879): 1074–77.

Galor, O., and O. Moav. 2007. "The Neolithic Revolution and Contemporary Variations in Life Expectancy." *Brown University, Department of Economics Working Papers*.

Garland, C. F., F. C. Garland, E. D. Gorham, M. Lipkin, H. Newmark, S. B. Mohr, and M. F. Holick. 2006. "The Role of Vitamin D in Cancer Prevention." *American Journal of Public Health* 96 (2): 252–61.

Gates, B., N. Myhrvold, and P. Rinearson. 1996. *The Road Ahead*. New York: Penguin Books.

Gibbons, A. 2012. "An Evolutionary Theory of Dentistry." *Science* 336: 973–75.

Gilbert, G. M. 1947. *Nuremberg Diary*. Cambridge, MA: Da Capo.

Giovannucci, E., Y. Liu, B. W. Hollis, and E. B. Rimm. 2008. "25-hydroxyvitamin D and Risk of Myocardial Infarction in Men: A Prospective Study." *Archives of Internal Medicine* 168 (11): 1174–80.

Glasenapp, C. F., and W. A. Ellis. 1908. *Life of Richard Wagner. Vol. 6*. London: Kegan Paul, Trench, Trübner and Company.

Gluckman, P., A. Beedle, M. Hanson. 2009. *Principles of Evolutionary Medicine*. New York: Oxford University Press.

Goebbels, J. 1948. *The Goebbels Diaries*. Edited by L. P. Lochner. New York: Doubleday.

Grandin, T., and C. Johnson. 2010. *Animals Make Us Human: Creating the Best Life for Animals*. Boston, MA: Mariner Books.

Griffith, J., and H. Omar. 2003. "Association Between Vegetarian Diet and Menstrual Problems in Young Women: A Case Presentation and Brief Review." *Journal of Pediatric and Adolescent Gynecology* 16 (5): 319–23.

Groark, K. P. 1997. "To Warm the Blood, to Warm the Flesh: The Role of the Steambath in Highland Maya (Tzeltal-Tzotzil) Ethnomedicine." *Journal of Latin American Lore* 20 (1): 3–96.

———. 2005. "Vital Warmth and Well-being: Steambathing as Household Therapy Among the Tzeltal and Tzotzil Maya of Highland Chiapas, Mexico." *Social Science and Medicine* 61 (4): 785–95.

Gurven, M., and H. Kaplan. 2007. "Longevity Among Hunter-Gatherers: A Cross-Cultural Examination." *Population and Development Review* 33 (2): 321–65.

Haidt, J. 2012. *The Righteous Mind: Why Good People Are Divided by Politics and Religion*. New York: Knopf Doubleday.

Hamilton, M. T., D. G. Hamilton, and T. W. Zderic. 2007. "Role of Low Energy Expenditure and Sitting in Obesity, Metabolic Syndrome, Type 2 Diabetes, and Cardiovascular Disease." *Diabetes* 56 (11): 2655–67.

Hancocks, D. 2001. *A Different Nature: The Paradoxical World of Zoos and Their Uncertain Future*. Berkeley, CA: University of California Press.

Hannuksela, M. L., and S. Ellahham, S. 2001. "Benefits and Risks of Sauna Bathing." *American Journal of Medicine* 110 (2): 118–26.

Harper, G. 2008. *Creative Writing Guidebook*. New York: Continuum International Publishing Group.

Harris, M. 1998. *Good to Eat: Riddles of Food and Culture*. Long Grove, IL: Waveland Press.

Harrison, P. 2004. *South Africa's Top Sites: Spiritual*. Kenilworth, Cape Town: New Africa Books.

Hart, B. L. 1988. "Biological Basis of the Behavior of Sick Animals." *Neuroscience and Biobehavioral Reviews* 12 (2): 123–37.

Hart, M. B. 2007. *The Healthy Jew: The Symbiosis of Judaism and Modern Medicine*. Cambridge, UK: Cambridge University Press.

Hatfield, J. H. 2009. *Why Call Me God?: The Gospel Seen with a Single Eye*. Cheshire, UK: Capabel Press, Limited.

Hawks, J., E. T. Wang, G. M. Cochran, H. C. Harpending, and R. K. Moyzis. 2007. "Recent Acceleration of Human Adaptive Evolution." *Proceedings of the National Academy of Sciences of the United States of America* 104 (52): 20753–58.

Healy, G. N., D. W. Dunstan, J. Salmon, J. E. Shaw, P. Z. Zimmet, and N. Owen. 2008. "Television Time and Continuous Metabolic Risk in Physically Active Adults." *Medicine and Science in Sports and Exercise* 40 (4): 639–45.

Held, M. R., R. D. Bungiro, L. M. Harrison, I. Hamza, and M. Cappello. 2006. "Dietary Iron Content Mediates Hookworm Pathogenesis in Vivo." *Infection and Immunity* 74 (1): 289–95.

Hemingway, E. 1917. *Ernest Hemingway Selected Letters 1917–1961*. Edited by C. Baker. New York: Scribner.

Herodotus. 1889. *The History of Herodotus*. Edited by G. Rawlinson, H. C. Rawlinson, et al. New York: D. Appleton and Company.

Hibbeln, J. R., L. R. G. Nieminen, and W. E. M. Lands. 2004. "Increasing Homicide Rates and Linoleic Acid Consumption Among Five Western Countries, 1961–2000." *Lipids* 39 (12): 1207–13.

Hill, K., H. Kaplan, K. Hawkes, and A. M. Hurtado. 1987. "Foraging Decisions Among Ache Hunter-Gatherers—New Data and Implications for Optimal Foraging Models." *Ethology and Sociobiology* 8 (1): 1–36.

Hirota, Y., D. Kang, and T. Kanki. 2012. "The Physiological Role of Mitophagy: New Insights into Phosphorylation Events." *International Journal of Cell Biology* 2012.

Hobrink, B. 2011. *Modern Science in the Bible: Amazing Scientific Truths Found in Ancient Texts*. New York: Simon & Schuster.

Hoenselaar, R. 2012. "Saturated Fat and Cardiovascular Disease: The Discrepancy Between the Scientific Literature and Dietary Advice." *Nutrition* 28 (2): 118–23.

Hoggan, R. 1997. "Considering Wheat, Rye, and Barley Proteins as Aids to Carcinogens." *Medical Hypotheses* 49 (3): 285–88.

Holick, M. F. 1989. "Phylogenetic and Evolutionary Aspects of Vitamin D from Phytoplankton to Humans." In *Vertebrate Endocrinology: Fundamentals and Biomedical Implications,* edited by P. Schreibman and M. Pang. San Diego: Academic Press.

———. 2004. "Sunlight and Vitamin D for Bone Health and Prevention of Autoimmune Diseases, Cancers, and Cardiovascular Disease." *American Journal of Clinical Nutrition* 80 (6 Suppl): 1678S–88S.

———. 2010. *The Vitamin D Solution: A 3-Step Strategy to Cure Our Most Common Health Problem.* New York: Penguin.

Holick, M. F., S. A. Holick, and R. L. Guillard. 1982. "On the Origin and Metabolism of Vitamin D in the Sea." In *Comparative Endocrinology of Calcium Regulation,* edited by C. Oguro and P. Pang, 85–91. Tokyo: Sci Soc Press.

Hood, L., and D. Galas. 2003. "The Digital Code of DNA." *Nature* 421 (6921): 444–48.

Horne, B. D., H. T. May, J. L. Anderson, A. G. Kfoury, B. M. Bailey, B. S. McClure, D. G. Renlund, D. L. Lappé, J. F. Carlquist, P. W. Fisher, R. R. Pearson, T. L. Bair, T. D. Adams, and J. B. Muhlestein. 2008. "Usefulness of Routine Periodic Fasting to Lower Risk of Coronary Artery Disease in Patients Undergoing Coronary Angiography." *The American Journal of Cardiology* 102 (7): 814–19.

Hosey, G., V. Melfi, and S. Pankhurst. 2009. *Zoo Animals: Behaviour, Management, and Welfare.* Oxford, UK: Oxford University Press.

Howell, L. D. 2010. *The Barefoot Book: 50 Great Reasons to Kick Off Your Shoes.* Berkeley: Hunter House.

Hyson, J. M. 2003. "History of the Toothbrush." *Journal of the History of Dentistry* 51 (2): 73–80.

Jablonski, N. G. 2004. "The Evolution of Human Skin and Skin Color." *Annual Review of Anthropology* 33 (1): 585–623.

Jacob, F. 1977. "Evolution and Tinkering." *Science* 196 (4295): 1161–66.

Jaminet, P., and S.-C. Jaminet. 2012. *Perfect Health Diet: Four Steps to Renewed Health, Youthful Vitality, and Long Life.* New York: Scribner.

Jensen, R. G. 1999. "The Lipids in Human Milk." *Lipids* 34 (12): 1243–71.

Johns, T. 1991. "Well-Grounded Diet." *The Sciences* 31 (5): 40.

Jönsson, T., Y. Granfeldt, B. Ahrén, U.-C. Branell, G. Pålsson, A. Hansson, M. Söderström, and S. Lindeberg. 2009. "Beneficial Effects of a Paleolithic Diet on Cardiovascular Risk Factors in Type 2 Diabetes: A Randomized Cross-over Pilot Study." *Cardiovascular Diabetology* 8 (1): 35.

Jönsson, T., Y. Granfeldt, C. Erlanson-Albertsson, B. Ahrén, and S. Lindeberg. 2010. "A Paleolithic Diet Is More Satiating Per Calorie Than a

Mediterranean-like Diet in Individuals with Ischemic Heart Disease." *Nutrition Metabolism* 7 (1): 85.

Kaplan, H., K. Hill, J. Lancaster, and A. M. Hurtado. 2000. "A Theory of Human Life History Evolution: Diet, Intelligence, and Longevity." *Evolutionary Anthropology* 9 (4): 156–85.

Katzenberg, M. A., V. I. Bazaliiskii, O. I. Goriunova, N. A. Savel'ev, and A. W. Weber. 2010. "Diet Reconstruction of Prehistoric Hunter-Gatherers in the Lake Baikal Region." In *Prehistoric Hunter-Gatherers of the Baikal Region, Siberia: Bioarchaeological Studies of Past Life Ways*, edited by A. W. Weber, M. A. Katzenberg, et al., 175–91. Philadelphia: University of Pennsylvania Press.

Katzmarzyk, P. T., T. S. Church, C. L. Craig, and C. Bouchard. 2009. "Sitting Time and Mortality from All Causes, Cardiovascular Disease, and Cancer." *Medicine and Science in Sports and Exercise* 41 (5): 998–1005.

Kellogg, J. H. 1891. *Plain Facts for Old and Young: Embracing the Natural History and Hygiene of Organic Life*. Burlington, IA: I. F. Senger and Company.

Kelly, K. 2010. *What Technology Wants*. New York: Viking.

Key, T. J., G. E. Fraser, M. Thorogood, P. N. Appleby, V. Beral, G. Reeves, M. L. Burr, J. Chang-Claude, R. Frentzel-Beyme, J. W. Kuzma, J. Mann, and K. McPherson. 1999. "Mortality in Vegetarians and Nonvegetarians: Detailed Findings from a Collaborative Analysis of 5 Prospective Studies." *The American Journal of Clinical Nutrition* 70 (3 Suppl): 516S–524S.

Keys, A., J. Brozek, A. Henschel, O. Mickelsen, and H. L. Taylor. 1950. *The Biology of Human Starvation*. University of Minnesota Press.

Khan, R., and B. S. R. Khan. 2010. "Diet, Disease and Pigment Variation in Humans." *Medical Hypotheses* 75 (4): 363–67.

Killanin, B. M. M., and M. V. Duignan. 1967. *The Shell Guide to Ireland*. London: Ebury Press.

Kitchener, A., and A. A. Macdonald. 2005. "The Longevity Legacy: The Problem of Old Animals in Zoos." In *Proceedings of the EAZA Conference 2004 Kolmarden*, edited by B. Hiddinga, 132–37. Amsterdam: EAZA Executive Office.

Kluger, M. J. 1986. "Is Fever Beneficial?" *Yale Journal of Biology and Medicine* 59 (2): 89–95.

Kluger, M. J., W. Kozak, C. A. Conn, L. R. Leon, and D. Soszynski. 1998. *Role of Fever in Disease*. Edited by M. Kluger, J. Bartfai, et al. *Annals of the New York Academy Of Sciences*. Vol. 856. Wiley Online Library.

Kluger, M. J., and B. A. Rothenburg. 1979. "Fever and Reduced Iron: Their

Interaction as a Host Defense Response to Bacterial Infection." *Science* 203 (4378): 374–76.

Kollias, N., E. Ruvolo, and R. M. Sayre. 2011. "The Value of the Ratio of UVA to UVB in Sunlight." *Photochemistry and Photobiology* 87 (6): 1474–75.

Kukkonen-Harjula, K., and K. Kauppinen. 2006. "Health Effects and Risks of Sauna Bathing." *International Journal of Circumpolar Health* 65 (3): 195–205.

Landers, J. 2011. *The Beginner's Guide to Hunting Deer for Food.* North Adams, MA: Storey Publishing.

———. 2012. *Eating Aliens: One Man's Adventures Hunting Invasive Animal Species.* North Adams, MA: Storey Publishing.

Larsen, C. S. 1995. "Biological Changes in Human Populations with Agriculture." *Annual Review of Anthropology* 24 (1): 185–213.

Larsson, C. L., K. S. Klock, A. N. Astrom, O. Haugejorden, and G. Johansson. 2002. "Lifestyle-related Characteristics of Young Low-meat Consumers and Omnivores in Sweden and Norway." *Journal of Adolescent Health* 31: 190–198.

Lazovich, D., R. I. Vogel, M. Berwick, M. A. Weinstock, K. E. Anderson, and E. M. Warshaw. 2010. "Indoor Tanning and Risk of Melanoma: A Case-control Study in a Highly Exposed Population." *Cancer Epidemiology, Biomarkers & Prevention* 19 (6): 1557–68.

Lecerf, J.-M., and M. De Lorgeril. 2011. "Dietary Cholesterol: From Physiology to Cardiovascular Risk." *The British Journal of Nutrition* 106 (1): 6–14.

Lee, C., L. Raffaghello, S. Brandhorst, F. M. Safdie, G. Bianchi, A. Martin-Montalvo, V. Pistoia, M. Wei, S. Hwang, A. Merlino, L. Emionite, R. De Cabo, and V. D. Longo. 2012. "Fasting Cycles Retard Growth of Tumors and Sensitize a Range of Cancer Cell Types to Chemotherapy." *Science Translational Medicine* 4 (124): 124ra27.

Lee, C., L. Raffaghello, and V. D. Longo. 2012. "Starvation, Detoxification, and Multidrug Resistance in Cancer Therapy." *Drug Resistance Updates Reviews and Commentaries in Antimicrobial and Anticancer Chemotherapy* 15 (1–2): 114–22.

Lee, S.-H., and M. H. Wolpoff. 2003. "The Pattern of Evolution in Pleistocene Human Brain Size." *Paleobiology* 29 (2): 186–96.

Leonard, J. 2007. *Fishing and Hunting Recruitment and Retention in the U.S. from 1990 to 2005.* U.S. Fish and Wildlife Service.

Leonard, W. R., M. L. Robertson, J. J. Snodgrass, and C. W. Kuzawa. 2003. "Metabolic Correlates of Hominid Brain Evolution." *Compara-*

tive *Biochemistry and Physiology Part A: Molecular & Integrative Physiology* 136 (1): 5–15.

Less, E. H. 2012. "Adiposity in Zoo Gorillas (Gorilla Gorilla Gorilla): The Effects of Diet and Behavior." Case Western Reserve University.

Levine, J. A., M. W. Vander Weg, J. O. Hill, and R. C. Klesges. 2006. "Non-exercise Activity Thermogenesis: The Crouching Tiger Hidden Dragon of Societal Weight Gain." *Arteriosclerosis, Thrombosis, and Vascular Biology* 26 (4): 729–36.

Levy, S. 2010. *Hackers: Heroes of the Computer Revolution—25th Anniversary Edition.* Sebastopol, CA: O'Reilly Media.

Lieberman, D. 2013. *The Story of the Human Body: Evolution, Health, and Disease.* New York: Pantheon.

Lieberman, D., J. Tooby, and L. Cosmides. 2003. "Does Morality Have a Biological Basis? An Empirical Test of the Factors Governing Moral Sentiments Relating to Incest." *Proceedings of the Royal Society. Series B: Biological Sciences* 270 (1517): 819–26.

Lieberman, D. E., M. Venkadesan, W. A. Werbel, A. I. Daoud, S. D'Andrea, I. S. Davis, R. O. Mang'eni, Y. Pitsiladis, S. D. Andrea, R. Ojiambo, and M. Eni. 2010. "Foot Strike Patterns and Collision Forces in Habitually Barefoot Versus Shod Runners." *Nature* 463 (7280): 531–35.

Lindeberg, S., B. Ahrén, A. Nilsson, L. Cordain, P. Nilsson-Ehle, and B. Vessby. 2003. "Determinants of Serum Triglycerides and High Density Lipoprotein Cholesterol in Traditional Trobriand Islanders: The Kitava Study." *Scandinavian Journal of Clinical & Laboratory Investigation* 63 (3): 175–80.

Little, M. A. 1989. "Human Biology of African Pastoralists." *American Journal of Physical Anthropology* 32 (S10): 215–47.

Liu, P. T., S. Stenger, H. Li, L. Wenzel, B. H. Tan, S. R. Krutzik, M. T. Ochoa, J. Schauber, K. Wu, C. Meinken, D. L. Kamen, M. Wagner, R. Bals, A. Steinmeyer, U. Zügel, R. L. Gallo, D. Eisenberg, M. Hewison, B. W. Hollis, et al. 2006. "Toll-like Receptor Triggering of a Vitamin D–mediated Human Antimicrobial Response." *Science* 311 (5768): 1770–73.

Lloyd, J. C., J. A. Antonelli, T. E. Phillips, E. M. Masko, J.-A. Thomas, S. H. M. Poulton, M. Pollak, and S. J. Freedland. 2010. "Effect of Isocaloric Low Fat Diet on Prostate Cancer Xenograft Progression in a Hormone Deprivation Model." *The Journal of Urology* 183 (4): 1619–24.

Lu, W., Q.-J. Meng, N. J. C. Tyler, K.-A. Stokkan, and A. S. I. Loudon. 2010. "A Circadian Clock Is Not Required in an Arctic Mammal." *Current Biology* 20 (6): 533–37.

Luby, S. P., A. K. Halder, T. Huda, L. Unicomb, and R. B. Johnston. 2011. "The Effect of Handwashing at Recommended Times with Water Alone and with Soap on Child Diarrhea in Rural Bangladesh: An Observational Study." *PLoS Medicine* 8 (6): e1001052.

Lyon, J. L., and S. Nelson. 1979. "Mormon Health." *Dialogue* 12 (3): 84–96.

Marlowe, F. W. 2005. "Hunter-gatherers and Human Evolution." *Evolutionary Anthropology* 14 (2): 54–67.

Mayo Foundation for Medical Education and Research. 2010. *The Mayo Clinic Diet: Eat Well, Enjoy Life, Lose Weight.* Intercourse, PA: Good Books.

Meehan, T. P., and L. J. Lowenstine. 1994. "Causes of Mortality in Captive Lowland Gorillas: A Survey of the SSP Population." In *Proc. Am. Assoc. Zoo Vet. Annu. Meet. 1994,* 216–18.

Mench, J. A., H. James, E. A. Pajor, and P. B. Thompson. 2008. "The Welfare of Animals in Concentrated Animal Feeding Operations." *The Pew Commission on Industrial Farm Animal Production.*

Menczer, J. 2003. "The Low Incidence of Cervical Cancer in Jewish Women: Has the Puzzle Finally Been Solved?" *The Israel Medical Association Journal* 5 (5): 120–23.

Michalak, J., X. C. Zhang, and F. Jacobi. 2012. "Vegetarian Diet and Mental Disorders: Results from a Representative Community Survey." *The International Journal of Behavioral Nutrition and Physical Activity* 9 (1): 67.

Mink, J. W., R. J. Blumenschine, and D. B. Adams. 1981. "Ratio of Central Nervous System to Body Metabolism in Vertebrates: Its Constancy and Functional Basis." *American Journal of Physiology* 241 (3): R203–R212.

Mitra, D., A. Morgan, J. Lo, K. C. Robinson, S. P. Devi, D. E. Fisher, X. Luo, K. M. Haigis, and D. A. Haber. 2012. "An Ultraviolet-radiation-independent Pathway to Melanoma Carcinogenesis in the Red Hair/Fair Skin Background." *Nature* 497 (November): 449–53.

Morris, D. 2009. *The Human Zoo.* New York: Random House.

Morris, J. N., J. A. Heady, P. A. Raffle, C. G. Roberts, and J. W. Parks. 1953. "Coronary Heart-disease and Physical Activity of Work." *Lancet* 265 (6795): 1053–57.

Mummert, A., E. Esche, J. Robinson, and G. J. Armelagos. 2011. "Stature and Robusticity During the Agricultural Transition: Evidence from the Bioarchaeological Record." *Economics and Human Biology* 9 (3): 284–301.

Munger, R. G., J. R. Cerhan, and B. C. Chiu. 1999. "Prospective Study of Dietary Protein Intake and Risk of Hip Fracture in Postmenopausal Women." *The American Journal of Clinical Nutrition* 69 (1): 147–52.

Murphy, H. W., and M. Mufson. 2001. "The Use of Psychopharmaceuticals to Control Aggressive Behaviors in Captive Gorillas." *The Apes: Challenges for the 21st Century,* 157–60. Chicago Zoological Society.

National Research Council. 2003. *Nutrient Requirements of Nonhuman Primates.* Washington, D.C.: National Academies Press.

Nesse, R. M., and G. C. Williams. 2012. *Why We Get Sick: The New Science of Darwinian Medicine.* New York: Knopf Doubleday.

Nichol, J. P. 1893. *Victor Hugo; a Sketch of His Life and Work.* London: Swan Sonnenschein and Company.

Nietzsche, F. W., and W. A. Kaufmann. 1954. *The Portable Nietzsche.* New York: Viking.

Noble, K. G., W. P. Fifer, V. A. Rauh, Y. Nomura, and H. F. Andrews. 2012. "Academic Achievement Varies with Gestational Age Among Children Born at Term." *Pediatrics* 130 (2): e257–64.

Nuñez, M. A., S. Kuebbing, R. D. Dimarco, and D. Simberloff. 2012. "Invasive Species: To Eat or Not to Eat, That Is the Question." *Conservation Letters* 0 (865): 3–6.

Ogden, C. L., M. D. Carroll, B. K. Kit, and K. M. Flegal. 2012. *Prevalence of Obesity in the United States, 2009–2010. Centers for Disease Control and Prevention NCHS Data Brief.*

Öhman, A., and S. Mineka. 2001. "Fears, Phobias, and Preparedness: Toward an Evolved Module of Fear and Fear Learning." *Psychological Review* 108 (3): 483–522.

O'Keefe, J. H., R. Vogel, C. J. Lavie, and L. Cordain, L. 2011. "Exercise Like a Hunter-gatherer: A Prescription for Organic Physical Fitness." *Progress in Cardiovascular Diseases* 53 (6): 471–79.

Orta, G. da. 1903. *Colloquies on the Simples and Drugs of India.* Translated by C. H. Markham. London: Sotheran and Company.

Osterdahl, M., T. Kocturk, A. Koochek, and P. E. Wändell. 2008. "Effects of a Short-term Intervention with a Paleolithic Diet in Healthy Volunteers." *European Journal of Clinical Nutrition* 62 (5): 682–85.

Ostrer, H. 2012. *Legacy: A Genetic History of the Jewish People.* Oxford, UK: Oxford University Press.

Pan, A., Q. Sun, A. M. Bernstein, M. B. Schulze, J. E. Manson, M. J. Stampfer, W. C. Willett, and F. B. Hu. 2012. "Red Meat Consumption and Mortality: Results from 2 Prospective Cohort Studies." *Archives of Internal Medicine* 172 (7): 555–63.

Pedersen, B. K. 2009. "The Diseasome of Physical Inactivity—and the Role of Myokines in Muscle-fat Cross Talk." *The Journal of Physiology* 587 (Pt 23): 5559–68.

Pentikäinen, J. 2001. *The Finnish Sauna, the Japanese Furo, the Indian Inipi: Bathing on Three Continents.* Helsinki: Building Information Ltd.

Pinker, S. 2003. *How the Mind Works.* New York: Penguin.

———. 2011. *The Better Angels of Our Nature: Why Violence Has Declined.* New York: Penguin.

Pitchappan, R. M. 2002. "Castes, Migration, Immunogenetics and Infectious Diseases in South India." *Community Genetics* 5 (3): 157–61.

Plimpton, G. 1958. "Interview: Ernest Hemingway, The Art of Fiction No. 21." *The Paris Review,* 18:66–67.

Pollan, M. 2006. *The Omnivore's Dilemma: A Natural History of Four Meals.* New York: Penguin.

———. 2009. *Food Rules: An Eater's Manual.* New York: Penguin.

Pontzer, H., D. A. Raichlen, B. M. Wood, A. Z. P. Mabulla, S. B. Racette, and F. W. Marlowe. 2012. "Hunter-gatherer Energetics and Human Obesity." *PloS One* 7 (7): e40503.

Pop-Vicas, A. E., and E. M. C. D'Agata. 2005. "The Rising Influx of Multidrug-resistant Gram-negative Bacilli into a Tertiary Care Hospital." *Clinical Infectious Diseases* 40 (12): 1792–98.

Preuss, J. 1978. *Biblical and Talmudic Medicine.* Translated and edited by F. Rosner. Northvale, NJ: J. Aronson.

Promislow, J. H. E. 2002. "Protein Consumption and Bone Mineral Density in the Elderly: The Rancho Bernardo Study." *American Journal of Epidemiology* 155 (7): 636–44.

Quinn, D. 1995. *Ishmael: An Adventure of the Mind and Spirit.* New York: Random House.

Rabinowitz, J. D., and E. White. 2010. "Autophagy and Metabolism." *Science* 330 (6009): 1344–48.

Raffaghello, L., C. Lee, F. M. Safdie, M. Wei, F. Madia, G. Bianchi, and V. D. Longo. 2008. "Starvation-dependent Differential Stress Resistance Protects Normal but Not Cancer Cells Against High-dose Chemotherapy." *Proceedings of the National Academy of Sciences of the United States of America* 105 (24): 8215–20.

Raymond, E. 2008. *The Cathedral and the Bazaar: Musings on Linux and Open Source by an Accidental Revolutionary, Revised Edition.* Sebastopol, CA: O'Reilly Media.

Reynolds, N. C., and R. Montgomery. 2002. "Using the Argonne Diet in Jet Lag Prevention: Deployment of Troops Across Nine Time Zones." *Military Medicine* 167 (6): 451–53.

Rivera, C. A., L. Gaskin, M. Allman, J. Pang, K. Brady, P. Adegboyega, and

K. Pruitt. 2010. "Toll-like Receptor-2 Deficiency Enhances Non-alcoholic Steatohepatitis." *BMC Gastroenterology* 10: 52.

Roche, H., R. J. Blumenschine, and J. J. Shea. 2009. "Origins and Adaptations of Early Homo: What Archaeology Tells Us." In *The First Humans: Origin and Early Evolution of the Genus Homo*, edited by F. E. Grine, J. G. Fleagle, et al., 135. New York: Springer.

Rogers, A. R., D. Iltis, and S. Wooding. 2004. "Genetic Variation at the MC1R Locus and the Time Since Loss of Human Body Hair." *Current Anthropology* 45 (1): 105–8.

Roizen, M. F., and M. C. Oz. 2009. *YOU: On a Diet Revised Edition: The Owner's Manual for Waist Management*. New York: Free Press.

Rozin, P., J. Haidt, and C. R. McCauley. 2008. "Disgust." In *Handbook of Emotions*, 3rd ed., edited by M. Lewis, J. M. Haviland-Jones, et al., 757–76. New York: Guilford Press.

Rozin, P., M. Markwith, and C. Stoess. 1997. "Moralization and Becoming a Vegetarian: The Transformation of Preferences into Values and the Recruitment of Disgust." *Psychological Science* 8 (2): 67–73.

Safdie, F. M., T. Dorff, D. Quinn, L. Fontana, M. Wei, C. Lee, P. Cohen, and V. D. Longo. 2009. "Fasting and Cancer Treatment in Humans: A Case Series Report." *Aging* 1 (12): 988–1007.

Salk, J. 1972. *Man Unfolding*. New York: Harper & Row.

Sanger, F., G. M. Air, B. G. Barrell, N. L. Brown, A. R. Coulson, C. A. Fiddes, C. A. Hutchison, P. M. Slocombe, and M. Smith. 1977. "Nucleotide Sequence of Bacteriophage Phi X174 DNA." *Nature* 265 (5596): 687–95.

Sankararaman, S., N. Patterson, S. Mallick, S. Paabo, and D. Reich. 2012. "A Genomewide Map of Neandertal Ancestry in Modern Humans." In *Society for Molecular Biology & Evolution 2012*.

Sawchuk, L. A., L. Tripp, and U. Melnychenko. 2012. "The Jewish Advantage and Household Security: Life Expectancy Among 19th Century Sephardim of Gibraltar." *Economics and Human Biology*.

Saxton, K. B., and R. Wallack. 2011. *Barefoot Running Step by Step: Barefoot Ken Bob, the Guru of Shoeless Running, Shares His Personal Technique for Running with More Speed, Less Impact, Fewer Leg Injuries, and More Fun*. Beverly, MA: Fair Winds.

Schleifer, D. 2012. "The Perfect Solution: How Trans Fats Became the Healthy Replacement for Saturated Fats." *Technology and Culture* 53 (1): 94–119.

Schmidt, D. A., M. R. Ellersieck, M. R. Cranfield, and W. B. Karesh. 2006.

"Cholesterol Values in Free-ranging Gorillas (Gorilla Gorilla Gorilla and Gorilla Beringei) and Bornean Orangutans (Pongo Pygmaeus)." *Journal of Zoo and Wildlife Medicine* 37 (3): 292–300.

Semaw, S. 2000. "The World's Oldest Stone Artefacts from Gona, Ethiopia: Their Implications for Understanding Stone Technology and Patterns of Human Evolution Between 2·6–1·5 Million Years Ago." *Journal of Archaeological Science* 27 (12): 1197–1214.

Semmelweis, I. 1983. *Childbed Fever*. Translated by K. C. Carter. Madison: University of Wisconsin Press.

Sheridan, R. B. 1974. *Sugar and Slavery: An Economic History of the British West Indies, 1623–1775*. Kingston, Jamaica: Canoe Press.

Sherman, P. W., and G. A. Hash. 2001. "Why Vegetable Recipes Are Not Very Spicy." *Evolution and Human Behavior* 22 (3): 147–63.

Shinohara, J., and P. Gribble. 2009. "Five-toed Socks Decrease Static Postural Control Among Healthy Individuals as Measured with Time-to-boundary Analysis." In *American Society of Biomechanics Annual Meeting*, poster presentation.

Siegel, J. M. 2012. "Suppression of Sleep for Mating." *Science* 337: 1610–11.

Siegel, R., E. Ward, O. Brawley, and A. Jemal. 2011. "Cancer Statistics, 2011." *CA* 61 (4): 212–36.

Silbergeld, E., J. Graham, and L. B. Price. 2008. "Antimicrobial Resistance and Human Health." *The Pew Commission on Industrial Farm Animal Production*.

Siri-Tarino, P. W., Q. Sun, F. B. Hu, and R. M. Krauss. 2010. "Meta-analysis of Prospective Cohort Studies Evaluating the Association of Saturated Fat with Cardiovascular Disease." *The American Journal of Clinical Nutrition* 91 (3): 535–46.

Slater, M. 2009. *Charles Dickens: A Life Defined by Writing*. New Haven, CT: Yale University Press.

Smith, A. 1767. *The Theory of Moral Sentiments: To Which Is Added a Dissertation on the Origin of Languages*. 3rd ed. London: A. Millar, A. Kincaid, and J. Bell.

———. 1896. *An Inquiry into the Nature and Causes of the Wealth of Nations, Volume 1*. 6th ed. London: George Bell & Sons.

Smith, A. M. 2006. "Veganism and Osteoporosis: A Review of the Current Literature." *International Journal of Nursing Practice* 12 (5): 302–6.

Stanford, C. B. 2001. *The Hunting Apes: Meat Eating and the Origins of Human Behavior*. Princeton, NJ: Princeton University Press.

Stefansson, V. 1960. *The Fat of the Land*. New York: Macmillan.

Stoinski, T. S., and B. B. Beck. 2004. "Changes in Locomotor and Foraging Skills in Captive-born, Reintroduced Golden Lion Tamarins (*Leontopithecus rosalia rosalia*)." *American Journal of Primatology* 62 (1): 1–13.

Stuster, J. 2011. *Bold Endeavors: Lessons from Polar and Space Exploration*. Annapolis, MD: Naval Institute Press.

Su, K.-P., S.-Y. Huang, C.-C. Chiu, and W. W. Shen. 2003. "Omega-3 Fatty Acids in Major Depressive Disorder. A Preliminary Double-blind, Placebo-controlled Trial." *European Neuropsychopharmacology* 13 (4): 267–71.

Suedfeld, P. 1987. "Extreme and Unusual Environments." In *Handbook of Environmental Psychology*, edited by D. Stokols and I. Altman, 863–86. New York: Wiley.

———. 1997. "Homo Invictus: The Indomitable Species." *Canadian Psychology* 38 (3): 164–73.

Suedfeld, P., and W. E. Henley. 2012. "Are We Still Indomitable? Homo Invictus Fifteen Years Later." *Canadian Psychology* 53 (1): 21–31.

Sugimura, T., T. Fujimoto, H. Motoyama, T. Maruoka, S. Korematu, Y. Asakuno, and H. Hayakawa. 1994. "Risks of Antipyretics in Young Children with Fever Due to Infectious Disease." *Acta Paediatrica Japonica Overseas Edition* 36 (4): 375–78.

Taubes, G. 2010. *Why We Get Fat: And What to Do About It*. New York: Random House.

Taylor, J. E. 2004. "Review: The Archaeology of Qumran and the Dead Sea Scrolls." *Palestine Exploration Quarterly* 136 (1): 79–81.

Thomas, E. M. 2007. *The Old Way: A Story of the First People*. New York: Picador.

Tipton, M. J., I. B. Mekjavic, and C. M. Eglin. 2000. "Permanence of the Habituation of the Initial Responses to Cold-water Immersion in Humans." *European Journal of Applied Physiology* 83 (1): 17–21.

Trepanowski, J. F., and R. J. Bloomer. 2010. "The Impact of Religious Fasting on Human Health." *Nutrition Journal* 9 (1): 57.

U.S. Food and Drug Administration. 2011. "Defect Levels Handbook." http://www.fda.gov/food/guidancecomplianceregulatoryinformation/guidancedocuments/sanitation/ucm056174.htm (accessed March 11, 2012).

U.S. Navy. 1999. *U.S. Navy Diving Manual: Air Diving*. Darby, PA: DIANE Publishing.

U.S. Senate Select Committee on Nutrition and Human Needs. 1977. *Dietary Goals for the United States*. Washington, D.C.

Vaca, Á. N. C. de. 1993. *The Account: Alvar Núñez Cabeza De Vaca's Relación*. Translated by M. A. Favata and J. B. Fernández. Houston: Arte Publico Press.

Valentine, J. W., D. Jablonski, and D. H. Erwin. 1999. "Fossils, Molecules and Embryos: New Perspectives on the Cambrian Explosion." *Development* 126 (5): 851–59.

Van Gent, R. N., D. Siem, M. Van Middelkoop, A. G. Van Os, S. M. A. Bierma-Zeinstra, and B. W. Koes. 2007. "Incidence and Determinants of Lower Extremity Running Injuries in Long Distance Runners: a Systematic Review." *British Journal of Sports Medicine* 41 (8): 469–80.

Van Oort, B. E. H., N. J. C. Tyler, M. P. Gerkema, L. Folkow, A. S. Blix, and K.-A. Stokkan. 2005. "Circadian Organization in Reindeer." *Nature* 438 (7071): 1095–96.

Von Cramon-Taubadel, N. 2011. "Global Human Mandibular Variation Reflects Differences in Agricultural and Hunter-gatherer Subsistence Strategies." *Proceedings of the National Academy of Sciences* 108 (49): 7–12.

Vosko, A. M., C. S. Colwell, and A. Y. Avidan. 2010. "Jet Lag Syndrome: Circadian Organization, Pathophysiology, and Management Strategies." *Nature and Science of Sleep* 2: 187–98.

Vreeland, J. K., D. R. Diefenbach, and B. D. Wallingford. 2004. "Survival Rates, Mortality Causes, and Habitats of Pennsylvania White-tailed Deer Fawns." *Wildlife Society Bulletin* 32 (2): 542–53.

Vucetich, J. A., L. M. Vucetich, and R. O. Peterson. 2011. "The Causes and Consequences of Partial Prey Consumption by Wolves Preying on Moose." *Behavioral Ecology and Sociobiology* 66 (2): 295–303.

Vybíral, S., I. Lesná, L. Jansky, and V. Zeman. 2000. "Thermoregulation in Winter Swimmers and Physiological Significance of Human Catecholamine Thermogenesis." *Experimental Physiology* 85 (3): 321–26.

Wander, K., B. Shell-Duncan, and T. W. McDade. 2009. "Evaluation of Iron Deficiency as a Nutritional Adaptation to Infectious Disease: An Evolutionary Medicine Perspective." *American Journal of Human Biology* 21 (2): 172–79.

Ward, S. 1882. "Days with Longfellow." Edited by J. Sparks, E. Everett, et al. *The North American Review* 134 (306): 459.

Wattleworth, R. 2011. "Human Papillomavirus Infection and the Links to Penile and Cervical Cancer." *Journal of the American Osteopathic Association* 111 (3, Supplement 2): S3–10.

Wierzbicki, A. S., R. Poston, and A. Ferro. 2003. "The Lipid and Non-lipid Effects of Statins." *Pharmacology and Therapeutics* 99: 95–112.

Windsor, J. S., R. C. McMorrow, and G. W. Rodway. 2008. "Oxygen on

Everest: The Development of Modern Open-circuit Systems for Moun-taineers." *Aviation, Space, and Environmental Medicine* 79 (8): 799–804.

World Health Organization. 2012. "Cardiovascular Diseases (CVDs)." http://www.who.int/mediacentre/factsheets/fs317/en/index.html (accessed November 7, 2012).

Worsley, A., and G. Skrzypiec. 1998. "Teenage Vegetarianism: Prevalence, Social and Cognitive Contexts." *Appetite* 30: 151–70.

Wrangham, R. 2010. *Catching Fire: How Cooking Made Us Human.* New York: Basic Books.

Wu, X., C. Zhang, P. Goldberg, D. Cohen, Y. Pan, T. Arpin, and O. Bar-Yosef. 2012. "Early Pottery at 20,000 Years Ago in Xianrendong Cave, China." *Science* 336 (6089): 1696–1700.

Yam, D., A. Eliraz, and E. M. Berry. 1996. "Diet and Disease—the Israeli Paradox: Possible Dangers of a High Omega-6 Polyunsaturated Fatty Acid Diet." *Israel Journal of Medical Sciences* 32 (11): 1134–43.

You, M., R. V. Considine, T. C. Leone, D. P. Kelly, and D. W. Crabb. 2005. "Role of Adiponectin in the Protective Action of Dietary Saturated Fat Against Alcoholic Fatty Liver in Mice." *Hepatology* 42 (3): 568–77.

Young, S. L. 2012. *Craving Earth: Understanding Pica: The Urge to Eat Clay, Starch, Ice, and Chalk.* New York: Columbia University Press.

Zazpe, I., J. J. Beunza, M. Bes-Rastrollo, J. Warnberg, C. De La Fuente-Arrillaga, S. Benito, Z. Vázquez, and M. A. Martínez-González. 2011. "Egg Consumption and Risk of Cardiovascular Disease in the SUN Project." *European Journal of Clinical Nutrition* 65 (6): 676–82.

Zequi, S. de C., G. C. Guimarães, F. P. Da Fonseca, U. Ferreira, W. E. De Matheus, L. O. Reis, G. A. Aita, S. Glina, V. S. S. Fanni, M. D. C. Perez, L. R. M. Guidoni, V. Ortiz, L. Nogueira, L. C. De Almeida Rocha, G. Cuck, W. H. Da Costa, R. R. Moniz, J. H. Dantas, F. A. Soares, et al. 2012. "Sex with Animals (SWA): Behavioral Characteristics and Possible Association with Penile Cancer." *The Journal of Sexual Medicine* 9 (7): 1860–67.

Zhang, A. Q., S. Y. R. Lee, M. Truneh, M. L. Everett, and W. Parker. 2012. "Human Whey Promotes Sessile Bacterial Growth, Whereas Alterna-tive Sources of Infant Nutrition Promote Planktonic Growth." *Current Nutrition & Food Science* 8 (3): 9.

Acknowledgments

This is my first book, so I have a lot of people to thank.

It's hard to find a word or role that encompasses everything Michael Malice did for this book: editing each line (on a short timeline); contributing his considerable knowledge of alga; teaching me how to write. I would have been grateful for his help as a craftsman; I got a consigliere. The most valuable advice is often the advice we don't want to hear—and by that measure, my research assistant, Zoe Piel, was invaluable. She was relentlessly skeptical, and in addition to her exceptional work, I'm grateful that she frequently disagreed with me.

Not only did my editor, Sydny Miner, see the vision for this book, but she also fought for it. Many thanks to her and the rest of the team at Crown for their top-notch work. Within the first five minutes of our first meeting, my literary agent, Mel Berger, understood why this couldn't be a diet book. Also, thanks to David Sherman, my TV agent, and the team at WME.

I'm grateful to Steve Pinker for many things, but particularly for his sane encouragement while pursuing what felt like an insane obsession with obscure aspects of the Zoroastrian hygiene code. Dan Lieberman has been a friend and mentor, and kindly agreed to appear in the book. I wish I were half the scientist he is.

I owe a huge debt to my sister, Maggie Durant, for her tireless and selfless work on the New York City Barefoot Run and countless other projects, which allowed me to focus on writing. Needless to say, I would not be where I am today if it were not for my mother and father, Susan and Clark Durant, who not only instilled in me a lifelong love of books, but also taught me how to read in the first place. Thanks to the rest of my family: Clark, Taylor, Pepper, Hope, Mike, Susan, Caroline, and Charlie; Nana, Papa and Audrey (my favorite celiac); the Taylor and Sparks families; Mama Rose and Grumps; Aunt Eugénie (Tiger Stadium, third base); Uncle Richard (creator of the Bachelor Salad); the Rochester Durant families; the Page families; and the Heenan families.

Writing a book means spending a lot of time on the computer, which also means bombarding your friends with email. Thanks to John Barkett, Rob Cacace, Brandon Fail, Jon Gattman, Alex Grodd, John Harrington, Dale Parker, Eliah Seton, Ben Wells, and Mookie Wilson. My (many) roommates throughout this project patiently put up with my freezer chest, standing desk, and caveman misadventures: Sam Abbott, Meredith Baker, Ryan Bellinghausen, Mike Blumenthal, Puanani Brown, Greg Damis-Wulff, Steven Duque, Andrew Glancy, Ally Jane Grossan, Tim Heckscher, Tala Itani, Tracy Johnson, Adam Kalamchi, John Kochalka, Spencer Lazar, Graham Lazar, Winston Lazar, Jen Lee, Kevin Lin, Kaitlyn Muns, Brandon Presser, Kate Randall, Leah Seifu, Richie Serna, Adrienne Schmoeker, and Samantha Stockman. Matt Stern, Zander Rafael, and Lauri Tähtinen also commented on early drafts. Also, thanks to Mariya Campwalla, Sarah Connolly, Jesse Elzinga, Jane Hanks, Joseph F. Hickey, Erik Kissel, June Lockhart, Denelle O'Neil, Noah Smalley, and Kevin Travis. Brief but heartfelt thanks to my many terrific teachers at St. Paul's, Richard, Liggett, and Harvard.

The staff at the Cleveland Metroparks Zoo was phenomenal, particularly Elena Less, Kristen Lukas, and Pam Dennis. They gave me a tour of the zoo, introduced me to Mokolo and Bebac, and reviewed the chapter multiple times. Other zoo professionals were also generous with their time and help: Jon Coe, Ruth Glancy, Ron Kagan, Gary Lee, and David Towne. The monks and staff of the Abbey of Gethsemani were welcoming and gracious, especially Abbot Elias Dietz, Br. Allen, Fr. Damien Thompson, Fr. Patrick Hart, and Br. Paul Quenon. Also, thanks to fellow traveler Tom Willis, as well as to Marc Fulkerson for tips on BBQ joints and bourbon distilleries. What's cooler than being cool? The Coney Island Polar Bear Swim Club. Special thanks to Dennis Thomas and Tony Nastro (who has a striking physical resemblance to an actual polar bear). Many thanks to the breeders I spoke with at the Westminster Kennel Club Dog Show (even though that part didn't make the final cut), especially Donna and David Smith, and Holly Horton.

Jackson Landers and Joe Cella taught me how to hunt, and both gave helpful comments on that chapter. Jay Hemker let me use his gun and lucky stand, and then talked me through dressing the deer. Many thanks to Kristen Cella, the Harrington family (Jim Sr., Chris, and Jim Jr.), and the Hemker clan (Bob, Jan, Josh, Tony, and Rita). Marta and Bob Miller kindly hosted a gun safety course at their cottage and reviewed an early book proposal. Other hunting buddies: Andy Anuzis, Zev Averbach, Andrew Frankel, Doug Ghizzoni, Geoff Hamilton, Nick Hamilton, Mee-Lise Robinson, and Jerry Stilianessis. An epic persistence hunt in Wyoming didn't make the final cut (we have to bag an antelope next time), but thanks to Philip Stark for conceiving and organizing the trip, and to Ulrich Honighausen, Barefoot Ted McDonald, Dennis Shaver, Bookis Smuin, Scott Smuin, and Patrick Sweeney.

Of all the awesome people I've met through Paleo NYC, I need to thank Melissa McEwen first and foremost. She led intro seminars, organized meat shares, set up my first blog, and even enlisted friends to review book chapters. Thanks to all the other members, particularly Vlad Averbukh, Uji Bluet, Richard Chin, Rahsaan Chisolm, Lisa Hammer, Grant Macaulay, Sam Mapp, Drew and Matt Sanocki, Christian Wernstedt, Don Wiss, and Levi Wilson. Thanks to food entrepreneurs Jordan Brown of Hu Kitchen (NYC restaurant), Ken Kleinpeter of Glynwood Farm (sustainable farming), Randy Hartnell and Craig Weatherby of Vital Choice (wild seafood), Heath Putnam of Møsefund Mangalitsa (heritage pork), and John Wood of U.S. Wellness Meats (grass-fed beef).

A big shout-out to all the members of Barefoot Runners NYC, plus the participants, volunteers, kudus, and sponsors who helped make the New York City Barefoot Run a huge success. A very incomplete list of members and volunteers includes Sanjay Amin,

Melissa Bybee, Jeff Cramblit, Kathryn "KC" Cusumano, Jeanne Davis, Lindsey Goble, Chris Hawson, Joe Maller, Rob Matthews, Chris Moffett, Dan Scanfeld, Trey Shelton, and Kris Wood. Lee Rawlings and Ira Rohde also commented on a chapter. Our terrific kudus included Mark Cucuzzella, Daniel Howell, Jason Robillard, Michael Sandler, and Barefoot Ken Bob Saxton. Thanks to our sponsors: Barefoot Wine, Injinji, JackRabbit Sports, Luna Sandals, Merrell, Paleonola, Smuttynose Brewing Company, Tip Top Shoes, Vita Coco, and Vivobarefoot.

The CrossFit community kicks ass. Thanks to everyone at Cross-Fit NYC, particularly Allison Bojarski, Joshua Newman, and Court Wing, each of whom contributed to the movement chapter, and Hari Singh. Thanks to Keith Wittenstein and Samantha Orme at Cross-Fit Virtuosity; Josh Hunnicutt at CrossFit New Species; the folks at CrossFit Transformation; and Geoff Tudisco, Justin Osborne, and the crew at CrossFit Bogotá. I'd like to recognize those who generously contributed to Fight Gone Bad 6: U.S. Wellness Meats, Calvin Ford, Lydia Guthartz, Philip Jonat, Skylee Jane Robinson, Lee Rawlings, Jim Meyer, Sue "Albino Barracuda" Durant, Alex Grodd, Sydny Miner, anonymous, John Harrington, Ryan Browne, Stacey Doering, Zach Puchtel, Matt Stern, Sam Teller, Kris Wood, and Molly Marco. Thanks to Will Dean and the Tough Mudder team.

My in-house legal team—my uncle, Peter Durant—has advised me to publicly and profusely thank him for his advice (sound counsel, as always). Thanks also go to my lawyer, Stephane Levy, who has been extremely helpful even though I can't actually afford him. David El Achkar was incredibly helpful as a research assistant and tech wizard. Erin Tyler did some amazing design work on an insanely short timeline. For contacts and conversations, thanks to Sven Beckert, Howard Berman, Jaime Davila, Wade Davis, Bob and Antonie Ewing, Cynthia Ford, Dan Fox, Chris and Kat Frank, Chuck Grimmett, Tucker Max, Tony Post, Matthew Stillman, Michael Strong, and Magatte Wade. Perpetual good karma is owed to Lee Teslik, Kate Ryder, and Kim Holmes. I'd also like to acknowledge Joe

Goldstein, who profiled Paleo NYC for the *New York Times,* as well as the staff of *The Colbert Report* for taking a risk on an unknown guest, then helping to make it a great show.

In the start-up world, I'm indebted to a number of people for introductions and advice: Michael Fishman, Peter Hopkins, Jonathan Hudson, Jim Moran, Ramit Sethi, Vin Vacanti, Patrick Vlaskovits, Mike Williams, and the crew at General Assembly. I'm deeply appreciative to my former co-workers at Mindset Media, who helped their amateur caveman go pro. Hollie Sehrt was incredibly generous with her impeccable design skills (thedesign23.com); Ryan Browne helped me get my website up at a critical moment; Sarah Welch has been a mentor on entrepreneurship (and life); and Jim Meyer not only tolerated my caveman antics when it was just a quirky hobby, but also made it possible for me to pursue the opportunity full-time. Also, thanks to Dan Armendariz, Rosemary Biagioni, J. B. Brokaw, Nicole Dugan, Steven Duque, Liz Gruszkievicz, Lauren Hudson, Michael Jordan, Brian Lee, John Lee, Howie Liu, Kerry and Desmond Lyons, David Malan, Amy O'Hara, Tom Pierce, Maggie Riso, Christiana Sudol, Jordan Tigani, and Stephanie Wang. Additional thanks to all the terrific people at Novantas, where I first started this adventure. Their caveman jokes were unceasing and merciless—invaluable training for what was to come.

For ideas and inspiration, I'm grateful to many of the thought (and action) leaders in ancestral health: the Ancestral Health Symposium, Dave Asprey, Aaron Blaisdell, Loren Cordain, Art De Vany, Erwan Le Corre, Michael and Mary Dan Eades, Esther Gokhale, Stephan Guyenet, Fred Hahn, Kurt Harris, Clifton Harski, Chris McDougall, Richard Nikoley, Brent Pottenger, Steve Rinella, Seth Roberts, Mark Sisson, Gary Taubes, Robb Wolf, and too many more to list. My blog readers and Twitter followers are the best.

For conversations or correspondence, I'm appreciative to Rebecca Bourke, Irene Davis, Akash Goel, Nicole George, John Hawks, Jonathan Haidt, Mitchell Hart, A. J. Jacobs, Aaron Kowalski, Geoffrey Miller, Tom Naughton, Michael Rose, Jack Stuster, Peter Suedfeld, and Nassim Taleb. For giving feedback on a chapter, my thanks go to Elan Barenholtz, Aleta Davies, Emily Deans, Henry Harpending, Michael Holick, Razib Khan, Dan Lieberman, Denise Minger, Kamal Patel, Steve Pinker, Lee Saxby, Steve Sailer, Rhys Southan, Philip Stark, Randy Thornhill, and Patrick Vlaskovits. For giving feedback on two or more chapters, I'm grateful to Jae Chung, Adam Crafter, Maggie Durant, Tucker Goodrich, Paul Jaminet, Chris Masterjohn, Melissa McEwen, and J. Stanton (Gnolls.org).

Sincere apologies (and gratitude) to anyone whom I may have inadvertently left out.

Any errors in the work are mine and mine alone.

Index

galactose, 134
Gandhi, Mohandas K. (Mahatma), 148
"garbage in, garbage out" (GIGO),
    90–91
Gates, Bill, 85
gathering, 256–78
GEICO, 1
genes, 84
genetic code, 85
genetic modification, 284
genetic selection, 47
genome, 84, 85
genome sequencing, 88, 140, 144
genomics, 85
geophagy, 132, 152
germ theory of disease, 56, 62, 67
ghee, 128, 292
Gibraltar, death statistics in, 66–67
Glaisher, James, 68–70, 71
Glassman, Greg, 169
Glisson, Francis, 75
glucose, 133–34, 135, 152, 154
gluten, 126, 136–37
glycogen, 134, 154
Goebbels, Joseph, 265
gorillas:
    diets for, 22–24, 27, 28
    life spans of, 26
    teeth of, 25
    in zoos, 15–24, 27, 28, 222–23
Gracie family, 177
Graham, Paul, 88
grains, 34, 129, 136–37, 141, 292
    see also specific grains
Grandin, Temple, 277
grazing, 145, 147
Green Revolution, 284
Greiter, Franz, 226
guanine (G), 84
gut, 136
gym design, 182–83
gym membership, 166–68

habitat, 279–90
    ancestral, 81

and behavior, 281
    constant features of, 78, 79, 81
    cyclical features of, 78, 79–80, 81
    definition of, 281
    designing from scratch, 81, 280
    and ecological niche, 28
    living outside, 25
    matching organisms' needs, 78
    natural, for humans, 33, 78, 280
    natural, living in, 28
    varied features of, 78, 80–81
    womb as, 98–99, 101
    and zoo design, 27, 182, 279–82
HACE (high altitude cerebral edema),
    76
hackers, 85–90
    biohackers, 88–89
    open systems sought by, 87–88
Hacker's Manifesto (The Mentor), 86
Hadza tribe, Tanzania, 119
Haidt, Jonathan, 262, 263
Hancocks, David, 280
Hands-On Imperative, 86, 89
hand washing, 47, 57, 59, 63, 64–65, 67
HAPE (high altitude pulmonary
    edema), 76
Harris, Marvin, 55
Hartman, Phil, 1
Hawthorne, Nathaniel, 190
healer-priests, 48–49
Health Professionals Follow-up Study,
    109
heart disease, see cardiovascular
    disease
heat, 106, 207, 215–16
heliotherapy, 225
Hemingway, Ernest, 191, 194
Henley, William Ernest, "Invictus,"
    82, 83
herbal medicines, 220
herder-farmers, 289
    diets of, 115, 118
    and infectious diseases, 224–25
    movement of, 164–65
    in Paleolithic Age, 34, 38, 42–43

About the Author

JOHN DURANT is a leader of the growing ancestral health movement. Durant studied evolutionary psychology at Harvard prior to founding Paleo NYC and Barefoot Runners NYC, the largest paleo and barefoot running groups in the world. He has been featured in the *New York Times* and on *The Colbert Report* and NPR. He blogs at HunterGatherer.com.